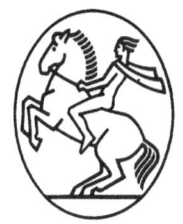

The Vertebral Artery

Pathology and Surgery

Bernard George

———

Claude Laurian

Springer-Verlag Wien New York

Bernard George, M.D.
Department of Neurosurgery, Hôpital Lariboisière, Paris, France

Claude Laurian, M.D.
Department of Vascular Surgery, Hôpital Saint Joseph, Paris, France

© 1987 by Springer-Verlag/Wien

The use of registered names, trademarks, etc in the publication does not imply, even in the absence of a specific statement, that such names are exempt from the relevant protective laws and regulations and therefore free for general use

Product Liability The publisher can give no guarantee for information about drug dosage and application thereof contained in this book In every individual case the respective user must check its accuracy by consulting pharmaceutical literature

With 97 Figures

Library of Congress Cataloging-in-Publication Data.
George, Bernard, 1948–   The vertebral artery Biblio-
graphy p. Includes index 1 Vertebral artery–Surgery I
Laurian, Claude, 1944–   II. Title [DNLM 1 Vertebral
Artery–surgery   WG 595 V3   G 346v]   RD 598 6 G46 1987
617' 413   87-9521

ISBN-13:978-3-7091-7454-8   e-ISBN-13:978-3-7091-6967-4
DOI: 10.1007/978-3-7091-6967-4

PREFACE

Our common interest in surgery of the vertebral artery was born in 1976, when as residents in the same hospital, we attended an attempt by two senior surgeons to treat an aneurysm of the vertebral artery at the C3 level. Long discussions had preceded this unsuccessful trial, to decide if surgery was indicated and to choose the surgical route. Finally a direct lateral approach was performed, but access was difficult and correct treatment was impossible, resulting in only partial reduction of the aneurysmal pouch. Following this experience, we decided to seek a regular and well defined approach for exposition of the vertebral artery.

Review of the literature indicated some surgical attempts, but the descriptions did not give the impression of safety and reproducibility. No landmark on the described surgical route appeared sufficiently reliable. Henry's anatomical work (1917) gave the only accurate description on vertebral artery anatomy, and it became the basis for our work.

When the same patient was referred again one year later, after a new stroke in the vertebro-basilar system, we had behind us repetitive experience on cadavers of an original approach to the distal vertebral artery.

We are very indebted to Dr. P. Derome and Dr. D. Guilmet for having accepted the proposals of the two young surgeons we were at the time, thus enabling us to perform our first revascularization of the distal vertebral artery. With juvenile enthusiasm, we had proposed and performed what can now be considered the most difficult technique, i.e. subclavian to distal vertebral artery by-pass because of absence of both posterior communicating arteries. This first encouraging result was the beginning of a fruitful and friendly collaboration.

Our increasing experience reported before the French, European and World societies of neurosurgery and vascular surgery has led many colleagues to consult us on cases with vertebral artery related lesions. Some referred their patients to us, others invited us to perform surgery in their center. We were very honored by their requests for consultation; and our grateful thanks are due to all.

We would also like to express our appreciation for the comprehensive attitude shown by our head surgeons, Prof. R. Houdart and J. Cophignon in the Neurosurgery Department of Lariboisière Hospital and Prof. J. M. Cormier in the Vascular Surgery Department of Saint Joseph Hospital, who not only permitted us to initiate and develop the vertebral artery techniques in their departments, but also gave us their encouragement throughout the past nine years.

We thank for their valuable assistance all our colleagues in Neurology, Neuro-radiology, Functional Investigations, Otolaryngology and Anesthesiology, who participated in exploring and treating our patients.

Finally, compliments and thanks are due to our two secretaries, Jacqueline Maurice and Martine Randon, for their inestimable help in preparing the manuscript, and equally to Mrs. J. Innes for her great assistance in translating and reviewing the text.

Bernard George
Claude Laurian

Paris, March 1987

CONTENTS

1. INTRODUCTION

Within the long history of vascular surgery, the vertebral artery (V.A.) does not occupy a large place. The relatively minor importance attributed to the V.A., together with its infrequent pathology, deep location, and difficult access for exploration and surgery has led to the accessory place of V.A. surgery. Compared to the carotid artery, developments in physiopathology, investigation and surgery of the V.A. have always appeared later. Today, while carotid artery surgery is routinely performed, V.A. surgery remains a challenge for most surgeons.

However, as early as 1929, Chiari tried to treat a V.A. lesion. Although he failed, since he ligated the carotid artery with subsequent death, this was nevertheless the first recognition of the need to treat a V.A. lesion (**Tables 1 and 2**).

Subsequently, Dietrich (1831) and Velpeau (1833) attempted ligation of the first and the third part of the V.A., but without success. Following these failures, Sanson in 1836, thought the vertebral arteries were so hidden and inacessible that "they were beyond the reach of surgery".

However, in 1853, Maisonneuve disproved Sanson's pessimism by ligating the first portion of the V.A. for treatment of a traumatic lesion. This was, to our knowledge, the first successful attempt to treat a V.A. lesion.

Some other successes followed: Smyth (1864), Barbieri (1867), Kocher (1871). Fenger (1881) was apparently the first to carry out successful ligation of the distal V.A. when he treated a traumatic aneurysm in a 19-year-old man.

Soon after, in 1888, R. Matas described the first direct attack on an aneurysm of the distal part of the V.A. through a posterior approach.

Initially and for long after, V.A. surgery was limited to traumatic lesions, and there was debate about the relative merits of packing of these lesions as opposed to ligation. Best results seemed to be achieved with packing. As an example, Matas's patient had repeated packing with ice and placement of a 5 lb. bag of lead shot for compression; then, since the patient was still bleeding, he was reoperated and three swabs were left in the wound area.

However, even these traumatic lesions were very rare, probably because of poor recognition. Matas noted that his patient was the only case of V.A. injury reported among 46 400 patients treated in Charity Hospital of New Orleans between 1832 and 1862. Only two V.A. injuries were recorded during the American Civil War (Shumacker, 1946); 40 cases during World War I by

Table 1. Traumatic aneurysms of the vertebral artery from Matas

No.	Age	Sex	Situation	Cause	Treatment	Author	Result
1	23	m	cervical	puncture	cold application	Moebus 1827	recovered
2	28	m	C1 C2	puncture	ligature of CCA	Chiari 1829	died
3	20	m	C2 C3	puncture	—	Ramaglia 1834	died
4	—	m	Jaw angle	puncture	ligature of CCA	Cattolica 1836	died
5	—	m	Jaw angle	puncture	compression	Cattolica 1836	died
6	30	m	mastoid apex	stab	cold + compression	Yppolito 1838	died
7	40	m	C4 C5	idiopathic	ligature of CCA	Stubb 1846	died
8	—	m	upper cervic.	wound?	ligature of CCA	South 1847	died
9	23	m	below mastoid	puncture	ligature of CCA	Kluyskens 1848	died
10	30	m	back of neck	stab	plugging	Stone 1849	recovered
11	29	m	C2 C3	puncture	ligature of CCA	Branco 1862	died
12	23	m	above C1	puncture	ligature of CCA	Lucke 1867	died
13	—	m	C4 C5	gunshot	plugging	Stroppa 1867	died
14	20	f	C1 C2	stab	ligature of CCA	Gherini 1867	died
15	42	m	C5 C6	puncture	plugging	Kocher 1871	recovered
16	33	f	mastoid	puncture	cold pressure	Verardini 1872	died
17	28	m	below earlobe	puncture	compression	Weir 1884	recovered
18	19	m	C1 C2	gunshot	ligature of VA	Fenger 1881	recovered
19	41	f	C5	gunshot	ligature of CCA	Simes 1888	died
20	21	m	C1 C2	gunshot	plugging	Matas 1888	recovered

Table 2. Injuries of the vertebral artery from Matas

No.	Age	Sex	Situation	Cause	Treatment	Author	Result
1	Ad	m	above C1	stab	—	Fabricius 1750	died
2	Ad	m	upper portion	gunshot	—	Sanson 1830	died
3	31	m	C2	stab	ligature of CCA	Voisin 1841	died
4	58	m	C2 C3	gunshot	—	Jolly 1841	died
5	Ad	m	upper cervic.	stab	ligature of CCA	Thurat 1848	died
6	Ad	m	C1	gunshot	—	Stromeyer 1850	died
7	Ad	f	C6	gunshot	ligature of VA	Maisonneuve 1852	died
8	Ad	f	C6	stab	ligature of CCA	Watson 1853	died
9	25	m	C3 C4	stab	—	Carter 1854	died
10	18	m	C5	gunshot	plugging	Van Buren 1857	died
11	11	m	C2 C3	gunshot	plugging	Waren 1861	recovered
12	Ad	m	C4	tuberculosis	plugging	Perrin 1861/62	died
13	Ad	m	C4	gunshot	plugging	Kade 1862	died
14	30	m	above C1	stab	ligature of CCA	Prichard 1863	died
15	Ad	m	C6	gored by OX	—	Pirogoff 1864	died
16	27	m	C5	gunshot	compression	Peters 1865	died
17	20	f	C1 C2	stab	ligature of CCA	Barbieri 1867	died
18	30	m	C3 C4	stab	—	Saviotti 1867	died
19	Ad	m	C4 C5	stab	—	Caspar-Liman 1871	died
20	11	m	C2	tuberculosis	—	Neuretter 1873	died
21	25	m	upper cervic.	stab	plugging	King 1885	recovered
22	35	f	C2	tuberculosis	plugging	Kuster 1883	died

Perrig (1931) and no cases during World War II among 2471 cases of battle arterial injuries by De Bakey and Simeone (1946).

Following its use for treatment of traumatic aneurysm, V. A. ligation was then proposed in different cases with some various and surprising indications: epilepsy, Alexander (1982); brain tumor, Dandy (1944), and arteriovenous fistulas, Elkin and Harris (1946). Contributing to these two last indications, a major advance in the diagnosis of V. A. lesions had been made with the first vertebral angiography using Thorotrast performed by E. Moniz in 1927. Accurate recognition of V. A. lesions could then be achieved; but until the end of the fifties, surgery remained mainly directed to arteriovenous fistulas and aneurysms of traumatic origin.

In 1957, Cate and Scott performed the first endarterectomy of the proximal V. A., followed in 1958 by Crawford and De Bakey.

At the same time, pathophysiology progressed with anatomopathologic studies of patients who died from vertebro-basilar ischemia: Hutchinson and Yates (1956), Martin et al. (1960), Stein et al. (1961), Fischer (1965, 1970). Relations between extracranial vessel pathology and cerebral ischemia became clearly established.

Vertebro-basilar insufficiency, manifested by intermittent symptoms, was recognized by Denny-Brown (1960) and further defined by Powers (1961) and Marshall (1964).

Causes of vertebro-basilar insufficiency could then be identified and proposals for adequate treatment be given. In fact, most of them had been suggested far earlier. For instance, the subclavian steal syndrome so christened by Fischer in 1961 and reported by Reivich et al. (1961), was first described by Smythe in 1864. External compression of the V. A. associated with spondylosis, reported by Bauer et al. (1960) and demonstrated angiographically for the first time by Meyer et al. (1960) and Sheehan et al. (1960), had been described by Barre in 1926; moreover, intermittent V. A. compression from rotation of the head had been anatomically proven by Gerlach in 1884 and then by De Kleyn and Versteegh in 1933.

Since that time, other pathologic conditions involving the V. A. have been identified, such as tumor (Love and Dodge, 1952 and Kriss and Schneider, 1968), dysplasia and dissection.

Following the general development of vascular surgery, V. A. surgery also improved, and techniques to preserve or to revascularize the V. A. were developed: anastomosis between the common carotid artery and the subclavian artery (De Bakey, 1965), between the common carotid artery and the V. A. (Wyllie and Ehrenfeld, 1970), between the subclavian artery and the V. A. (Carney, 1976); anastomosis to the distal V. A. (Clark and Perry, 1966 and Corkill et al., 1977), and saphenous vein by-passes to the proximal V. A. (Berguer et al., 1976, Cormier and Laurian, 1976) or the distal V. A. (Carney and Anderson, 1978, George and Laurian, 1979) from various arterial trunks.

Decompression of the V. A. was performed on its proximal portion by

Powers *et al.* in 1963 and on its second portion with removal of osteophytic spurs by Hardin *et al.* (1960) and then by Gortvai (1964) and Keggi *et al.* (1966).

Although descriptions of lesions involving the V. A. are now numerous, V. A. surgery remains exceptional. In fact, except for the proximal portion of the V. A., most surgeons, if faced with V. A. lesions, are still hesitant. As written by A. J. Walt: "the V. A. remains for many surgeons, a reclusive vessel with some of the features of a hedgehog, hinding behind the cervical foramina, difficult to get close to and always ready to attack". However in recent years, some surgeons have changed their minds and are attempting to render V. A. surgery as common as any other vessel surgery. Among them, as early as 1976, the two authors of this book associated their experience to define anatomically and then surgically the best ways to approach every type of lesion on any part of the cervical V. A. The benefits of this association of two surgeons coming from the complementary specialities of neurosurgery and vascular surgery have never ceased throughout the past ten years. As a consequence, patients referred exhibit a large variety of pathologic conditions, covering both specialities.

It must be underlined that close collaboration with the neuroradiologic team (Merland J. J.) and the E. N. T. team (Freyss) has greatly contributed to the development of V. A. surgery in this hospital. At the same time that their notoriety has increased the number of patients referred, further enlarging the spectrum of V. A. lesions, they have contributed their own expertise in exploring and treating these patients. Embolization is by far the best example of the interest and the need for such collaboration.

Thus this book is not only the result of the development of surgical techniques for the V. A. but also the fruit of collaboration among several specialists with a common pole of interest.

As proven by its historical background, V. A. surgery has numerous applications. Therefore this book is not only devoted to recent progress in vertebro-basilar insufficiency pathophysiology, but also to the surgical treatment of every type of lesion which may compromise flow in the vertebro-basilar system. Basic knowledge of V. A. anatomy and of the different causes of V. A. flow compromission is a prerequisite for contemplating the different techniques of V. A. surgery and their indications and these subjects are treated in depth.

Many classic specialities such as neurosurgery, vascular surgery, E. N. T. surgery, orthopaedic surgery and neuroradiology may be involved in V. A. surgery. However, frontiers between these specialities interpenetrate and are becoming blurred. Some surgeons interested in skull base tumor surgery now call their speciality *head and neck surgery*. V. A. surgery is another field which can obviously be included in this new speciality overlapping several others.

2. ANATOMY

2.1 Introduction

The vertebral artery (V. A.) is anatomically divided into four portions from its origin to its intracranial junction with the controlateral V. A. (**Fig. 1**).

First Portion

This portion includes the proximal or ostial segment, from the artery origin to its entry into the bony transverse canal, which is usually at the level of C 6.

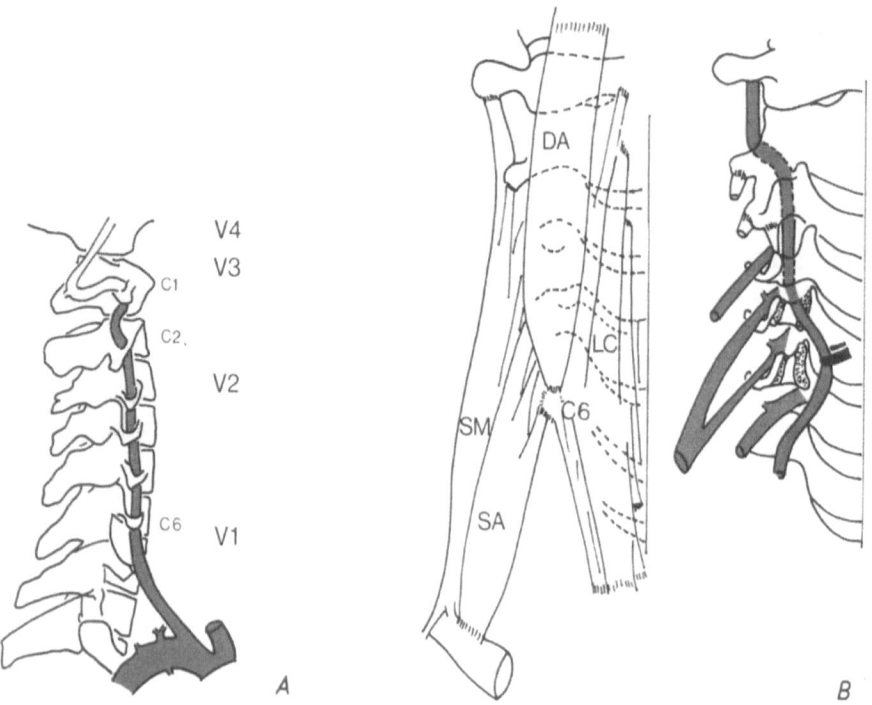

Fig. 1. A) Anatomical division of the cervical V. A. **B)** Anatomical relationship of the cervical V. A. Left: deep muscles covering anteriorly the V. A. *LC* Longus colli M. *DA* Anterior rectus M. *SM,* *SA* Scalenus M. Right: nerve roots merging posteriorly to the V. A. The transverse canal is opened at C 5 C 6

Second Portion

This portion consists of the transverse segment from its entry at the C 6 level to the transverse foramen of C 2.

Third Portion

This portion is the suboccipital segment and extends from C 2 up to penetration of the dura meter at the foramen magnum.

Fourth Portion

This intracranial segment extends from the foramen magnum to the junction of the V. A. with the controlateral V. A., forming the basilar trunk.

This text concerns only the cervical V. A., excluding the fourth intracranial portion.

2.2 Embryology

According to D. H. Padget (1948–1954), the V. A. trunk appears late in the evolution of the embryo, at the 7 to 12 mm stage. It results from anastomoses of the cervical and dorsolateral intersegmentary arteries above the seventh, from which the subclavian artery (S. C. A.) will develop.

In fact, these anastomoses lead to formation of 3 arterial trunks:

1. Pre-costal anastomosis: the thyrocervical trunk.
2. Post-transverse anastomosis: the deep cervical artery.
3. Post-costal anastomosis: the vertebral artery.

The common embryologic origin of these 3 trunks explains their normal anastomotic connections, which develop if one of them is occluded (Bosniak, 1964, Francke *et al.*, 1980) or which may appear during embolization (Spetzler *et al.*, 1980).

As the intersegmentary arteries are connected to the future carotid artery, it also explains the normal anastomoses between the external carotid artery via the occipital artery and these three cervical trunks (Bosniak, 1964, Spetzler *et al.*, 1980).

This mode of formation also explains the persistence of congenital anastomoses between the common or the internal carotid artery (proatlantal artery), and the V. A., or the persistance of fenestration or duplication.

The seventh intersegmentary artery remains patent to give the S. C. A., from which the 3 above-mentioned arterial trunks take origin.

2.3 Structure

The V. A. has a very thin wall in proportion to its size and when compared with arteries of similar diameter elsewhere in the body, but the structure of the V. A. wall is quite similar to that of any other artery. Comparison has been made with the internal carotid artery by Fang (1958) and by Wilkinson (1952). On the extracranial part of the internal carotid artery as well as the V. A., a well developed external elastic lamina and media are observed. After

penetration of the dura, for both arteries, the adventitia is much reduced,
the external elastic lamina disappears
and elastic fibrils in the media become
very rare.

2.4 Description

2.4.1 Diameter

The average diameter of the V. A. is
4.5 mm; 4.3 mm for the right V. A. and
4.7 mm for the left V. A., as established
by Francke *et al.* (1980) from 11 reports
on 1 256 cases collected in the literature
between 1916 and 1971.

As is well known, the vertebral arteries
are frequently asymmetric; the larger is
called the *dominant* artery and the smaller controlateral one is called the *minor*
artery.

The *minor* V. A. is sometimes very
small and does not participate in formation of the basilar trunk. Actually, it
is often difficult on angiographic data to
be certain that a small V. A. which

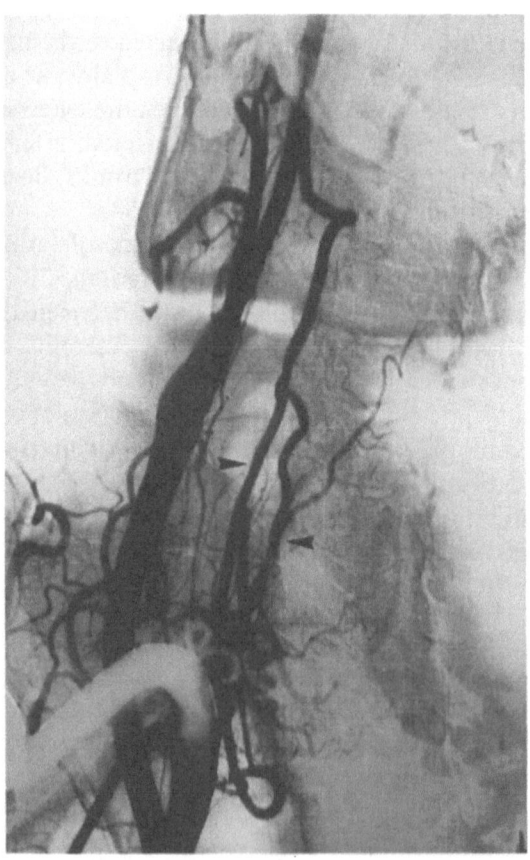

Fig. 2. V. A. origin by two separate roots from the subclavian artery

seems to end at the posterior inferior cerebellar artery (P. I. C. A.), does not fill the basilar trunk. Only the injection of the V. A. during compression or occlusion of the dominant V. A. can confirm the lack of connection of a minor V. A. with the basilar trunk.

The term *hypoplastic* V. A. usually refers to this type of minor V. A., but it supposes that a connection with the basilar trunk exists.

The term *atretic* V. A. usually refers to a minor V. A. which does not inject the basilar trunk (**Fig. 3**).

Finally, one or both V. A. may be *absent*; in that case, they are frequently replaced by a persistant congenital anastomosis (Tsai *et al.*, 1975).

Table 3 indicates the frequency in

Table 3

Dominant	left V. A.	35.8%
	right V. A.	23.4%
Equivalent		40.8%
Hypoplastic	left V. A.	5.7%
or atretic	right V. A.	8.8%
	bilateral	0.7%
Absent	left V. A.	1.8%
	right V. A.	3.1%

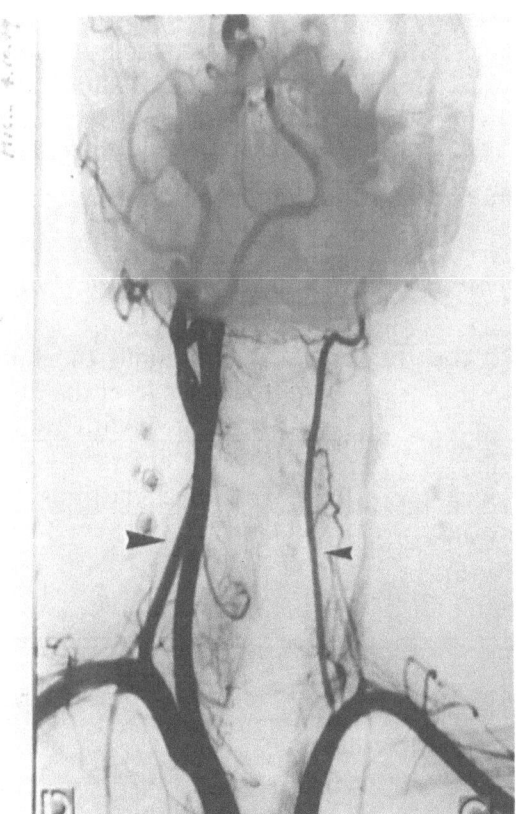

Fig. 3. Dominant V. A. on right side. Atretic V. A. ending at PICA and not filling the basilar trunk on left side

which each type of V. A. is encountered: dominant, hypoplastic or atretic (as they are not well differentiated in the literature) and absent.

2.4.2 First Portion—Ostium

2.4.2.1 Origin

The V. A. takes origin most frequently from the subclavian artery (S. C. A.), usually at the junction of its vertical and horizontal portions.
Many variations of origin are possible but rare:
— from the vertical part of the S. C. A.,
— or from the horizontal part of the S. C. A. more or less distally,
— from the thyrobicervicoscapular trunk (Sarter *et al.*, 1980),
— or from the cervicointercostal trunk,
from the inferior thyroïdian artery,
from the common carotid artery,
from the innominate artery,

— from the aorta, usually between the left carotid artery and the S. C. A. This is the most frequent anomaly of origin and represents about 4% of the cases,
— from two or three roots of various origin which join before the V. A. entry into the transverse canal (Suzuki, 1979) (**Fig. 2**).

2.4.2.2 Course

The V. A. runs vertically, a little inwards and backwards. In fact, direction of the proximal part of the V. A. depends on its origin. Moreover, tortuosity is frequent around the ostium (**Fig. 4**).

2.4.3 Second Portion — Transverse Canal C 6–C 2

2.4.3.1 Entry into the Transverse Canal

The V. A. entry into the transverse canal is usually located at C 6: 89,8% of 2642 cases collected in the literature (Francke *et al.*, 1980) but it may vary from C 7 to C 2 (**Fig. 5**).
This entry is symetric in 85% of the cases analyzed and asymetric in 15%. There are never more than two vertebrae between the entry level on each side; the right V. A. always has the lowest entry.
In case of V. A. origin from the aorta, the entry into the transverse canal is most frequently at C 5 or C 4.

Entry into the transverse canal at a higher level than C 6 is sometimes associated with duplication; an atretic V. A. enters at C 6 and joins the main trunk in the transverse canal (**Table 4**).

Table 4

Entry	%
C 7	3
C 6	89.8
C 5	6.3
C 4	0.9
C 3	0.1

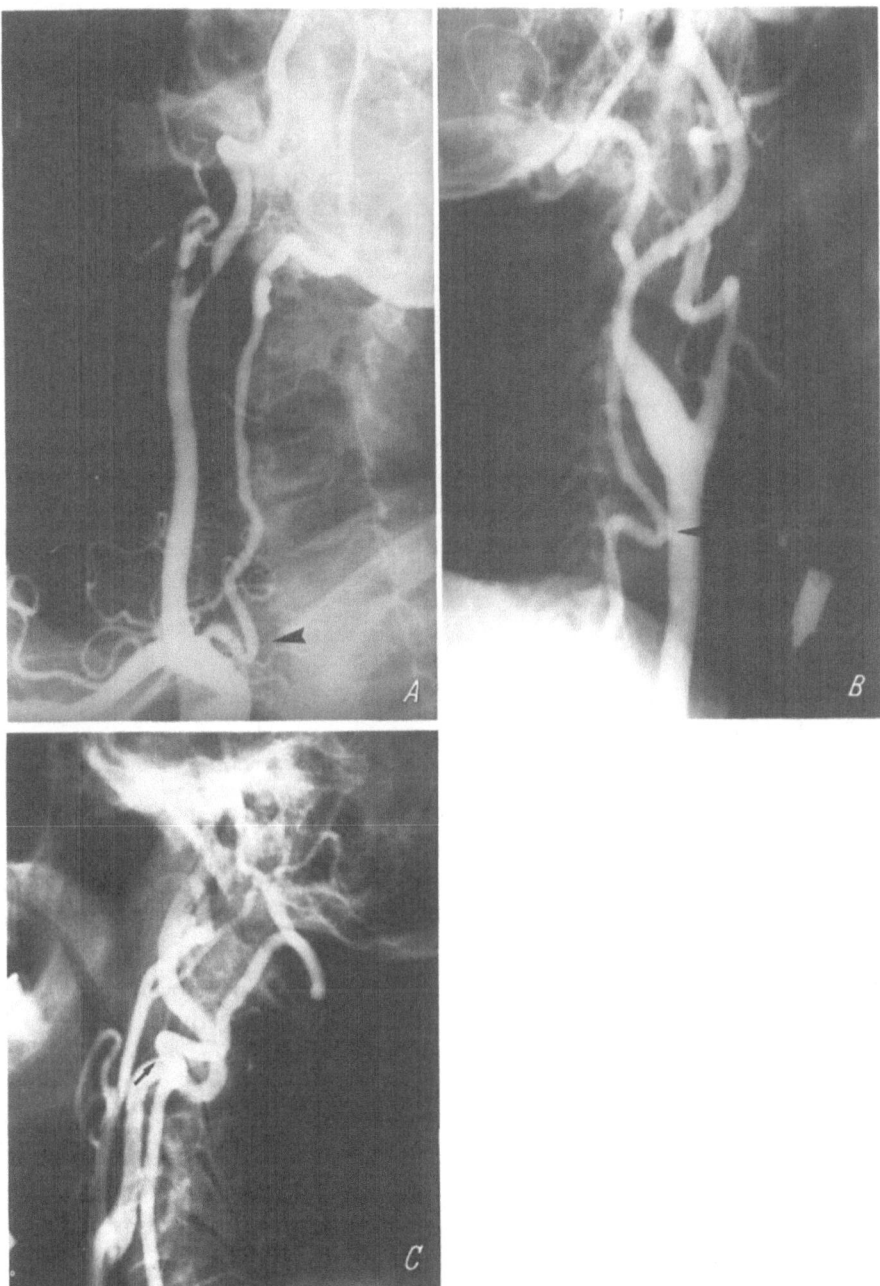

Fig. 4. V. A. loops. **A)** In the first portion, **B)**–**C)** in the second portion

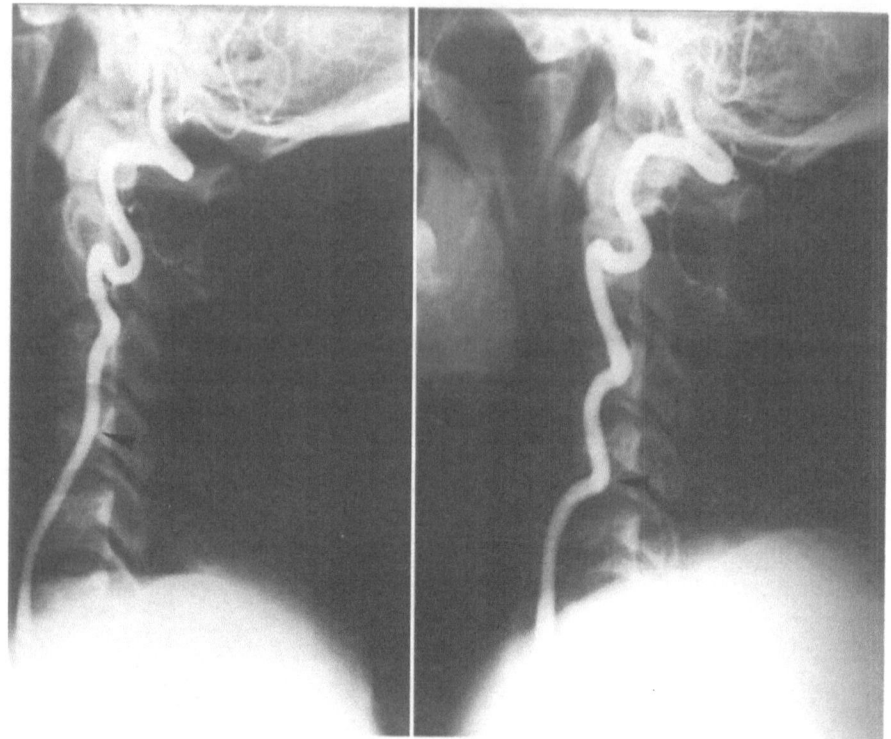

Fig. 5. V. A. abnormal entry in the transverse canal at C 4 on both sides (associated to fibromuscular compression at this level in head extension)

2.4.3.2 Course

In the transverse canal, the V. A. runs linearly and vertically from one transverse foramen to the following one up to C 2.

Tortuosity between two transverse foramina may be observed; its frequency increases with age (**Fig. 4**).

a) Transverse Canal

From C 6 to C 2, the V. A. runs in the transverse canal. It is a true canal which is formed by the transverse foramina and between them, by the overlying muscles (the anterior and posterior intertransverse muscles with the overlying scalenus and longus colli muscles) and by the lateral border of the vertebrae and the articular processes, mainly the superior facets.

This canal can be measured at the transverse foramen level; its antero-posterior diameter decreases slightly and progressively from C 6 to C 2. It varies with the size of the V. A. So, obviously, the left transverse canal is usually a little bigger than the right: from 5.6 mm to 6.4 mm on the right and 5.7 mm to 6.5 mm on the left, on average.

It should be noted that between the average diameter of the transverse canal and the V. A. diameter, there is a small difference of 1 to 2 mm.

b) Periosteal Sheath

Inside the transverse canal, the V. A. is surrounded by a continuous periosteal sheath adherent to the bony foramen and the deep surface of the muscles. This forms nevertheless an anatomically and surgically distinct plane which enables separation of the V. A. inside its periosteal sheath from the surrounding structures.

Therefore, the V. A. is protected by a periosteal sheath which is in turn, surrounded by the transverse osteomuscular canal.

2.4.4 Third Portion—Suboccipital

2.4.4.1 Course

The third portion extends from the transverse foramen of C 2 to the foramen magnum, where the artery becomes intracranial. Four parts can be distinguished on this portion according to Fischer:

a) Transverse foramen of C 2: this forms a true canal with two different curves; the first in a horizontal plane on its inferior side (foramen entry) and the second, oblique, backward, and outward at its entry, becomes horizontal inside the foramen and again runs vertically after its exit.

b) Between C 2 and C 1: the V. A. runs vertically up to the foramen of C 1, still surrounded by the same periosteal sheath as in the transverse portion, and covered by the levator scapulae and inferior oblique muscles.

c) Transverse foramen of C 1: at this level, the V. A. bends backwards and inwards. The transverse foramen of C 1 is noticeably prolonged by a process much larger than at any other level. This serves as a very good surgical landmark.

d) Groove above C 1: the artery runs around the lateral mass of the atlas in a horizontal groove above the posterior arch of C 1. The end of this groove is marked by a small increase in the height of the posterior arch. At this point, the V. A. bends forward, upward and a little inward to reach the dura on the lateral aspect of the foramen magnum. In this portion, the periosteal sheath is reinforced laterally by the transverse

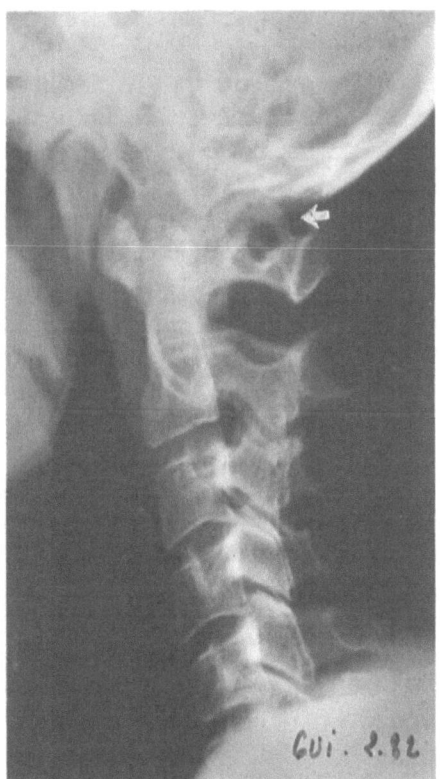

Fig. 6. Bony canal around the V. A. above the arch of atlas

ligament and posteriorly by the retro-glenoid ligament. These ligaments may be ossified, either on the external portion or over the entire length of the posterior groove. In the latter case, the groove becomes a completely osseous canal (Radojevic and Negovanovic, 1963) (**Fig. 6**).

2.4.5 Intracranial Penetration

The V. A. passes through the dura mater at the foramen magnum level between 12 and 15 mm from the midline. The periosteal sheath is in continuity with the dura and even extends intracranially for 4 to 6 mm.

2.5 Relation to Vascular and Nervous Structures

2.5.1 Vertebral Veins and Plexus

Throughout its course, the V. A. is accompanied by the vertebral veins.

1. In the first portion: the main vertebral vein runs anteriorly to the artery. An accessory vein is frequently observed on the posterior aspect of the artery.

2. In the second and third portion: the vertebral veins are usually described as a network around the artery, and the words "plexus" or "sinus" are used instead of veins. For Francke *et al.* (1981), the vertebral veins in the transverse portion can be compared to the cavernous sinus. In fact, under surgical microscope, veins with a true wall can always be individualized. Therefore it is preferable to say that the vertebral veins are densely interconnected above the first portion and can no more be described as two separate venous trunks.

The vertebral veins are more developed at both extremities of the transverse canal, particularly above C 1. They predominate on the anterior and lateral sides of the V. A.

Wherever the vertebral veins are considered, the important point is that they are always included in the periosteal sheath with the V. A. Therefore, as long as the periosteal sheath is preserved, injury of these veins should not occur. The vertebral veins are joined by radicular veins connecting with the venous extradural plexus through the intervertebral foramen and by transversal veins connecting with the posterior jugular vein.

2.5.2 Sympathetic Nerves

The posterior vertebral nerve originates from the inferior cervical or stellate ganglion or the ansa subclavia. The anterior vertebral nerve, usually smaller than the posterior, originates from the intermediate or vertebral ganglion or the middle cervical ganglion (Hoffman and Kuntz, 1957, Mitchell and Netsky, 1962).

As the nerves ascend through the transverse foramina, they are interconnected by fine branches forming the periarterial plexus which is reinforced by rami arising from the cervical nerves. The vertebral nerve runs posteriorly to the V. A., usually in the transverse canal in the same periosteal furrow as the V. A. and its surrounding veins and sympathetic plexus. However, in about 15% of cases, the vertebral nerve passes either in a posterior groove on the posterior root of the transverse process or even in a separate foramen. This separate foramen disappears above the C 4 transverse foramen, where the vertebral nerve can no longer be identified. The function of these vertebral nerves is still a subject of debate. As noted by Nagashima and Iwana (1972), the deep or posterior cervical sympathetic system is functionally different from the cervical sympathetic nerve, induces dizziness, posterior headache and various pupillary changes but it does not seem to produce a significant effect on blood flow of the brain stem vessels or the V. A. (Schmidt and Pierson, 1934, Meyer et al., 1967).

2.5.3 Nerve Roots

At each level, the corresponding spinal nerve root crosses the posterior aspect of the V. A. (**Fig. 1 B**).

In the first portion, the V. A. is located at some distance anterior to the brachial plexus.

In the second portion, the nerve roots are in contact with the posterior aspect of the V. A., but outside the periosteal sheath. Each root emerges from the intervertebral foramen above the transverse process; then it passes obliquely behind the artery. The anterior branch spins around the postero-lateral aspect of the artery and then crosses the posterior tip of the transverse process.

Between C 1 and C 2, the anterior branch of the second cervical nerve turns around the lateral aspect of the V. A. and remains above the transverse process of C 2. This anterior branch is a good landmark in the lateral anterior approach of the V. A. between C 1 and C 2, since it appears just in front of the vessel.

Above C 1, the small first cervical nerve passes under and then behind the horizontal portion of the V. A., above the arch of the atlas.

2.5.4 Other Structures

In the first portion, *lymphatic vessels* are frequently encountered in close vicinity to the V. A. On the left side, the thoracic duct may cross the V. A. on either side.

The *inferior thyroïdian artery* crosses the V. A. anteriorly at some distance in the usual case, but if the V. A. entry into the transverse canal is at C 4 or above, it may pass closely behind the V. A.

In the second portion, no other vascular

or nervous structures are in close relation with the V. A., but of note here is the proximity of the V. A. with the superior articular facet of each vertebra and with the unco-vertebral joint; respectively 1.5–8 mm and 1 mm for Kovacs (1955) and Francke *et al.* (1981).

2.6 Branches

The cervical V. A. gives origin to many small branches supplying different structures (**Fig. 7**):
— muscular branches,
— osteo-articular branches,
— meningeal branches,
— radicular and radiculo-medullary branches.

We shall only dwell on a few of the characteristic points in some of them.
Posterior meningeal artery: This artery arises either above C 1 or at the dura

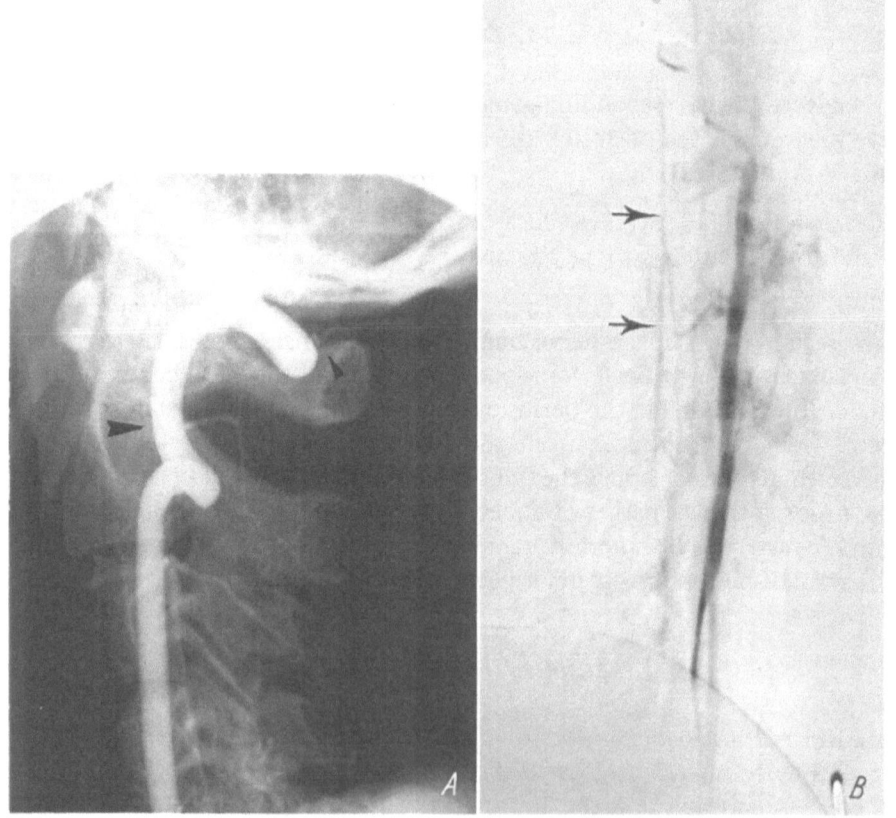

Fig. 7. A) V. A. muscular branches at C1, C2, and C3, **B)** anterior radiculo-medullary branch arising at C 4

penetration or intracranially. It supplies the dura of the posterior fossa in its medial part.

Radicular arteries: Among all the radicular branches which accompany each spinal nerve root through the intervertebral foramen, some are also medullary branches. Most are posterior medullary branches, but one and sometimes even two anterior medullary branches may arise from one or both V.A. When an anterior medullary branch exists, it originates from one of the lowest radicular branches, below C4. When no anterior medullary branch arises from the V.A., it comes from one of the other S.C.A. branches: mainly the costo-cervical trunk or the ascending cervical artery. The origin of these branches is entirely unpredictable: for example, one anterior medullary branch may arise from the V.A., while a controlateral one may originate from the ascending cervical artery. Therefore, the entire length of both V.A.'s must be seen on angiography to assess whether or not an anterior medullary branch arises from it.

Muscular branches: Of note also are the muscular branches which pass between the V.A. and the occipital and cervical arteries. Two are particularly important and constant in their location: one between C1 and C2, the atlanto-axial branch; and one above C1 at the point where the V.A. bends towards the dura: the suboccipital artery of Salmon. They are sometimes called anastomoses of the first and second interspace, recalling the primitive intersegmentary arteries (Lasjaunias *et al.*, 1978).

3. CONGENITAL ABNORMALITIES

Congenital abnormalities and variations are frequent in the V.A. They must be particularly well known and recognized if any surgical approach to the V.A. is being considered.

Some of these abnormalities have already been presented in the previous chapter (Anatomy):

— variations in diameter; hypoplastic, atretic and absent V.A.,
— variations in origin,
— variations in the level of the transverse canal entry.

Some other anomalies need further description:

3.1 Duplication

This anomaly probably results when a primitive intersegmental artery persists during embryologic development (Kadyi, 1886, Wackenheim and Babin, 1969, Makahashi et al., 1970, Lasjaunias et al., 1980, Hasegawa et al., 1986).

It is a very rare anomaly except in Japan, where it occurs in 1% of cases (Kawada et al., 1972).

In the second portion, V.A. duplication is associated with an abnormal level of entry into the transverse canal. The main trunk runs outside the transverse canal, while a hypoplastic trunk enters as the C6 level and joins the main trunk at its higher entry (Adachi, 1928, Skopakoff, 1964).

In the third portion, reported cases of V.A. duplication indicate either a main trunk penetrating the dura at the C1–C2 level with an atretic or hypoplastic trunk following the normal course, or two trunks of equal size, one intradural and the other in the transverse canal. At this level, this anomaly has been reported as the cause of vertebral artery injury after lateral puncture for myelography, with severe consequences (Rogers, 1983). It may also be responsible for spinal cord symptoms due to pulsatile compression (Hasegawa et al., 1983) (**Fig. 11**).

Mizukami et al. (1972) reported 10 cases of duplication at the level of the atlas which he labeled "diastematoarteria". One trunk follows the normal V.A. course, and the other is posteromedial outside the arch of the atlas.

3.2 Tortuosity and Kinking

These are frequently observed on the first portion of the V. A. and much more rarely on the second and third (**Fig. 4**).

It may be difficult to assess their congenital origin, since tortuosity has been shown to increase with age (Clarisse *et al.*, 1977, Hadley, 1958, Krayenbühl and Yaşargil, 1957). Anatomic and microradiological studies on the internal carotid artery by Macke and Macke-Ribet (1978) confirmed the lenghtening and the progressive dilatation of the artery throughout life, often accompanied by thinning of its walls. Head and neck movements of rotation and extension may play a role in these changes of the cervical arteries. Other factors may intervene in the development of V. A. deformities: the sympathetic ganglion and nerves or an abnormal cervical rib, on the first portion; osteophytic spurs, fibrous bands and tumors on the second portion.

They all imply external compression of the V. A. and will be detailed in a further chapter.

These tortuosities rarely have hemodynamic consequences, as they are not usually associated with significant stenosis. V. A. loops may be symptomatic in two ways: by radicular compression (Anderson and Shealy, 1970) or by spinal fracture secondary to bone erosion (Cooper, 1980). This latter feature has been reported by several authors; but most frequently, bone erosion by the V. A. raises the problem of diagnosis of a widened cervical intervertebral foramen (Danziger and Bloch, 1975, Wilckbom and Williamson, 1980, Beraneck, 1984, Gabella *et al.*, 1981, Gatti *et al.*, 1983) or of a radiolucent cervical spinal defect (Cooper, 1980, Roy-Camille *et al.*, 1982). Neurinomas and osseous tumors are usually evoked prior to the angiographic examination.

3.3 Persistent Primitive Arteries

Primitive arteries are embryonic anastomoses between the carotid and basilar circulatory systems. These intersegmental arteries normally disappear by the time the embryo reaches a length of 14 mm (35th to 40th day of gestation). In certain cases, one or even two of them persists longer and can be identified on angiograms performed to investigate vascular pathology (Sutton, 1950, Parkinson *et al.*, 1979, Tanaka *et al.*, 1983) or at autopsy (Gottschau, 1885, and Oertel, 1922).

Four main primitive arteries exist, among which three are intracranial: the trigeminal, otic and hypoglossal arteries, and one is extracranial: the proatlantal artery (**Figs. 8** and **9**).

From the embryologic point of view, the proatlantal artery is as important as the trigeminal artery but the former persists far less frequently than the latter. According to Lasjaunias *et al.* (1978), the proatlantal artery is a rudimentary channel with should have become the proximal portion of the

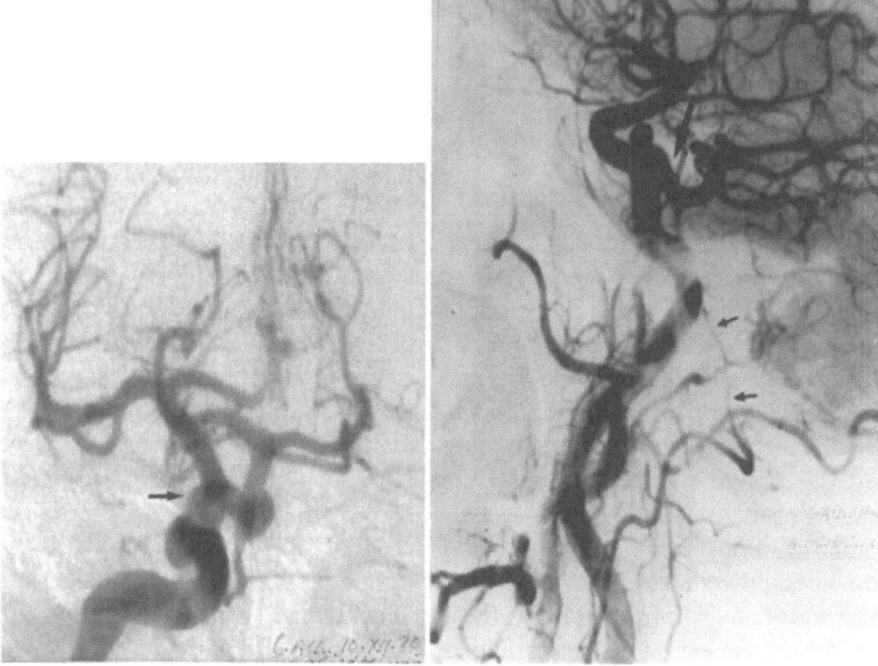

Fig. 8. Bilateral hypoplastic V. A. associated with persistent trigeminal artery

occipital artery. Initially, the occipital artery originates from the internal carotid artery and connects later with the external carotid artery. This fact may explain that two types of proatlantal artery may be observed (Rao and Sethi, 1975): type E arising from the external carotid artery and type I arising from the internal carotid artery.

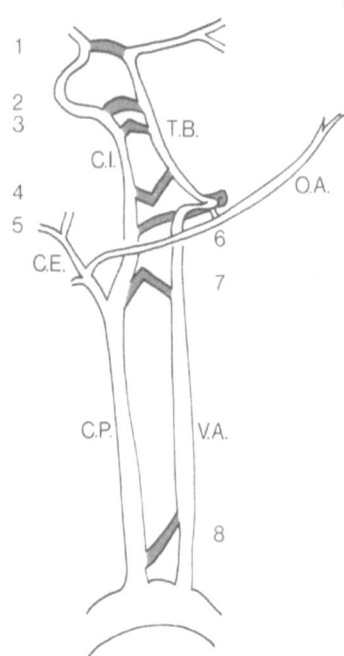

Fig. 9. Peristent congenital anastomoses between the carotid and the vertebro-basilar system. *C. E.* External carotid artery, *V. A.* vertebral artery, *O. A.* occipital artery, *C. I.* internal carotid artery, *T. B.* basilar trunk. *1* Posterior communicating artery, *2* trigeminal artery, *3* otic artery, *4* hypoglossal artery, *5* proatlantal artery, *6* occipital artery anastomosis, *7, 8* cervical intersegmentary arteries

In both types, the differentiating features are:

1. Sharp curve after origin to rest upon the superior aspect of the transverse process of C 1; the artery does not pass through the transverse foramen of any vertebrae.

2. Entry into the skull through the foramen magnum, since it joins the normal course of the V. A.

The proatlantal artery may be associated with other congenital anomalies: other primitive artery or/and intracranial aneurysm (Tanaka *et al.*, 1983). In every reported case, the vertebral arteries are absent or hypoplastic, suggesting that the proatlantal artery persisted because of the failure of normal V. A. development.

Other persistent cervical intersegmental arteries connecting the internal or the common carotid artery and the V. A. at a lower level than the proatlantal artery may be observed but are extremely rare (Lie, 1972).

3.4 Branches

— Variations in origin of the anterior medullary artery have been discussed previously (Chapter Anatomy).

— Variations in origin of the posterior inferior cerebellar artery (P. I. C. A.) are possible. Ordinarily, the P. I. C. A. emerges from the intracranial V. A. at about 1.5 cm below the vertebro-basilar

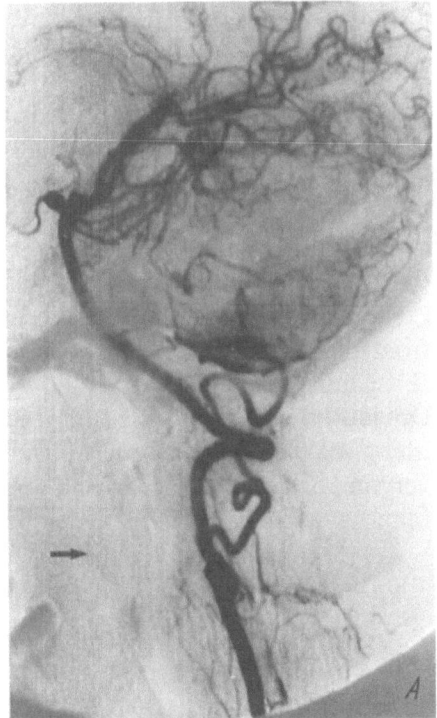
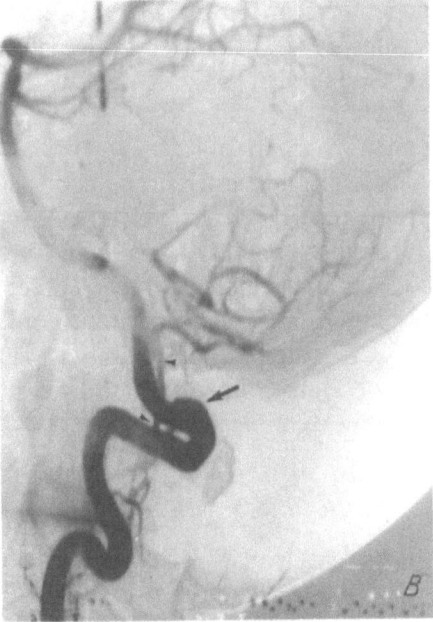

Fig. 10. Abnormal origin of the PICA. **A)** Between C 1 and C 2, **B)** above C 1

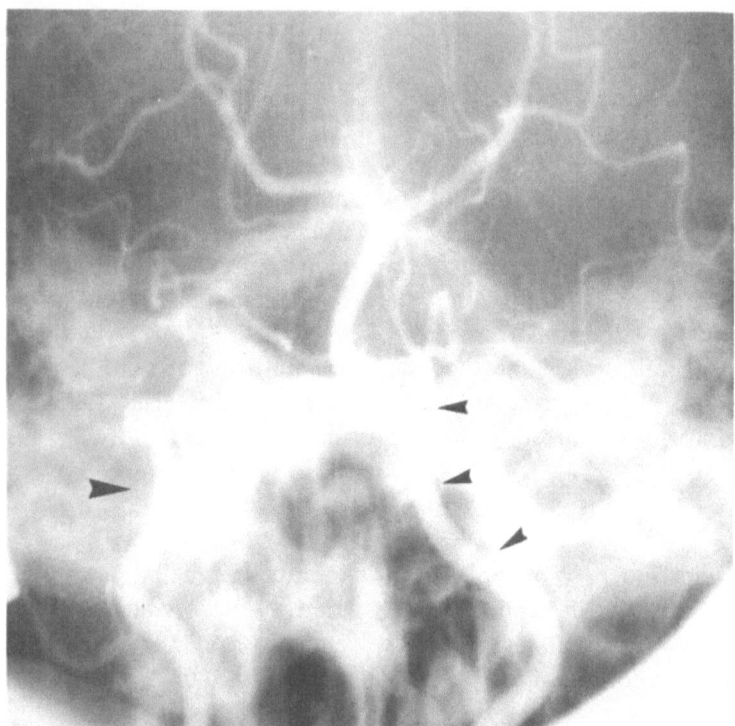

Fig. 11. Intradural course of the left V. A.

junction. According to Margolis and Newton (1972), the artery originates within the skull in 57% of cases, outside the skull in 18% and at the level of the foramen magnum in 4% (Fig. 10).

When it originates from the cervical portion, the P. I. C. A. penetrates the dura rapidly and then runs along the cord. It may rejoin a second root emerging at the normal site of P. I. C. A. origin. For Frankhauser et al. (1979), this type of origin by two roots shows a similarity to some cases of

V. A. duplication. In fact, in the case reported by Fankhauser, the main root of P. I. C. A. arises exactly at the site of origin of the atlanto-axial artery between C 1 and C 2.

Other variations in P. I. C. A. origin are exceptional but possible, such as origin from the ascending pharyngeal artery (Lasjaunias et al., 1981).

Obviously, correct analysis and recognition of such vascular variations are very important in order to avoid vessel injury at surgery.

4. WALL LESIONS

4.1 Atherosclerosis

Wall lesions involving the V. A. are of multiple causes, among which atherosclerosis is largely predominant.
Pathologic studies, more frequent angiographic investigations, and operative data have contributed to better knowledge of the atherosclerotic lesions involving the extracranial V. A. and their clinical consequences.

4.1.1 Ostial Lesions

4.1.1.1 Frequency

Frequency of atherosclerotic lesions has been found to be equivalent in the carotid and vertebro-basilar system by Hutchinson and Yates (1957), from post-mortem studies on selected patients with cerebro-vascular disease.

Significant stenosis was observed principally on the first segment of the V. A. by Mitchell and Schwartz (1965). This data is confirmed by Fischer *et al.* (1965), who demonstrated that the main site of stenosis or occlusion was at the V. A. origin from the subclavian artery.

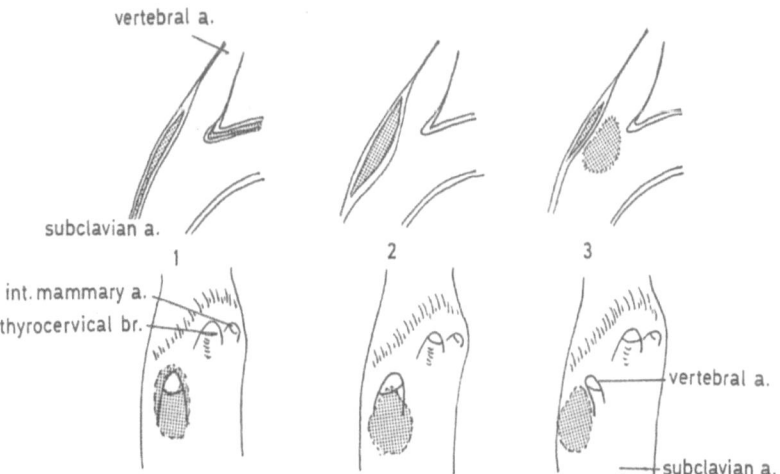

Fig. 12. Atherosclerotic lesion of the V. A. origin (see text). *1* Diaphragm stenosis, *2* fibrocalcified plaque, *3* subclavian artery plaque with external compression

Furthermore, Mitchell and Schwartz (1965) found a higher incidence of tight stenosis in the vertebro-basilar than in the carotid system, which may be explained by the smaller diameter of the V. A.'s.

4.1.1.2 Morphology

Fischer *et al.* (1965) described the ostial lesion as a ringshaped proliferation of atherosclerosis at the ostium. More rarely, the lesion formed a 5 to 10 mm long thickening of the posterior wall.

Usually, the lesion is a smooth plaque which may be calcified. Hemorrhage in the plaque was observed by Hutchinson and Yates (1957) and Duffy and Jacobs (1958), but ulceration of V. A. plaques is much less frequent than on the carotid artery and was estimated at 4% by Fisher *et al.* (1965).

On an autopsy series, Laurian (1977) studied the morphologic aspects of atherosclerotic lesions at the subclavian V. A. junction. Three different aspects were demonstrated (**Figs. 12** and **13**).

— The most frequent is a diaphragm stenosis at the ostium, resulting in fact from subclavian artery arteritis proliferation.

— A fibrocalcified plaque located in the V. A. implantation cone on the subclavian artery is the second feature. This proliferation at the level of the vertebral artery spur leads to ostial and juxtaostial stenosis with a posterior predominance.

— The third aspect results in fact from external compression rather than true stenosis, since it is due to plaque involving the subclavian artery dome which compresses and displaces the V. A. ostium. Some of the stenosing ulcerated lesions described by Fischer *et al.* (1965) might actually be on the subclavian artery.

The importance of atherosclerotic lesions located on the proximal V. A. is now being recognized. In fact, although certain post-mortem studies (Fisher *et al.*, 1965, Castaigne *et al.*, 1973) suggested that infarctions in the vertebro-basilar territory were most frequently related to distal V. A. lesions, implying that these lesions were more severe, these studies underestimated the main role played by the proximal lesions.

4.1.2 Transverse Portion Lesions

In the transverse canal, the atherosclerotic lesions are located on the second portion of the V. A., surprisingly avoiding the third portion above C 2.

Atheromatous plaques can be found on any part of the transverse portion, from C 6 to C 2 (Fisher *et al.*, 1965). This feature of V. A. lesions contrasts with the unifocal localization of carotid lesions. According to Mitchell and Schwartz (1965), atherosclerotic lesions of the transverse portion are less severe but as frequent as those around the ostium.

A particular aspect results from fibrous plaques of atherosclerosis opposite osteoarthritic spurs compressing the V. A. in the transverse canal. The possibility of multiple localizations at several

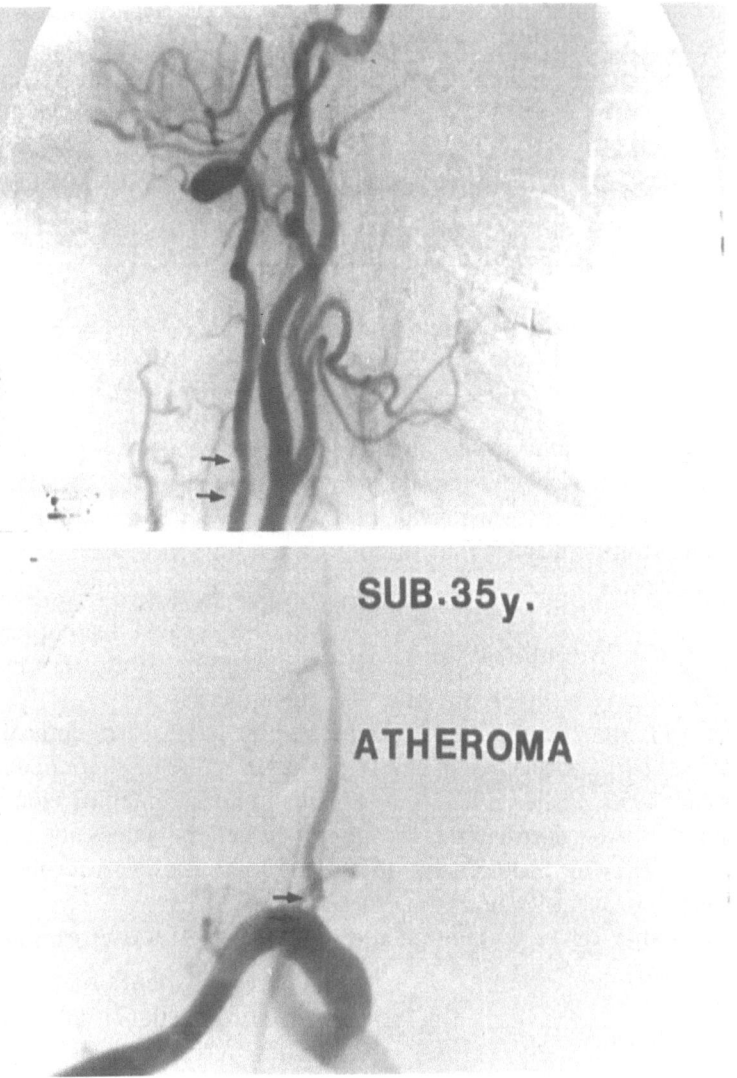

Fig. 13. Angiography: atherosclerotic stenosis at the ostium and in the transverse canal

transverse foramina levels determines what Meyer (1964) called "a rythmic distribution" of these lesions.

While these lesions may produce multi-focal stenosis, their exact clinical significance and natural course remain obscure.

4.1.3 Occlusive Lesions of the Extracranial V. A.

Thrombosis may occur in the context of stenosis whatever the anatomic level (Fisher *et al.*, 1965).

Three sites of thrombosis may be observed:

— proximal V. A. thrombosis in the

course of tight ostial stenosis, the extension of which is generally limited by the collateral branches arising from the transverse portion of the V. A. A muscular network at C1–C2 or above C1 reinjects the distal V. A. with variable efficacy,
— thrombosis at the transverse level (between C6 and C2) is exceptionally observed,

— distal V. A. thrombosis (from C2 to the intracranial junction with the controlateral V. A.) predominates in the series of Castaigne *et al.* (1973). It represents retrograde thrombosis extension from an intracranial atherosclerotic stenosis.

4.1.4 Complications of Extracranial Atherosclerotic V. A. Lesions

The possible complications include local thrombosis, ischemia, embolism and reduction in V. A. flow producing inadequate supply distal to the atherosclerotic lesion.

4.1.4.1 Local Thrombosis

Thrombosis may occur at the site of stenosis and then extend throughout the artery or serve as a source of emboli (Castaigne, 1973, Fisher, 1965).
An intact V. A. controlateral to an occluded V. A., even if dominant, does not always prevent infarcts in the vertebro-basilar territory (George and Laurian, 1981).

4.1.4.2 Ischemia

Vertebro-basilar flow reduction may result from occlusion or stenosis of both V. A.'s or of one V. A. when the controlateral V. A. is hypoplasic or atretic. Proximal as well as distal lesions may

lead to a fall in vertebro-basilar flow with subsequent ischemia.

4.1.4.3 Embolism

Emboli in the vertebro-basilar system can be thrown from proximal V. A. stenoses or from the tail of V. A. thromboses.
In the latter case, clinical manifestations seem to be contemporary with the thrombosis; embolus from the thrombosis generally does not repeat after the completion of V. A. occlusion.

4.1.4.4 Reduction in V. A. Flow

There is evidence that ischemia in the vertebro-basilar circulation, like in any other territory, can occur distal to stenotic or occlusive lesions on the basis of compromised flow, but the episodic nature of the symptoms is more difficult to explain (see chapter Pathophysiology).

4.2 Dissection

Dissection of the V. A. is a recently recognized pathologic process. Its frequency has been revealed through the increasing use of angiographic investigations of the vertebro-basilar system.
V. A. dissection should be considered in the diagnosis of vertebro-basilar

ischemia, especially in young people or when usual risk factors are lacking.

The close relationship between the V. A. and the cervical spine explains that traumatic dissections are predominant.

V. A. dissections can be classified into:
1. traumatic,
2. associated with pre-existing arterial disease,
3. true "spontaneous".

4.2.1 Traumatic Dissection

4.2.1.1 Injury

Injury to the cervical spine producing V. A. dissection can be severe or minor and even forgotten by or unknown to the patient. A clear history of trauma is therefore not always directly available and must be carefully sought.

In fact, minor trauma of the neck without detectable changes of the cervical spine, or rotation alone (during neck manipulation or voluntary movements) without superimposed abnormalities can be responsible for such arterial trauma.

External mechanical factors may be associated with trauma in producing V. A. dissection:
— congenital or degenerative abnormality of bony structures,
— fascial bands or contraction of the cervical musculature,
— anomaly in the V. A. course (loops, tortuosity, high level of entry into the transverse canal).

Most commonly these anomalies are located below C 2 and compromise arterial flow during head and neck rotation (see chapter External Compression).

4.2.1.2 Location

The V. A. is most susceptible to external forces at the following four sites:

— near the V. A. entrance into the C 6 foramen,
— along the ascent into the transverse canal,
— at the C 1 transverse foramen,
— above C 1 at the V. A. dural penetration.

Therefore, with the exception of the juxta-ostial segment, dissecting arterial lesions can be found on any part of the extracranial V. A.

4.2.1.3 Causative Injury

a) Chiropractic Manipulation

Chiropractic manipulation has long been recognized as an origin of V. A. lesion, with more or less deleterious neurologic effects (Pratt-Thomas and Berger, 1947, Clark, 1956, Green and Joynt, 1959).

The third portion of the V. A., especially in the C 1–C 2 interspace, is the preferential site of dissection following chiropractic manipulation.

As a matter of fact, several studies on the effect of various head positions on V. A. flow have demonstrated that rotation is the most effective movement producing flow reduction, either at the C 6 level (Husni et al., 1966) or at the C 1–C 2 level (Outchi and Ohara, 1973, Barton and Margolis, 1975) (see chapter External Compression).

In most earlier reports, V. A. injury was linked to chiropractic manipulation because of a temporal relation: onset of neurological symptoms followed the manipulation after a short delay. However, in some cases, manipulation was indicated for headache or stiff neck appearing after a fall or an abrupt head rotation (Krueger and Okazaki, 1980, Sherman *et al.*, 1981, Katirji *et al.*, 1985). Therefore the true causative factor, manipulation or previous trauma, cannot be determined.

Unilateral V. A. involvement is most frequently observed, but bilateral dissection has also been reported by Krueger and Okazaki (1980) and Pamela *et al.* (1983).

Dissection observed in the newborn after delivery may be compared to that occurring after chiropractic manipulation, since in both, forced movements imposed on the neck produce the lesion. However, in infancy, dissection is due to tearing of a V. A. branch and not of the V. A. itself.

b) Spontaneous Change in Head Position

Volontary movements may produce V. A. injury with subsequent dissection. Excessive controlateral rotation alone, such as may occur while driving a vehicle (Schellhas *et al.*, 1980, Sherman *et al.*, 1981) or during gymnastic exercises (Nagler, 1973, Hanus *et al.*, 1977) may be responsible for V. A. dissection in the third portion (**Fig. 14**).

In childhood, rare cases of dissection at the C 2 level have been reported, the mechanism of which is trauma by re-peated subluxation due to bony anomalies or ligamentous laxity (see chapter Infancy and Childhood). At this age, head flexion—extension is the causative movement.

More abrupt movements with associated rotation and flexion-extension of the neck have been reported to produce V. A. dissection at the C 6 level. These dissections have been observed after sports activities: tennis (Roualdes *et al.*, 1985), soft ball (Katirji *et al.*, 1985, Goldstein, 1985), or after rapid orotracheal intubation (Alexander *et al.*, 1986), or after traffic accidents (Heilbrun and Ratcheson, 1972).

V. A. injury at the C 6 level during neck hyperextension occurs at the level of entry into the transverse canal and is due to compression by the tendinous digitations of the anterior scalenus and longus colli muscles attached to the rim of the canal.

More rarely, V. A. dissection involves the second portion. In the cases already reported, causative injuries were various, such as minor fall (Sherman *et al.*, 1981) or sustained compression (heavy bag over the shoulder in Katirji's case, 1985).

At this level, predisposing factors are more often identified: abnormally high level of V. A. entry into the transverse canal, or osteophytic spur.

c) Direct Cervical Trauma

The V. A. is far less protected in its passage from the atlas to the skull than at any other level. Moreover, the periosteal sheath is firmly attached to the dura, fixing the V. A. at its dural penetration.

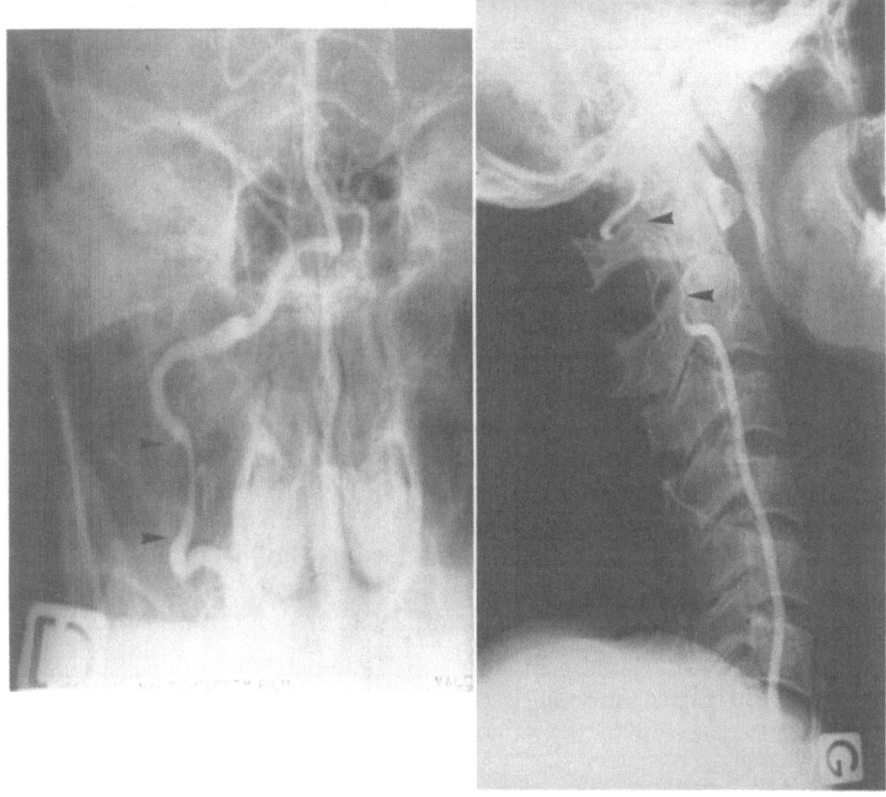

Fig. 14. Dissecting hematoma on both V. A.'s at C 1–C 2 level after mild cervical trauma

Consequently, direct cervical trauma at this level may lead to V. A. stretching (Sherman *et al.*, 1981, Hadley *et al.*, 1985).

4.2.1.4. Physiopathologic Aspects

a) Mechanism

Several different mechanisms have been advanced to explain the traumatic intimal disruption and subsequent dissection. Autopsy and operative reports have helped to understand them (Krueger and Okazaki, 1980, Hadley *et al.*, 1985, Alexander *et al.*, 1986).

a—1. V. A. stretching in the third portion, during head turning if sufficiently forced and rapid, or during head flexion in the particular form of the child.

a—2. Direct contusion of the V. A.:
— at the C 1–C 2 level by the anterior branch of the second cervical nerve, which may compress the V. A. during rotational movements,
— in the second portion, by an osteophytic spur,
— at the entry into the transverse canal by fascial bands or musculo-tendinous formations.

a—3. Tearing of the V. A. by muscular branches at each interspace is a possible mechanism, especially at the C1–C2 level. This is the mechanism advanced for dissection in the newborn.

b) Consequences

Intimal tear can lead to local thrombosis or dissecting hematoma with subsequent stenosis or occlusion.

Both may subsequently be the source of distal embolism or thrombotic extension up to the basilar trunk.

c) Evolution

The identical arteriographic aspects and evolution of dissections affecting the internal carotid artery and the extracranial V. A. may be explained by the similarity in their structural histology; in both vessels, the arterial wall contains a well developed musculoelastic medial sheath. Conversely, the changes in the intracranial portion of the V. A., with reduction of elastic fibers in the media and disappearance of the external elastic lamina (Wilkinson, 1972), explain the more frequent aneurysmal evolution on this portion.

4.2.1.5 Clinical Aspect

The clinical findings in patients presenting with V. A. dissection are usually suggestive of vertebro-basilar ischemia. Transitory deficits are less frequent than complete stroke, but they are probably underestimated, since only the more severe and persistant neurological complications have received sufficient attention until recently. In fact, isolated symptoms such as vertigo or dizziness may be the only manifestation, although head and neck pain, usually on the side of the involved V. A., are commonly associated.

The clinical course indicates a tendancy for delayed and progressive onset of symptoms. In most cases, a few minutes to several days elapse between trauma and clinical signs. The variability in the course of the illness is probably related to the nature of the pathologic process. Some reports indicate worsening of neurological status during roentgenographic procedures with specific head and neck positioning: flexion-extension for X-rays of the cervical spine, extension for brain C. T. scan (Katirji et al., 1985) or extension for angiography (Goodman and Crawford, 1983).

4.2.1.6 Angiographic Aspects

— Traumatic dissection is usually unilateral, but some bilateral cases after more severe trauma have been reported (Heilbrun et al., 1972, Katirji et al., 1985).

— Three main aspects may be observed:

— regular or irregular narrowing of the V. A., generally segmentary but sometimes involving the entire length of the second portion of the V. A. The exact location of the arterial damage from which the dissection has extended may be indicated by an aneurysm formed at the initial site of intimal tear;

— dissecting aneurysm located at an interspace and often associated with a short narrowing "de voisinage". Such aneurysms are usually described at the V. A. entry into the transverse canal (C6 level), or between C1 and C2 or above the C1 transverse foramen (Davidson et al., 1975, Sherman et al., 1981);

— occlusion of the V. A., more frequently observed on a non-dominant V. A., probably because of the small diameter.

Embolic occlusion or filling defects in branches of the intracranial vertebro-basilar system may be noted. They are usually associated with neurologic sequelae and features of infarction on C. T. scan. Unique or multiple areas of infarction, suggesting, in the latter case, repetitive emboli, located in the brain-stem or cerebellum have been reported by Krueger and Okazaki (1980) and Katirji *et al.* (1985).

4.2.1.7 Evolution

The natural history of V. A. dissection is still unknown.

a) Clinical Evolution

Most patients remain stable, frequently with neurologic sequelae. Katirji (1985) reported one case with recurrent attacks of occipital ischemia after interruption of anticoagulant therapy.

b) Arteriographic Evolution

Angiographic controls have shown that dissection of the V. A., like that of the internal carotid artery, is not a fixed lesion. Improvement or complete resolution is commonly observed on angiograms repeated 3 to 6 months after diagnosis.

In fact, resolution is the usual outcome when the initial lesion is an arterial narrowing, although small residual irregularities on the arterial wall are frequent.

Conversely, in the case of occlusion, repermeabilization is uncommon, probably because of the small size of the V. A.

If aneurysm is the initial feature, variable improvement in the form of a more regular wall and smaller ectasy, may be observed; but, as on the internal carotid artery, angiographic control at 3 months always reveals a persistent dissecting aneurysm.

In the case of resolution after initial narrowing, angiographic control may help find certain predisposing factors: V. A. loop, fibrous band, osteophytic spur ... The discovery of such factors may lead to surgical treatment in order to prevent recurrence of ischemic complications.

4.2.2 Treatment

Reported treatments generally consist of supportive care and rehabilitation. When dissection of the V. A. is suspected, neck manipulation of any kind should be avoided and extreme care should be taken when performing roentgenographic procedures that require specific head and neck positioning, such as roentgenograms of the cervical spine, C. T. scan or cerebral angiograms.

Treatment should be directed at reducing the danger of future extension and complications of the dissection.

Anticoagulation by intravenous heparin and then warfarin for at least three months has been suggested by some as rational therapy in the hope of preventing progressive brainstem infarction (Sherman *et al.*, 1981), but others prefer antiaggregant drugs in order to avoid the risk of anticoagulant therapy causing hemorrhage into infarcted brain.

Surgery has been proposed very rarely for initial treatment of this lesion (Goodman and Crawford, 1983, Hadley *et al.*, 1985, Alexander *et al.*, 1986). The aim of surgery is to eliminate the point of origin of the dissection; but since the natural course of the disease is usually benign, medical management is in most cases preferred initially.

However, distal embolism and repeated ischemic attacks under medical treatment have led to proposals for surgical exclusion of the lesion. In these cases, the dissection is in general not completely healed, and even after 6 months, an arterial lesion persists which explains the continuing embolic events. This is particularly observed when the initial lesion was an aneurysm, which "a priori" requires surgical treatment. Since experience in V. A. dissecting aneurysm is limited, it seems advisable to treat any form of dissection, conservatively in the initial stages. Surgery must not be considered before a minimum of 3 months in cases with arterial narrowing or occlusion. Faced with aneurysm, a shorter delay should be observed before deciding to occlude the V. A. under distal revascularization (Laurian *et al.*, 1983). Immediate surgery is indicated only in the rare cases where the diagnosis is made after several ischemic events.

4.2.3 Dissection on a V. A. with Pre-existing Arterial Disease

4.2.3.1 Fibromuscular Dysplasia (F. M. D.)

Occurrence of dissection in the course of F. M. D. affecting vascular axes in the neck is now well established and documented (Ojeman *et al.*, 1972, Fisher *et al.*, 1978).

It has been suggested that minor injuries to the neck could be sufficient to precipitate dissection of arteries involved by F. M. D. (Ringel *et al.*, 1978) and that hypertension due to renal F. M. D. could be a contributing factor. Diagnosis of F. M. D. may be easy when a "string of beads" angiographic appearance is seen on the cervico-cerebral or renal arteries; but in some cases it can only be made on histologic examination (Hugenholtz *et al.*, 1982).

However, pathologic samples of the V. A. are rarely obtained from autopsy studies, and therefore the diagnosis of dissection on preexisting F. M. D. is frequently inferred but seldom proven. Simultaneous involvement of several cervical and visceral arteries by F. M. D. associated with V. A. dissection has already been reported (Ringel *et al.*, 1977, Alpert *et al.*, 1982, Mas *et al.*, 1985, Chiras *et al.*, 1985).

The mechanism by which carotid and vertebral arteries are simultaneously affected by dissection, remains totally unclear. However, the angiographic similitude of this lesion with dissection of traumatic origin, and the elective involvement of the third portion of the V. A. suggest a more predominant role of traumatic factors than of the under-lying arterial disease.

4.2.3.2 Other Underlying Arterial Diseases

Several underlying diseases have been suggested as predisposing factors for V. A. dissection and aneurysm forma-tion: migraine (Bladin, 1974), Ehlers-Danlos syndrome (Edwards, 1969, Brodribb, 1970), infection (Ogilvic, 1940) or atheroma (Thompson *et al.*, 1979), but a clear demonstration of their relation to V. A. dissection is rarely made.

In 2 cases reported in the literature, V. A. dissection was associated with arterial dissection in other territories: bilateral dissection of the renal arteries (Bostrom and Lilliequist, 1967) or dis-section of the external carotid artery and the subclavian artery (Pilz, 1982). Pathologic exam of the cervical arteries revealed non specific idiopathic medial necrosis. These cases could be classi-fied in the group of spontaneous dis-section; but as several arteries were involved, one cannot help evoking diffuse arterial disease.

4.2.4 *Spontaneous Dissection—Fig. 15*

Spontaneous onset of cervical artery dissection is now commonly recog-nized. In these cases, no evidence of trauma, of predisposing factors, or of underlying arterial disease is demon-strated (Bradac *et al.*, 1981, Mas *et al.*, 1985, Chiras *et al.*, 1985). The diagnosis of these cases is generally reported under the name of cystic medianec-rosis, but some factors may have been underestimated or overlooked as possi-ble explanations:

1. A variety of circumstances associated with abrupt changes in head position can lead to hyperextension or rotation injury to the neck and induce arterial dissection. Such head and neck move-ments are generally not spontaneously reported by the patients and hence the traumatic origin of these cases is not recognized. A careful history, with maximum details on patient activities

preceding the onset of symptoms, should be taken before eliminating any traumatic influence.

2. Equally, some predisposing factors should be more thoroughly sought: cervical spine anomalies, whether con-genital or acquired, or anomaly of V. A. entry into the transverse canal.

3. Associated arterial disease may not be apparent on biologic and radiolog-ical investigations, and pathologic studies are rarely obtained, as already mentioned (Hugenholtz *et al.*, 1982).

In all "spontaneous" dissections of the V. A., iterative angiograms should be obtained at least as frequently as after internal carotid artery dissection. Tor-tuosity, loop, or plicature from external compression could probably be more frequently demonstrated and appro-priate prophylactic treatment under-taken where indicated.

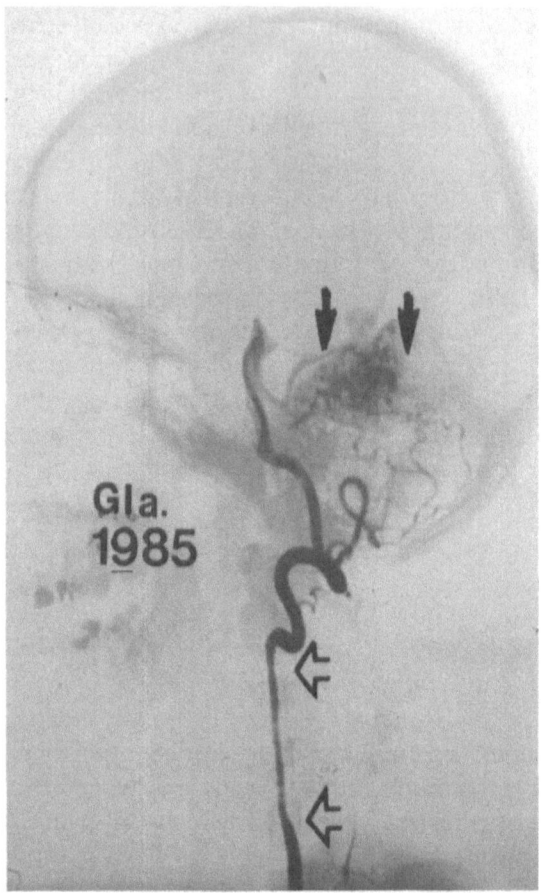

Fig. 15. Spontaneous dissection of the transverse portion (C 5–C 2) associated with cerebellar arteriovenous malformation

4.3 Fibromuscular Dysplasia

Fibromuscular dysplasia (F. M. D.) is the third most frequent structural lesion involving the V. A., after atherosclerotic lesion and dissection, as on the internal carotid artery.

4.3.1 Frequency

F. M. D. is often discovered incidentally during angiographic investigations performed on patients presenting with various neurological symptoms and, especially, with subarachnoïd hemorrhage.

It is generally estimated that changes due to F. M. D. can be expected in 0.25% to 0.77% of all cerebral angiograms (Stanley *et al.*, 1974, So *et al.*, 1981).

Extracranial V. A. involvement is observed in about 7 to 10% of the reported cases of cephalic F. M. D. (Frens *et al.*, 1974) but V. A. F. M. D. is undoubtedly more common than generally inferred from the paucity of existing cases. The reason is that extracranial dysplastic lesions have long remained unrecognized, since many of the angiographic studies, performed to seek intracranial aneurysm, were limited in most neuroradiological centers to the intracranial vessels, with resulting incomplete visualization of the cervical area.

4.3.2 Genetic Characteristics

F. M. D. is considered a hereditary vascular disease with a wide spectrum of cerebro-vascular accidents, including subarachnoïd hemorrhage from intracranial aneurysms. F. M. D. preferentially affects young and middle-aged patients, mainly female (Mettinger and Ericson, 1982).

4.3.3 Clinical Findings

Among clinical findings, cerebral ischemia is not the predominant feature, even in cases involving the cervicocephalic vessels. In their compilation from the literature, Mettinger and Ericson (1982) found that more than 50% had hemorrhagic neurological events. Symptoms of vertebro-basilar insufficiency were rarely reported.

4.3.4 Angiographic Features

1. The characteristic angiographic feature of F. M. D. is the "string of beads" appearance, corresponding to segments of vessel constriction alternating with dilatation. This feature may explain reduction in cerebral blood flow if it is sufficiently pronounced to induce significant stenosis on several cervical vessels.

It is very likely that F. M. D. lesions produce more significant stenosis than is usually estimated on angiography. Doppler effect should be more frequently used as an adjunct to angiography in order to more accurately assess the hemodynamic consequences of F. M. D. stenoses.

2. Atypical F. M. D., as named by Houser *et al.* (1971) and Mettinger and Ericson (1982), corresponds to angiographic changes with tubular narrowing or dissecting aneurysm. These aspects may represent a particular stage in the disease development; dissection is referred to as a possible complication in the course of F. M. D., but complete occlusion of the V. A. has not yet been reported. Nevertheless, one case with bilateral involvement by F. M. D. and complete occlusion on one side is reported in our series (see chapter Personal Experience) (**Fig. 17**).

3. F. M. D. mainly affects the first and third portions of the cervical V. A. The most frequent location is near the C 2 transverse foramen.

In one report by So *et al.* (1981), V. A. lesions extended intracranially but did not affect the basilar artery.

Bilateral involvement seems less common in the V. A.'s than in the internal carotid arteries.

4.3.5 *Associated Arterial Lesions*

4.3.5.1 Internal Carotid Artery

Most cases of V. A. F. M. D. are associated with concomitant carotid system involvement (Stanley *et al.*, 1974, Osborn and Anderson, 1977) **(Fig. 16)**.

4.3.5.2 Intracranial Aneurysm

Correlation between F. M. D. and intracranial aneurysm is now well established. Mettinger and Ericson (1982) report a frequency of 21% of associated intracranial aneurysm.

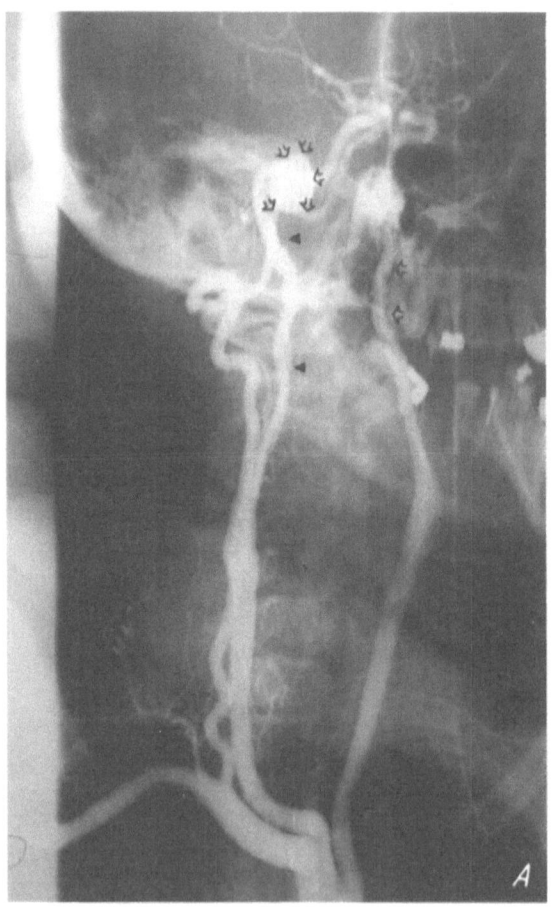

Fig. 16. A) Fibromuscular dysplasia affecting both carotid arteries and the right V. A. Aneurysm on the intracranial V. A. **B)** Fibromuscular dysplasia with multiple ectasias on the right carotid and V. A.

Aneurysms when associated with F. M. D. are more frequently multiple or located on the supraclinoid internal carotid artery. Actually, this percentage is probably underestimated, as the cervical area is generally omitted in the angiographic studies; some studies with complete angiography indicate a true incidence of more than 50%. This suggests the possibility of two different diseases producing intracranial aneurysm, with separate characteristics regarding sex, topography and multiplicity (George et al., 1986) (Fig. 16).

4.3.5.3 Other Associated Dysplastic Lesions

F. M. D. involvement of other arteries has been found to occur with low frequency among patients having carotid and vertebral F. M. D.. Renal and visceral vessels are the most frequently reported arteries simultaneously involved by F. M. D. (Stanley et al., 1974, So et al., 1981, Mas et al., 1985).

A rare case of widespread F. M. D. was reported by Bellot et al. (1985). F. M. D. was found to affect the extracranial vessels (internal carotid artery, V. A., external carotid artery and subclavian artery) as well as intracranial vessels, the aorta and visceral branches.

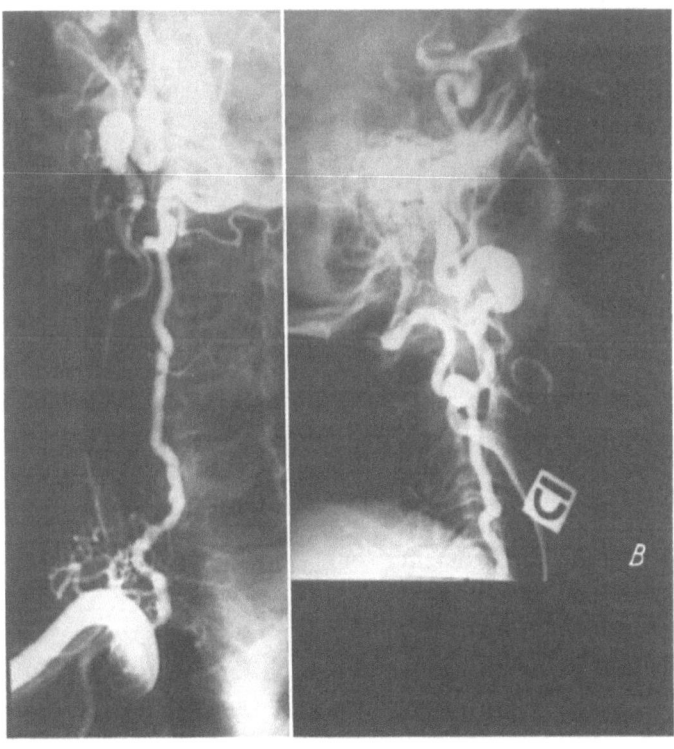

Fig. 16 B

4.3.6 Evolution

Follow up studies reported by Mettinger and Ericson (1982) give evidence of both progressive and stationary evolution on the internal carotid artery, whereas regression has not been reported.

Conversely, the natural history of V. A. F. M. D. is still not well known.

4.3.7 Complications

In the course of F. M. D., several complications may occur, explaining the rare clinical manifestations related to the disease: dissection and aneurysm, thromboembolism, arterio-venous fistula and cerebral blood flow reduction. Besides these pathologic conditions, the particular complications of other localizations of the disease (systemic hypertension, cerebral hemorrhage) must not be forgotten.

4.3.7.1 Dissection and Aneurysm

Arterial dissection and dissecting aneurysm of the V. A. is an already discussed complication related either to medial anomalies or to traumatic factors (see chapter Dissection) (**Fig. 17**).

4.3.7.2 Thromboembolism

a) At the time of diagnosis, most patients with V. A. as well as internal carotid artery F. M. D., are probably asymptomatic; in the reported cases where neurologic deficits have been attributed to extracranial cerebrovascular dysplasia, the existence of F. M. D. in general correlates poorly with the clinical symptoms. Although there is a real possibility for F. M. D. to be the source of cerebral emboli, since thrombus has been shown to be present in carotid artery F. M. D. (So *et al.*,

1981); this has not yet been observed in V. A. F. M. D..

Despite this fact, in older patients, atherosclerosis is frequently associated with F. M. D. and can be sufficient to explain onset of cerebral ischemia.

Finally, there is the possibility of em-

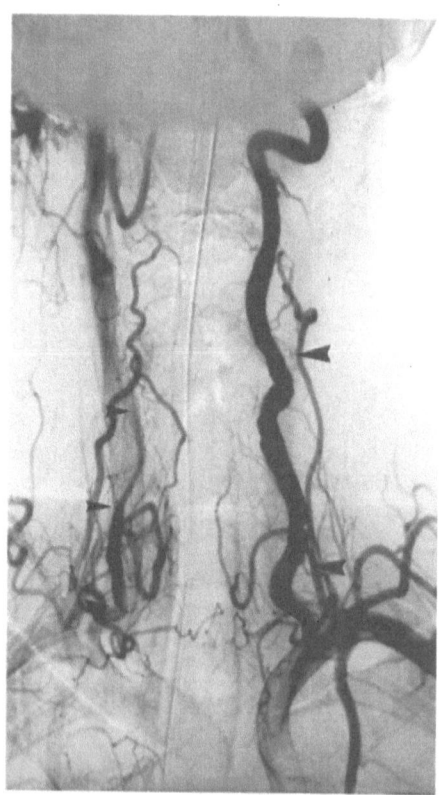

Fig. 17. Fibromuscular dysplasia affecting both V. A.'s. Dissecting hematoma with occlusion on the right side

bolus migration from a dissection or an aneurysm developed in the course of F. M. D..

b) Occlusion has been thought to result from progressive evolution of the disease (Stanley et al., 1974). Dissection is more probably responsible, but this has never been demonstrated.

4.3.7.3 Arteriovenous Fistula (Fig. 18)

Rupture of a dissection or, more likely, of a dissecting aneurysm into the perivertebral venous plexus explains the rare but possible occurrence of an arterio-venous fistula in the course of F. M. D.. Clinical features depend on the location and size of the fistula. Most cases have been discovered as an incidental finding in asymptomatic patients with a cervical bruit (Robles, 1968, Bonduelle et al., 1973, Geraud et al., 1973). Rarely, progressive neurological deficit leads to diagnosis (Reddy et al., 1981).

Arteriovenous fistulas are usually found at C 2–C 4 level and most of the cases present as low flow fistulas.

Very few have been treated by surgical procedures (Reddy et al., 1981).

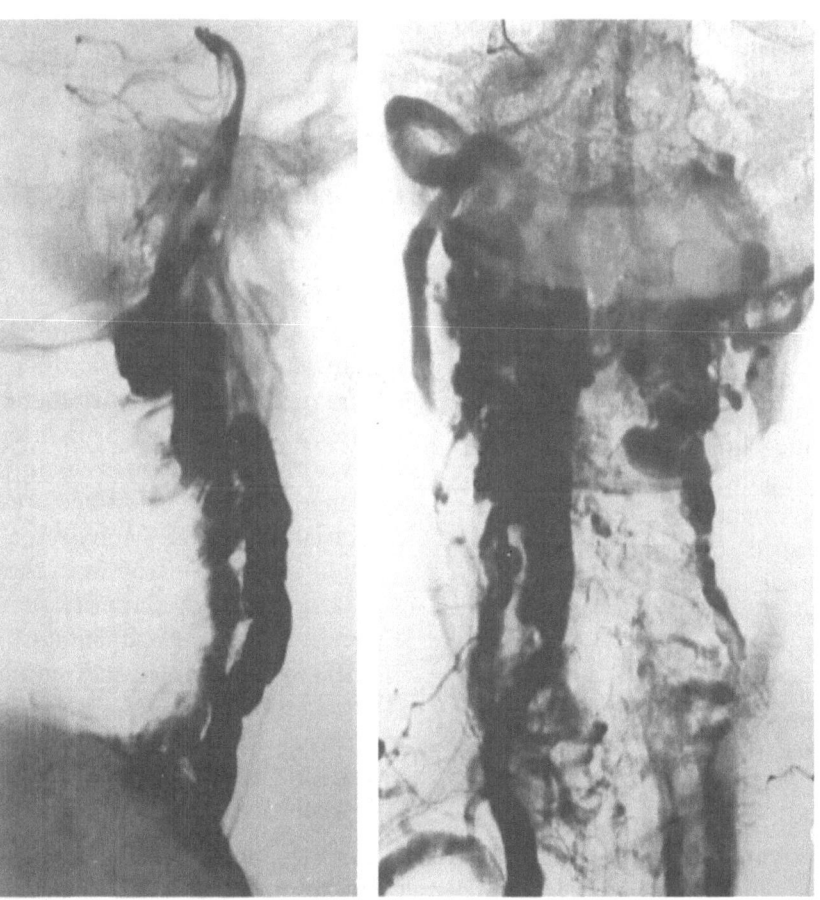

Fig. 18. Fibromuscular dysplasia affecting both V. A.'s. Arteriovenous fistula on both sides

Spontaneous closure after angiography has been seen in some cases (Sher *et al.*, 1966, Bonduelle *et al.*, 1973).

4.3.7.4 Cerebral Blood Flow Reduction

F. M. D. involvement of up to four extracranial vessels may cause signifi- cant reduction of cerebral blood flow if F. M. D. lesions of carotid and ver- tebral arteries lead to severe stenosis. Doppler examination more accurately evaluates the hemodynamic conse- quences, as emphasized above. Surgical indications must be discussed in such cases.

4.4 Unusual Lesions of the V. A.

Unusual diseases involving the ver- tebral artery may produce either occlusive or aneurysmal lesions. Occlusion is mainly observed in giant cell arteritis (Horton's disease in French literature). Extracranial aneurysms are essentially traumatic in origin; other causes such as neurofi- bromatosis, Ehlers-Danlos syndrome, atherosclerosis or mycosis are very rare.

4.4.1 Giant Cell Arteritis

4.4.1.1 Pattern of Arterial Involvement

During the acute phase of giant cell arteritis, there appears to be a very high incidence of severe involvement of the V. A. However this statement is based on pathologic studies and not on sys- tematic clinical and angiographic in- vestigations. The pattern of arterial involvement is reflected by the high incidence of monocular blindness, occipital blindness and brain stem stroke in the course of this arteritis. Some pathologic studies have shown the pattern of arterial involvement (Crompton, 1959, Wilkinson and Russel, 1972, Voordecker *et al.*, 1972):
— The most consistently and severely involved arteries are: first, the super- ficial temporal and, second, the ver- tebral, ophthalmic and posterior ciliary arteries.

— The mode of V. A. involvement is always the same; characteristic features of the disease are observed throughout the extracranial segment from the origin up to a sharply defined upper limit located 5 mm above the point of dural penetration. It must therefore be stressed that evidence of arteritis is never observed above this point, where changes in histologic structure of the arterial wall occur. Moreover, a corre- lation can be found between the sever- ity and extent of the arteritic process on the V. A. and the amount of elastic fibers in the media and adventitia in the extracranial portion.

4.4.1.2 Clinico-pathologic Correlation

The striking incidence of ischemic strokes and autopsy findings of infarct in the cerebellum, occipital lobe or brain stem correlates well with post-mortem evidence of severe V. A. involvement.

Cerebral infarcts can occur as a result of direct extension of thrombosis or embolization from the segment involved by disease.

It seems likely that arteritic thickening of the V. A. is quite common in giant cell arteritis, but most often it has little or no effect on the hemodynamic supply of the vertebro-basilar system. This explains the frequent absence of symptoms and, consequently, the low number of angiographically investigated patients.

4.4.2 Neurofibromatosis

In addition to tumoral manifestations, vascular lesions are well recognized but uncommon features of Recklinghausen's disease.

Arterial lesions are known to affect the renal and gastro-intestinal vessels and, more rarely, the large intracranial vessels.

The most common abnormality is arterial stenosis, particularly on the proximal portion of the renal artery. Aneurysms are less common lesions.

Four cases of aneurysm on the extracranial V. A. are reported in the literature (Schubiger and Yaşargil, 1978, Pentecost et al., 1981, Deans et al., 1982). The diagnosis was never evoked initially, since in all cases the referring symptoms were those of progressive or sudden compression of the cervical nerve roots or the spinal cord. Solid tumor, because of its far higher frequency, was always the primary diagnosis. One should be aware of the possibility of an aneurysm in the course of neurofibromatosis so as to perform an angiography when a tumoral process is not demonstrated.

The diagnosis of neurofibromatosis was made in 3 adult patients on the basis of "café au lait" spots on the skin or subcutaneous neurofibromas.

In the fourth patient, a child, diagnosis was made after histologic examination. The arterial lesion was a saccular aneurysm of the first portion of the V. A. in one case, and the second portion in the others, with an associated arterio-venous fistula in 2 cases.

An angiographic follow up was available in the child case; over a period of 7 years, aneurysmal dilatation of the thoracic aorta and subclavian artery appeared.

In every case, cervical spine films showed enlargement of one intervertebral foramen, and myelography revealed an extradural defect with spinal cord displacement.

In neurofibromatosis, angiography should be more routinely performed; in cases where an hour-glass neurofibroma is suspected, the relation between tumor and the V. A. is important pre-operative information (see chapter Tumor); in addition, angiography may discover an aneurysm, which obviously will alter the surgical procedure. Adequate treatment should include exclusion of the V. A., followed by resection of the aneurysm in order to decompress the spinal cord or the nerve root. Associated revascularization of the V. A. above the distal exclusion should be considered.

4.4.3 Other Aneurysmal Lesions

Blunt or penetrating trauma is the most common cause of aneurysm, whether it is a "true" or a "false" one.

Non-traumatic aneurysms have been attributed to fibromuscular dysplasia (see Fibromuscular Dysplasia), atherosclerosis (Thompson *et al.*, 1979) or mycotic lesions due to osteomyelitis of the spine (Ogilvic, 1940).

Cases of aneurysm in the course of Ehlers-Danlos syndrome have also been described (Edwards, 1969, Brodribb, 1970). This condition might be more common than is generally thought, particularly in its mildest forms.

Spontaneous aneurysm, especially in a young patient, should lead to investigations directed towards connective tissue disorders.

In some cases, no explanation can be found, as in the case reported by Kikuchi and Kowada (1983), and congenital origin must be assumed.

5. ARTERIOVENOUS MALFORMATIONS

Vertebral arteriovenous malformations are defined by the presence of abnormal communications between the extracranial V. A. or one of its muscular or radicular branches and the neighboring veins (**Fig. 19**).

Several different types of V. A. arteriovenous malformations can be described, according to their nature and mode of occurrence:

1. Spontaneous vertebro-vertebral fistulas, in fact frequently occurring on pre-existing arterial disease.
2. Arteriovenous fistulas following trauma of various types.
3. Congenital regional arteriovenous malformations, or what will be termed here "angiodysplasia".

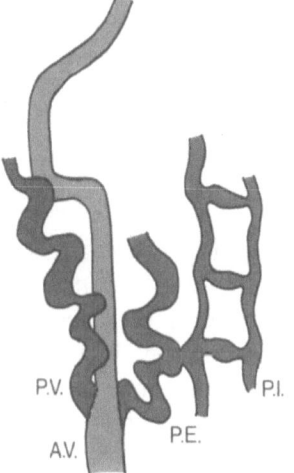 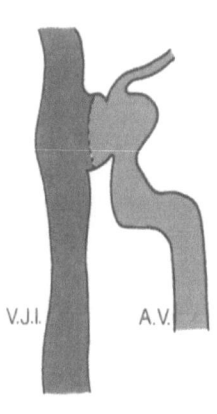

Fig. 19. Arteriovenous fistula. Left: arteriovenous fistula between the V. A. and the peri-vertebral venous plexus. *P. I.* Intraspinal venous plexus; *P. E.* extraspinal venous plexus; *P. V.* perivertebral venous plexus. Right: arteriovenous fistula between the V. A. and the internal jugular vein with an interposed false aneurysm

5.1 Spontaneous Vertebro-vertebral Fistulas

Congenital arteriovenous fistula (A. V. F.) is a rare lesion, generally discovered incidentally in childhood during routine examination, but sometimes also at an older age. This explains the usual confusion in the terminology between spontaneous and congenital A. V. F. (Reizine *et al.*, 1985).

Congenital vertebro-vertebral A. V. F. is discussed in the chapter on Infancy and Childhood. This chapter will therefore be devoted solely to A. V. F. associated with fibro-muscular dysplasia (F. M. D.).

In parallel with improvements in cerebral angiography, F. M. D. has been diagnosed with increasing frequency. Association of F. M. D. involving the cerebral vessels and intracranial aneurysms and/or arterio-venous fistulas in the intracranial carotid system or the extracranial vertebral system is now well established (Bellot *et al.*, 1985, Reizine *et al.*, 1985, Hieshima *et al.*, 1986).

5.1.1 Clinical Symptoms

A. V. F. is discovered in a variety of settings:

— Most frequently, the complaint is occipital or cervical pain associated with a bruit in the homolateral ear.

— Another frequent circumstance is incidental discovery of a cervical bruit in asymptomatic patients.

— More rarely, patients present with spinal cord dysfunction due to compression by a markedly engorged epidural venous plexus (Reddy *et al.*, 1981, Reizine *et al.*, 1985).

In all reported cases, symptoms have appeared spontaneously in adult female patients.

5.1.2 Angiographic Features

Most of the fistulas are located at the C 2–C 3 level and are directly supplied by the V. A. All have very small orifices of communication, implying that the source of fistula is a tiny rupture in the arterial wall (Reddy *et al.*, 1981, Bahar *et al.*, 1984, Hieshima *et al.*, 1986).

Dissecting aneurysm of the extracranial V. A. may be observed in the course of F. M. D. associated with A. V. F. (Geraud *et al.*, 1973). In this case, rupture of the aneurysm is the likely cause of A. V. F.

Venous communication is into the perivertebral venous plexus, and drainage involves epidural and paravertebral veins.

5.1.3. Pathophysiology

As previously mentioned, rupture of a dissecting aneurysm is a possible explanation, but association between F. M. D. and spontaneous A. V. F. could be purely coincidental. Actually, minor trauma may precipitate such a complication. F. M. D. probably appears before the onset of A. V. F. and may be considered as a predisposing factor by weakening the arterial wall.

This hypothesis has not yet been clearly demonstrated, since there are no reported cases with repetitive angiography showing pre-existing F. M. D. at the site of a subsequent arterio-venous fistula. Similarly, there is no available evidence of the relation between F. M. D. and A. V. F. from pathologic studies.

However, some cases have been reported (Robles, 1968—see also **Fig. 18** in the chapter Wall Lesion) with a long standing history of arterio-venous fistulas and an enlarged and tortuous appearance of the proximal V. A., quite similar to that observed in F. M. D.

5.1.4 Treatment

5.1.4.1 Endovascular Technique

Detachable balloon embolization by femoral or brachial route is now the initial treatment of choice.

However, some difficulties related to the changes induced by F. M. D. in the arterial wall may be encountered. Catheterization of the V. A. and stabilization of the balloon at the exact fistula site may be difficult and sometimes impossible. In case of failure by this route, the balloon may be positioned through either an anastomotic collateral artery such as the occipital artery, or a dilated venous channel, with the balloon released on the venous side of the fistula (Reizine et al., 1985).

5.1.4.2 Surgical Technique

Direct surgical closure is indicated only after failure of the endovascular procedure. V. A. control below and above the fistula generally allows exposure and occlusion of the arterial orifice.

5.1.4.3 Indication

Spontaneous cure of a vertebro-vertebral fistula is a possibility already reported (Reizine et al., 1985), but usually, the natural evolution is progressive and very slow. This explains why some patients have never been treated (Geraud et al., 1973, Bonduelle et al., 1978). Today, endovascular techniques in well-trained hands are quite reliable and in most cases successful. Surgery is to be considered only after failure of invasive radiological techniques in symptomatic patients.

5.2 Traumatic Arteriovenous Fistulas

5.2.1 Iatrogenic A. V. F.

Iatrogenic vertebro-vertebral A. V. F.'s have now become very infrequent, raising the question of whether this complication may not be more common than is reported in the literature.

Direct intentional puncture of the V. A. is no longer performed, but fistulas may develop after attempts of common carotid artery puncture. In fact, the most frequent cause today is unintentional puncture of the V. A. during routine insertion of internal jugular and subclavian venous catheters.

Interventional radiology with endovascular procedures is now the treatment of choice, and surgery is confined to cases in which endovascular techniques have failed to achieve correct closure of the fistula.

5.2.1.1 Etiology

The first identified cause of iatrogenic A. V. F. was the direct puncture of the V. A. for vertebral angiographic injection (Olson *et al.*, 1963, Chou and French, 1965, Jamieson, 1965, Lester,

1966, Sher *et al.*, 1966, Veneken, 1970, Bergquist, 1971).

The exact incidence of the onset of A. V. F. following direct vertebral angiography is difficult to establish, since spontaneous closure is possible and unrecognized cases because of mild symptoms were probably numerous.

Vertebral A. V. F. may also be observed after attempts at carotid artery puncture; this is more likely to occur in a technically difficult exam or if performed by inexperienced radiologists (Bergstrom and Lodin, 1966, Bjork, 1966, Marelli, 1967, Maroun *et al.*, 1983, Stecken *et al.*, 1983).

The wide use of the internal jugular

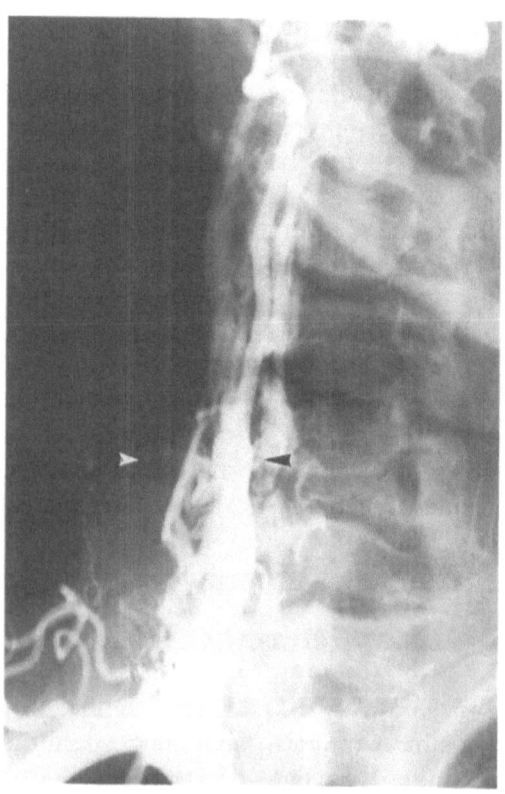

Fig. 20. Arteriovenous fistula at C6 between the V. A. and the perivertebral venous plexus, following puncture (attempts of venous catheterism)

vein to place central catheters explains the reported cases of cervical arterial trunk injuries, including the V. A. in its first portion (Dodson *et al.*, 1980, Reizine *et al.*, 1985) (**Fig. 20**).

Surgery on neighboring structures has also induced, in rare cases, V. A. injury with subsequent A. V. F.: cervical spine surgery (Weinberg and Flom, 1973), mastoidectomy or cervical sympathectomy (Reizine *et al.*, 1985).

5.2.1.2 Physiopathology

The mechanism of injury by puncture explains some particularities of these A. V. F.

a) V. A. Injury

Whether the arterial puncture is intentional or not, the V. A. is generally transfixed by the needle, and double opposing fistula sites are therefore possible.

Moreover, repeated puncture attempts may lead to multiple arteriovenous fistulas, the identification of which is generally not possible, since the early filling of the venous plexus hides them (Stecken *et al.*, 1983).

b) A. V. F.

Punctiform communication is usually the result of iatrogenic A. V. F., since the puncture is usually performed at the transverse canal level where the arterial and venous walls are in contact. In such cases, the fistulas were never identified during surgery and the V. A. was merely isolated from the venous channels (Chou and French, 1965).

Conversely, in first portion of the V. A., the vertebral veins are slightly more distant from the V. A., and a false aneurysm is usually interposed.

c) A. V. F. Site

A. V. F. in the transverse canal after vertebral or carotid artery puncture is observed more frequently between C 4 and C 6.

A. V. F. after venous catheterization attempts is seen at the lowest level of the transverse canal (C 5–C 6) or in the first portion of the V. A.

5.2.1.3 Clinical Aspects

The small communication explains the low flow observed in these A. V. F. and consequently the lack of symptoms, except for a bruit sometimes perceived by the patient.

5.2.1.4 Angiographic Aspects

Selective injection of the V. A. confirms the vertebro-vertebral fistula and determines its level, site of communication, and venous drainage. Frequently these data cannot be obtained without selective injection below or above an occlusive balloon.

This technique, generally performed in the first step of endovascular treatment, may reveal multiple fistula sites or, conversely, a single fistula where standard injection shows an apparently complex malformation.

5.2.1.5 Treatment

a) Endovascular Technique

Endovascular technique is the treatment of choice because of its relative simplicity and overall efficacy.

However some cases may raise certain difficulties:
— difficulty in entering the fistula if it is punctiform,
— difficulty in the case of multiple fistulas,
— difficulty in treating successfully in the case of false aneurysm, since a residual pouch may persist on the arterial wall (Reizine et al., 1985). However, for the authors just cited, few complications have been observed with these residual aneurysms.

b) Surgery

Cure of these low flow fistulas has been obtained by proximal ligation only (Bergstrom and Lodin, 1966, Bergquist, 1971) or by trapping between double proximal and distal ligation (Olson et al., 1963).

However, the preferable objective of preservation of V. A. flow can only be achieved by direct operative approach and closure of the fistula (Jamieson, 1965, Chou and French, 1965).

c) Indications

Since these iatrogenic fistulas are pauci or asymptomatic, their treatment remains debatable.

Continuous and poorly tolerated bruit or evidence of A. V. F. enlargement are the sole reasons justifying treatment of these A. V. F.

Treatment must always start with embolization techniques, and surgery is discussed only after failure of the radiological treatment attempts.

5.2.2 A. V. F. Following Nonpenetrating Trauma

Occurrence of vertebral A. V. F. following blunt trauma to the neck is extremely rare.

Several mechanisms have been proposed to explain their development.

5.2.2.1 Physiopathology

a) Mechanism

Severe hyperextension injury to the cervical spine, associated with fracture luxation or fracture of the transverse process may cause V. A. tearing and subsequent rupture of the arterial wall. V. A. compression or contusion may also follow blunt trauma to the neck and evolve into an A. V. F.

These lesions are observed either in the first portion, at the level of V. A. entry into the transverse canal (Quatromoni et al., 1979, Berguer et al., 1982) or in the third portion.

b) A. V. F.

Hyperextension injury may produce 2 different types of A. V. F.:
— A. V. F. involving the trunk of the V. A., which is the most frequent type,
— A. V. F. involving V. A. branches and not the V. A. itself, which is particular to the C 1–C 2 level, probably because of the rich collateral arterial and venous pathways in the nucal muscles. Tearing of one of these V. A. collaterals is probably the point of origin of this type of A. V. F. (Aronson, 1961, Faeth and Ducker, 1961, Guena

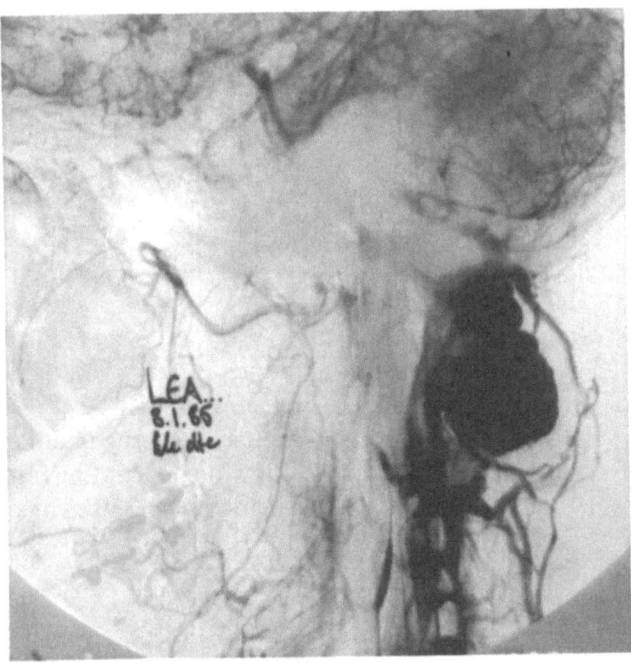

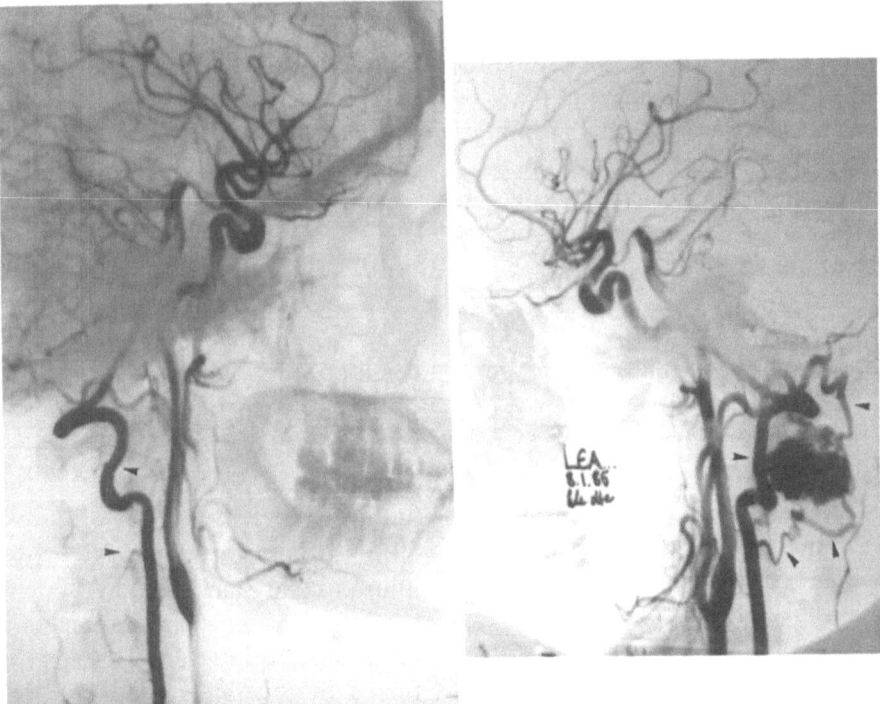

Fig. 21. Arteriovenous malformation of the C1–C2 intervertebral space, four years after hyperextension cervical trauma. Vascular supply from one branch of the V. A. between C1 and C2, one at C3 and one from the occipital artery. Lower: post-operative control

et al., 1978), one case in our own series **(Fig. 21)**.

5.2.2.2 Clinical Aspect

Clinical aspects are not specific; in most cases, nucal or occipital pain and audible bruit are the presenting symptoms. In 2 cases, neurological symptoms were predominant and led to patient referral (Avellanosa *et al.*, 1977, Ohanessian *et al.*, 1980).

Clinically, it is frequently difficult to relate the A. V. F. to trauma because of the paucity of symptoms and the long delay of discovery after trauma.

5.2.2.3 Angiographic Aspects

Angiographic features are those of high or low flow fistula through either direct communication or interposed false aneurysm (Quatromoni *et al.*, 1979, Miller *et al.*, 1984) or V. A. branches at the C 1–C 2 level. The distal V. A. may be occluded (Guena *et al.*, 1978).

5.2.2.4 Treatment

Treatment will be discussed simultaneously with the treatment of A. V. F. following penetrating trauma, since the general attitude is similar.

5.2.3 A. V. F. Following Penetrating Trauma

This was the most frequent V. A. lesion in the past. Direct wounds of the V. A. were mainly observed in the military practice (see chapter Introduction). Large defects in the arterial wall, high flow fistulas, and frequent associated lesions are the main features.

5.2.3.1 Physiopathology

a) Traumatic Agents

Many agents have been reported to produce a penetrating injury of the V. A.: bullets, shell fragments, knives, bayonnets, or non-metallic missiles, such as glass fragments.

b) A. V. F.

Transection or partial section is the most common lesion, and false aneurysm is frequently associated.

The first and third portions of the V. A. are the most frequently involved (Elkin and Harris, 1946, Jefferson *et al.*, 1956, Shumacker *et al.*, 1966).

Venous drainage utilizes the perivertebral venous plexus and epidural veins; but above C 2, the close proximity of the internal jugular vein explains that vertebro-jugular fistula is not uncommon (Goodman *et al.*, 1975, Nagashima *et al.*, 1977, Benhamou *et al.*, 1979) **(Fig. 22)**.

c) Associated Lesions

Other structures in the neck may be injured at the same time; in particular, associated traumatic aneurysm of the common carotid artery has been mentioned by several authors (Sher *et al.*, 1966, Chou *et al.*, 1967, Tsuji *et al.*, 1968, Rothman *et al.*, 1974). Simultaneous injury to the spinal cord and

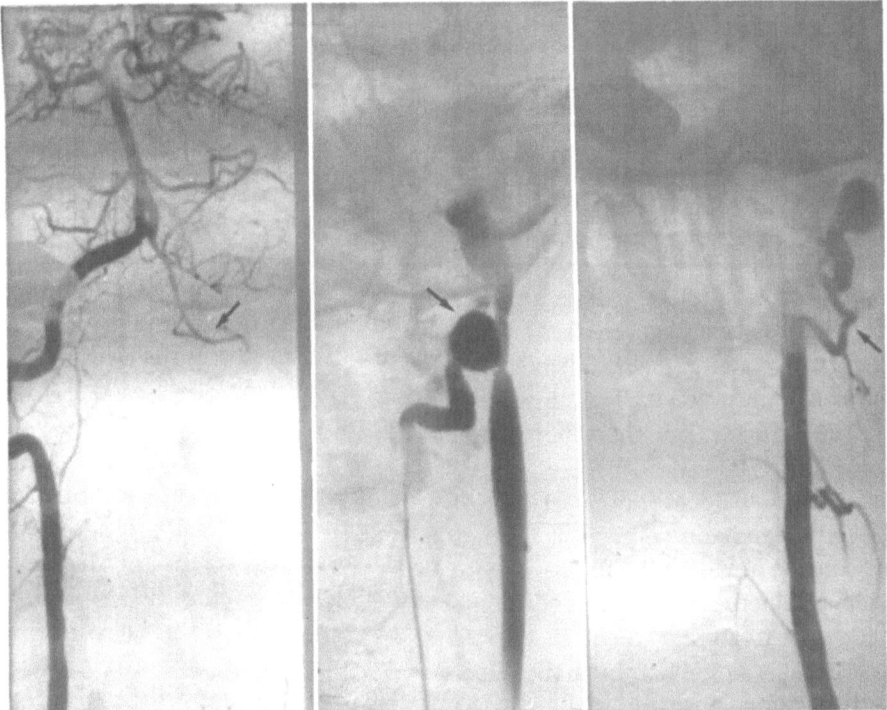

Fig. 22. Arteriovenous fistula between the V. A. and the internal jugular vein with a false aneurysm (gunshot wound)

cervical nerve roots may also, not surprisingly, be observed (Sher *et al.*, 1966, Linde *et al.*, 1970). However, explanation of neurologic symptoms by traumatic A. V. F. may be equivocal, since spinal cord compression by distended epidural veins is another reported possibility (Nagashima *et al.*, 1977).

5.2.3.2 Clinical Aspects

A pulsating mass is the most common finding. However, the A. V. F. may be discovered only on angiography performed for hemorrhagic problems or routinely performed after a penetrating wound to the neck or in the presence of a paravertebral foreign body.

5.2.3.3 Radiological Aspects

— Angiography generally demonstrates a high flow fistula through a large communication, frequently with an interposed aneurysm (**Fig. 22**).

In some cases, external carotid and subclavian artery branches also supply the A. V. F.

The patency of the distal V. A. must be evaluated, but the high flow deviated by the fistula usually results in an important steal from the vertebrobasilar circulation. The best way to differentiate distal occlusion from a complete steal is to inject the V. A. beyond an occlusive balloon placed just distal to the A. V. F. The use of a balloon may also help determine the exact site and importance of the fistula.

— C.T. scan of the cervical spine may be useful, since it can demonstrate cervical spine fractures, false aneurysms and their extension intra and extraspinally, and even dilated epidural veins.

5.2.3.4 Treatment

Many factors, including type and size of the fistula, interposed false aneurysm, patency of the distal V.A. and size of the involved V.A., intervene in the choice of the therapeutic procedure.

In addition, the degree of experience of the radiologist and surgeon, as well as the context in which the fistula is seen, such as emergency, may modify the method of treatment.

In general, a single fistula can be selectively occluded with preservation of the V.A.; on the contrary, a large fistula with false aneurysm requires trapping between proximal and distal V.A. occlusions, with distal revascularization.

a) Surgical Methods

Many different surgical procedures have been proposed in the past. Although some were successful, more often incomplete results or repetitive failures were reported (Elkin and Harris, 1946, Jefferson et al., 1956, Shumacker et al., 1966):

— Simple ligation of the V.A. proximal to the A.V.F. may decrease but not occlude this type of fistula.

— Trapping between distal and proximal ligations must be accomplished as close as possible to the communication in order to avoid recruitment of muscular and radicular collaterals, and sub-

sequent failure (Aronson, 1961, Avellanosa et al., 1977, Ohanessian et al., 1986). However, complete closure of the fistula by this technique cannot be expected, except in some low flow A.V.F.'s.

— Direct surgical closures of the A.V.F. have been attempted with success by some authors (Chou and French, 1965, Verbiest, 1981, Berthelot et al., 1982), but correct results were more likely in the case of small communications.

— Intra-operative balloon occlusion.

A Fogarty balloon catheter introduced through a proximal arteriotomy has been used to occlude the distal V.A. (Bainkley and Wilie, 1973).

A Fogarty catheter has also been utilized to occlude a fistula previously unsuccessfully trapped between proximal and distal ligatures (Goodman et al., 1975, Herrman et al., 1975).

Today, progress in interventional radiology and new surgical techniques offer more reliable means of treatment.

b) Endovascular Methods

— Various materials may be used to occlude a fistula (blood clot, I.B.C., coil, balloon). In the case of A.V.F. following penetrating trauma, detachable balloon is certainly the most appropriate.

The aim of treatment by endovascular methods should be the same as that of surgery. A.V.F. closure with preservation of V.A. flow.

However, this goal cannot always be reached, since it is sometimes impossible to pass the balloon across the fistula or to stabilize it at the proper level.

These difficulties are particularly encountered in the following settings:

— Large fistula with false aneurysm. Sometimes one or several balloons placed inside the aneurysm can correctly treat this form of A. V. F., but most frequently, endovascular treatment either leaves an ectasy on the arterial wall or encroaches upon the arterial lumen. Therefore it may be preferable to deliberately occlude the V. A. and to trap the fistula between 2 balloons. The distal balloon, which must be placed first, sometimes cannot cross the fistula site when passed in anterograde fashion. Retrograde approach through the controlateral V. A. is sometimes feasible in these cases. However the fistula and the V. A. are occluded, the need for V. A. revascularization must be evaluated. As usual, this is decided according to the importance of the involved V. A. in the total cerebral vascular supply.

— A. V. F. on V. A. branches. Occlusion of these branches, precisely at their junction with the fistula, is sometimes impossible; this can result in the development of new collateral branches reinjecting the A. V. F.

— A. V. F. supplied by external carotid and subclavian arteries. These arteries must be embolized first; then the balloon occlusion technique is applied on the V. A. fistula itself.

c) Indications

These traumatic A. V. F. should be treated, as they are generally high flow fistulas with important vertebral steal. Furthermore, symptomatic forms are largely predominant, with at minimum a poorly tolerated bruit.

c—1. Emergency treatment is sometimes required for hemorrhagic problems. Endovascular technique with trapping is the most appropriate procedure in this case.

c—2. A. V. F. without false aneurysm. Direct surgical closure can suppress the fistula if embolization has failed (Kormesser and Bergan, 1974, Fairman et al., 1984). The small size of this type of A. V. F. should pose no particular problems.

c—3. A. V. F. with false aneurysm.

— On the first portion of the V. A., surgical approach may be preferred, since revascularization of the V. A. distal to the lesion can easily be performed using a saphenous vein graft. The fistula and aneurysm are then resected.

— On the third portion, A. V. F. occlusion with a detachable balloon can rarely be achieved without sacrifying the V. A. Closure of the A. V. F. is therefore generally realized by trapping.

If an adequate collateral blood supply to the posterior fossa can be demonstrated, there is no need for distal revascularization. Conversely, in the case of a dominant V. A., by-pass implanted beyond the fistula is performed first, associated with exclusion of the involved V. A. and followed by embolization of the A. V. F.

Direct surgical approach of the fistula is exceptionally indicated, when complete closure of the fistula cannot be achieved by endovascular techniques. However, in large fistulas localized distally near the base of the skull, control of the V. A. above the fistula is often very difficult. Finally, for all V. A. arteriovenous malformations, whatever the therapeutic procedure, close collaboration between well-experienced radiologists and surgeons is mandatory. In all cases, those methods which preserve or restore V. A. flow are to be preferred.

5.3 Congenital Regional Arteriovenous Malformation or Angiodysplasia

Angiodysplasia is a rare disease with a protracted course which presents a major therapeutic problem. Only those lesions supplied principally by the V. A. will be considered here.

The combination of embolization and complex vascular surgery affords new therapeutic possibilities.

5.3.1 Physiopathology

V. A. angiodysplasia is entirely confined to the cervical area, frequently extending to the base of the skull, with major contributing vessels from branches of the external carotid, subclavian and V. A.'s.

Three different types of congenital regional arteriovenous malformation can be distinguished:

I) Angiodysplasia located in the paravertebral soft tissues and posterior cervical muscles (**Fig. 23**).

II) Angiodysplasia located in or around the cervical spine, supplied by branches of both V. A.'s

III) Multiple vertebro-vertebral fistulas located in the transverse and suboccipital portions (C 6–C 1), supplied by muscular and radicular branches of the V. A. This form is quite distinct from the other two, as it does not present as an angiomatous mass in the neck.

From a clinical and therapeutic point of view, this form of multiple fistulas is rather akin to previously described A. V. F. following non-penetrating trauma or F. M. D.; but since it is a congenital anomaly involving several levels of the V. A., it is classified among congenital and regional arteriovenous malformations.

To distinguish these lesions, we prefer to keep the term angiodysplasia for types I and II. This chapter will be devoted only to angiodysplasia.

5.3.2 Clinical Aspects

Patients are most frequently referred for cosmetic reasons because of a cervical mass. Sometimes ulceration of the skin around the ear is the reason for referral.

Very rarely, congestive heart failure ensues from angiodysplasia.

In our experience, one unusual circumstance was observed: spinal cord compression with tetraparesis, due to

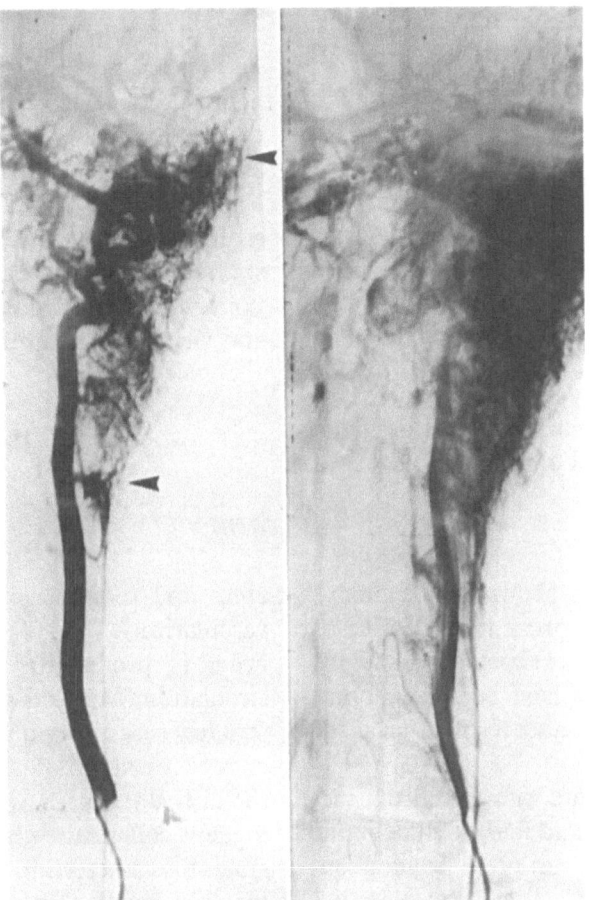

Fig. 23. Angiodysplasia involving the paravertebral muscles from C 4 to the occipital bone

angiodysplasia involving the cervical spine.
On physical examination, a pulsating mass with systolic souffle is confirmed. The overlying skin may also have an angiomatous appearance.

5.3.3 Radiological Aspects

The extent of arteriovenous malformations can be evaluated by angiography and C. T. scan. The first identifies the primary feeding arteries, and the second evaluates the extension in the cervical tissues.

5.3.3.1 Angiography

Global and selective injection of the vertebral, external carotid and subclavian arteries identifies the feeding branches. Some problems may arise when embolization is contemplated:

— Previous ligature of arterial trunks, particularly the external carotid artery, which necessitates, if possible, puncture distal to the ligature.

— Branches of the V. A. cannot be embolized safely without distal protection of vertebral flow by V. A. occlusion. Prior distal V. A. revascularization should be considered even in a minor V. A., since these patients are generally young.

— The origin of V. A. branches supplying the spinal cord must be identified before embolization.

5.3.3.2 C. T. Scan

C. T. scan is more demonstrative and helpful than angiography to determine the true extent of the angiodysplasia and its surgical accessibility.

Extension to certain areas and structures is of particular importance: skull base, upper thoraco-cervical area, upper mediastinal area, cervical spine and visceral structures.

5.3.4 Treatment

Experience has shown that angiodysplasia is highly prone to recur unless it is completely extirpated. Generally, surgical results have been disappointing because of underestimation of the true extent.

Selected patients with significant local complications and fairly well delimited malformations can profit from a combination of embolization and surgical therapy (Rappaport and Rappaport, 1977).

In recent years, embolization therapy alone has been proposed as an alternative form of treatment for inoperable or inaccessible angiodysplasia (Kuhne and Helmke, 1982).

5.3.4.1 Method

a) Embolization

Embolization of the external carotid and subclavian artery branches is performed with various materials. V. A. branch embolization poses the hazard of backflow into functionally important areas and requires exclusion and revascularization of the distal V. A. in order to protect the vertebro-basilar circulation (Merland et al., 1979).

In a few cases, previous surgical failure or repeat embolizations have increased the difficulties because of development of new collaterals which are inaccessible to catheterism since the main trunk is occluded. Percutaneous or peroperative direct puncture and embolization may be discussed in such cases.

b) Surgery

Two techniques can be proposed: excision after embolization, and exclusion plus distal V. A. revascularization before embolization and excision. Postoperative angiographic control must be systematically performed, since persisting residual arterio-venous shunts necessitate re-operation.

c) Indications

Angiodysplasia raises therapeutic problems of varying degrees of magnitude. It must be kept in mind that partial embolization or excision is always a very dangerous procedure. Rapid and sometimes more disabling recurrence is to be feared, with increasing therapeutic problems.

Palliative embolization should be limited to those patients with hemorrhagic or neurologic complications when surgery cannot reasonably be undertaken.

In asymptomatic cases, close follow-up is sufficient. In the face of cosmetic demands, surgery is frequently inadvisable, since the necessary resection of involved muscles and soft tissues may lead a worse result, even more so if complete resection cannot be achieved.

6. TUMOR

6.1 Introduction

The relation of cervical tumors to the V.A. seems not to have been considered before 1967, when Kriss and Schneider reported on the value of vertebral angiography in the treatment of cervical neurofibromas. Before this report, all published studies had been confined almost exclusively to lesions related to the extracranial carotid arteries in the neck. Carotid angiography had been performed to study carotid body tumors, glomus jugulare tumors, and primary and metastatic neoplasms, but there was almost no information and angiography in neurogenic cervical tumors, with the exception of a report by Putney et al. (1964) on a neurilemnoma of the vagus nerve compressing the carotid bifurcation. No data was available from vertebral angiography in cases of intra or paraspinal tumors.

Since that time, the angiographic aspects of every type of tumor that can be observed in the neck have been studied, but the surgical implications of data obtained from vertebral angiography have been stressed by only a few authors. In most reports, even recent, no mention is made of controlling the V.A. Hour-glass tumors are still removed through a posterior approach which progresses blindly towards the V.A. As stated by Kriss and Schneider (1967) in the case of neurinoma, the most frequent tumor, "the vessel is invariably adherent to the capsule anterior to the tumor mass and thus not directly visualized by the surgeon". Love (1952) seems to have been the first to emphasize the interest of the V.A. control in cervical tumor removal. Although he did not attempt V.A. control, he considered it to be a troublesome and dangerous technical problem, as proven by his following comment: "The V.A. can occasionally pose a serious problem since sacrifice of this artery or severe hemorrhage from it may permanently handicap the patient and at times the removal of these lesions taxes the ingenuity of the surgeon to the utmost".

Subsequently, reports on single cases or short series have appeared in the literature, underlying the usefulness of the combined anterior and posterior approach for dumb-bell tumors (Kamano et al., 1980) or of the anterior approach alone (Hakuba et al., 1984) to treat paraspinal and foraminal tumors. Recently, George et al. (1983–1985) reported on a large series of various types of cervical tumors, with removal performed in every case after surgical control of the V.A.

6.2 Relation to the V. A.

Surgical control of the V. A. prior to tumor removal is required in two conditions, which may or may not be associated.

A. The V. A. is in close vicinity of the tumor. The tumor may be in contact with or adherent to the V. A.; at maximum, the V. A. is surrounded by or embedded in the tumor mass. Whatever the degree of involvement, tumor removal is more safely and often more completely achieved after V. A. control.

B. The tumor is highly vascularized and its vascular supply arises mainly from the V. A. In fact, most paraspinal, intraspinal or osseous tumors are supplied by the V. A., since the vertebral body, nerve roots, meningeal sheaths and part of the paravertebral soft tissues belong to the vascular bed of the V. A. It is a basic principle in surgery to begin the removal of a vascular lesion by dividing the main vascular feeders. The fact that the V. A. was considered too difficult and dangerous to expose and to control, led to an exception to this rule. Embolization could be considered, but this technique remains hazardous in the vertebral territory.

6.3 Location of Tumors Involving the V. A.

Any part of the cervical V. A. can be related to a tumor, but the second and third portions are more likely to be involved, since the V. A. is relatively fixed in these parts by the transverse canal (see chapter Anatomy). In the first portion, tumors must be large or extensive to cause a V. A. problem (**Fig. 24**).

Four different locations of tumor,

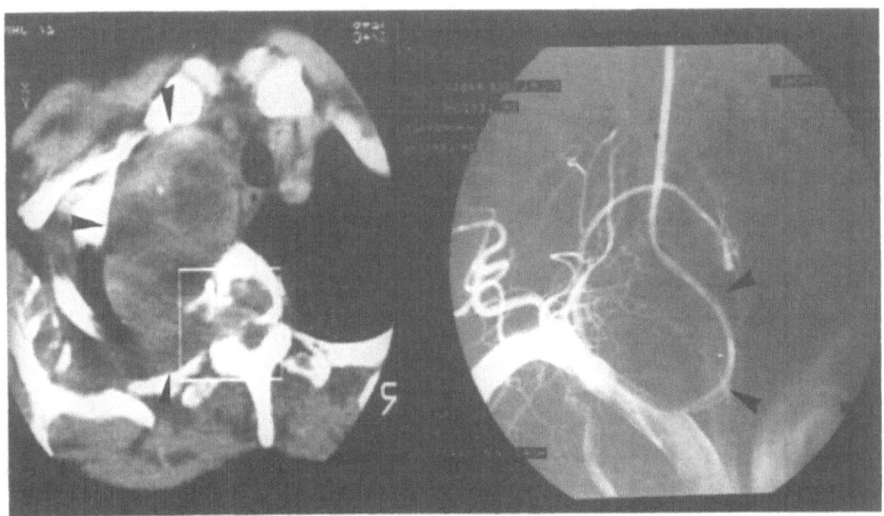

Fig. 24. Hour-glass neurinoma with intrathoracic prolongement

Table 5

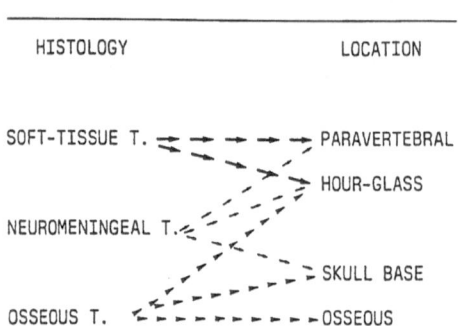

HISTOLOGY	LOCATION

whatever their histologic type, can be related to the V. A.: hour-glass tumor, para-vertebral tumor, osseous tumor of the vertebrae and skull base or foramen magnum tumor with cervical extension.

Table 5 indicates the relation between location and histologic type.

6.3.1 Hour-Glass Tumor

Hour-glass (or dumb-bell) tumors are tumors growing through the intervertebral foramen. Either they originate within the spinal canal and extend outwards towards the V. A., or they begin primarily outside the spinal canal and develop inwards through the foramen. In both cases, the V. A. is usually displaced anteriorly and medially. In rare instances, it may be shifted laterally (**Figs. 25** and **26**).

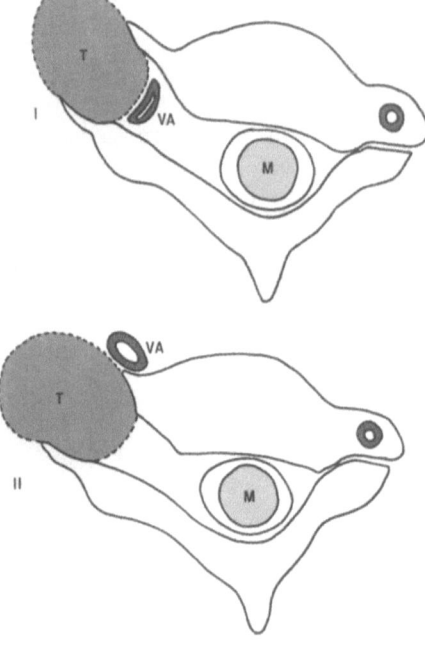

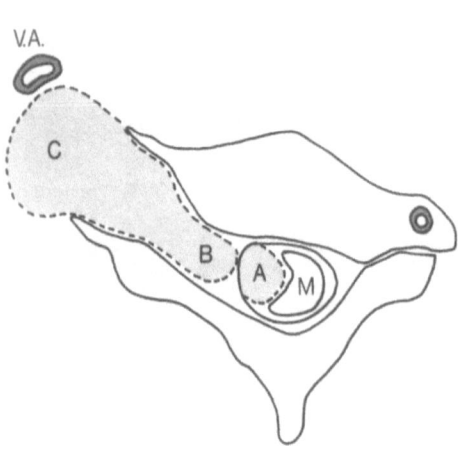

Fig. 25. Cervical hour-glass tumors: *A* intraspinal intradural part, *B* intraspinal extradural part, *C* extraspinal part, *M* spinal cord. Three types may be observed: *A* + *B*: (no relation with the V. A.); *A* + *B* + *C* and *B* + *C* related to the V. A.

Fig. 26. Cervical hour-glass tumors. I) V. A. displacement medially inside the intervertebral foramen. II) V. A. displacement medially and anteriorly. Feature II is the most commonly encountered

6.3.2 Paravertebral Tumor

These tumors remain entirely external to the intervertebral foramen and usually develop at the level of the transverse foramina. Some originate from the cervical soft tissues and reach the transverse canal during their growth. Displacement of the V.A. may be anterior or posterior but is usually medial.

6.3.3 Osseous Tumor

Any type of vertebral tumor may extend to the transverse processes. Most frequently, these tumors arise from the vertebral body or the laminae, but they may also originate from the transverse process itself. This type of tumor usually surrounds the V.A. with minimal displacement; however, compression with more or less marked stenosis or occlusion is frequent.

Osseous location must be clearly distinguished from osseous histologic type, since certain primary osseous tumors may present with an hour-glass form.

6.3.4 Skull Base Tumor

In addition to primary cervical tumors, some skull base and foramen magnum tumors may extend to the cervical area and involve the V.A. (**Fig. 27**). These

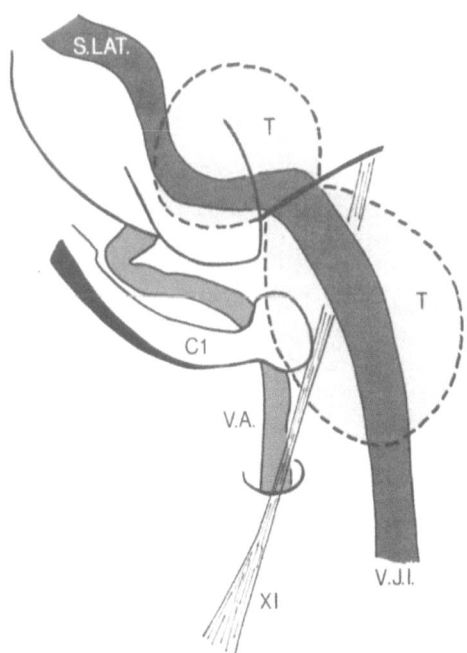

Fig. 27. Intra-extracranial hour-glass tumor. *T* Tumor, *C1* arch of atlas, *V.J.I.* internal jugular vein, *XI* accessory spinal nerve

produce a particular form of hour-glass tumor (intra and extracranial). Extension towards the neck of an intracranial tumor may pass through the jugulare foramen or be direct after invading the bony part of the skull base. Invasion of the base of the skull is most frequently seen with primary osseous tumors. The V. A. is usually displaced inferiorly and posteriorly, with stretching of its segment above the atlas and of its intracranial portion.

6.4 External Compression

Angiographic demonstration of external compression of the V. A. is very frequent in tumors involving the V. A. In our series of 58 tumors, V. A. displacement was noted in 25 cases and stenosis in 12 (George and Laurian, 1986) (**Figs. 28, 29, 30,** and **31**).

As far as we know, only a few symp-

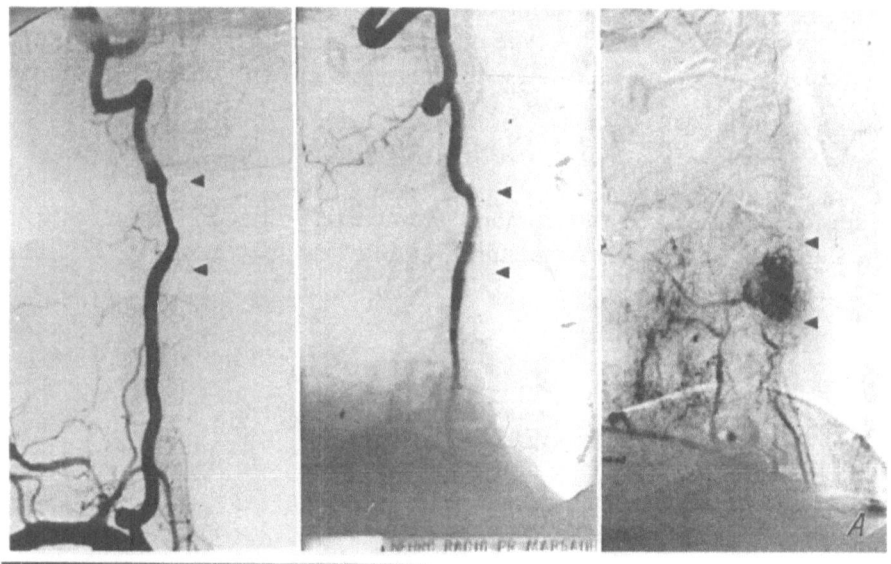

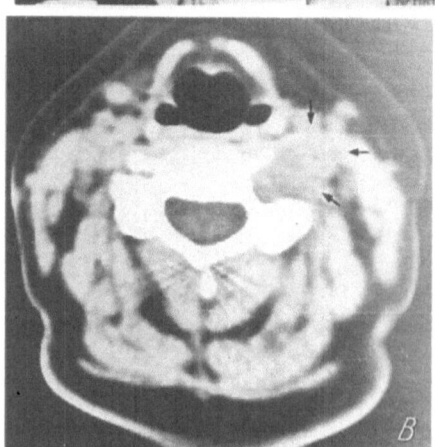

Fig. 28. **A)** Displacement and stenosis of the V. A. by an hour-glass extradural neurinoma at C 3–C 4. Tumoral blush on late phase. **B)** Widening of the intervertebral foramen

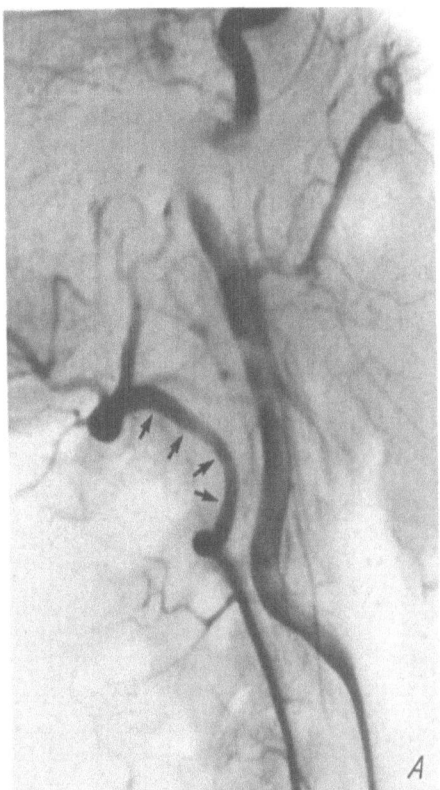 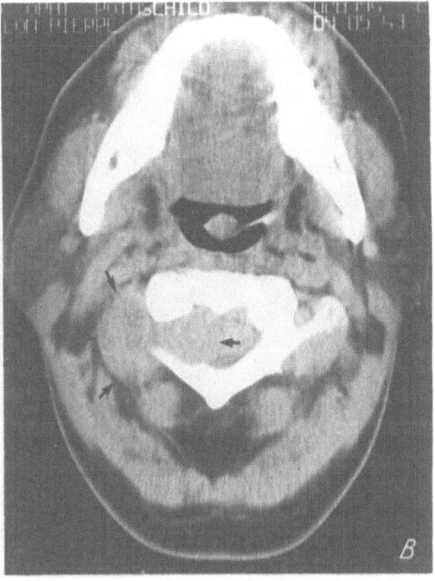

Fig. 29. A) Anterior shift of the V. A. by an hour glass intra and extradural neurinoma at C 1–C 2. **B)** C. T. scan showing intra and extraspinal prolongement in the same case

tomatic cases of external compression of the V. A. by a tumoral process have been reported: one case of a cervical aneurysmal cyst by Iraci *et al.* (1981), one case of neurinoma, by Geissinger *et al.* (1972), one chordoma at C 2 and one metastasis at C 6–C 7 by David *et al.* (1968). Symptomatic vertebral artery compression always produced intermittent signs. In the case of the aneurysmal cyst, at C 3, no clear explanation was given for the symptoms. Since they occurred during head rotation, dynamic V. A. flow compromise was suspected. In the case of the neurinoma at the C 3–C 4 level, transient symptoms appeared when the head was rotated to the left, due to occlusion of the right V. A. by the tumor. A similar case was observed by Fields *et al.* (1979), who mentioned marked stenosis on the left V. A. above C 3 due to V. A. compression by a neurinoma at the C 1–C 2 level; the V. A. became completely occluded when the head was turned to the right, but no mention is made of subsequent clinical symptoms.

In the last two cases reported by David *et al.*, no clinical or angiographic details are given. Mention is only made of symptoms of vertebro-basilar insufficiency.

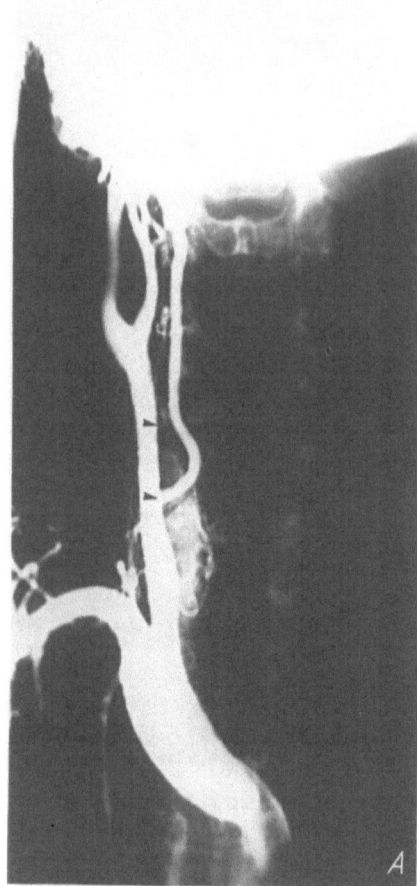
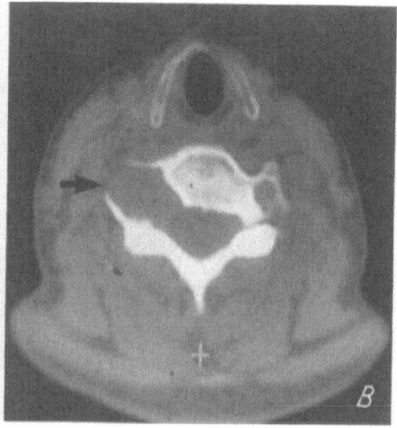

Fig. 30. A) Medial shift of the V. A. by an extradural neurinoma at C 6–C 7. **B)** Enlarged transverse foramen; compare with the opposite side

Verbiest (1970) reported 3 cases of cervical hour-glass neurinomas, with V. A. displacement in all cases and stenosis in one. Four cases of V. A. occlusion due to tumor were reported by George and Laurian (1982): one fibrous dysplasia, one Hodgkin's disease, one Paget's disease and one osteochondroma; none was symptomatic. All were located at the C 2 level. Slow tumor growth and possible compensation of homolateral V. A. flow through distal reinjection by the controlateral V. A. and muscular network explain the good tolerance of tumoral compressions of the V. A.

It must be underlined that most cases with severe V. A. stenosis or occlusion were located at the C 2 level. The lone exception was a metastasis at C 6–C 7 around the V. A. entry into the transverse canal.

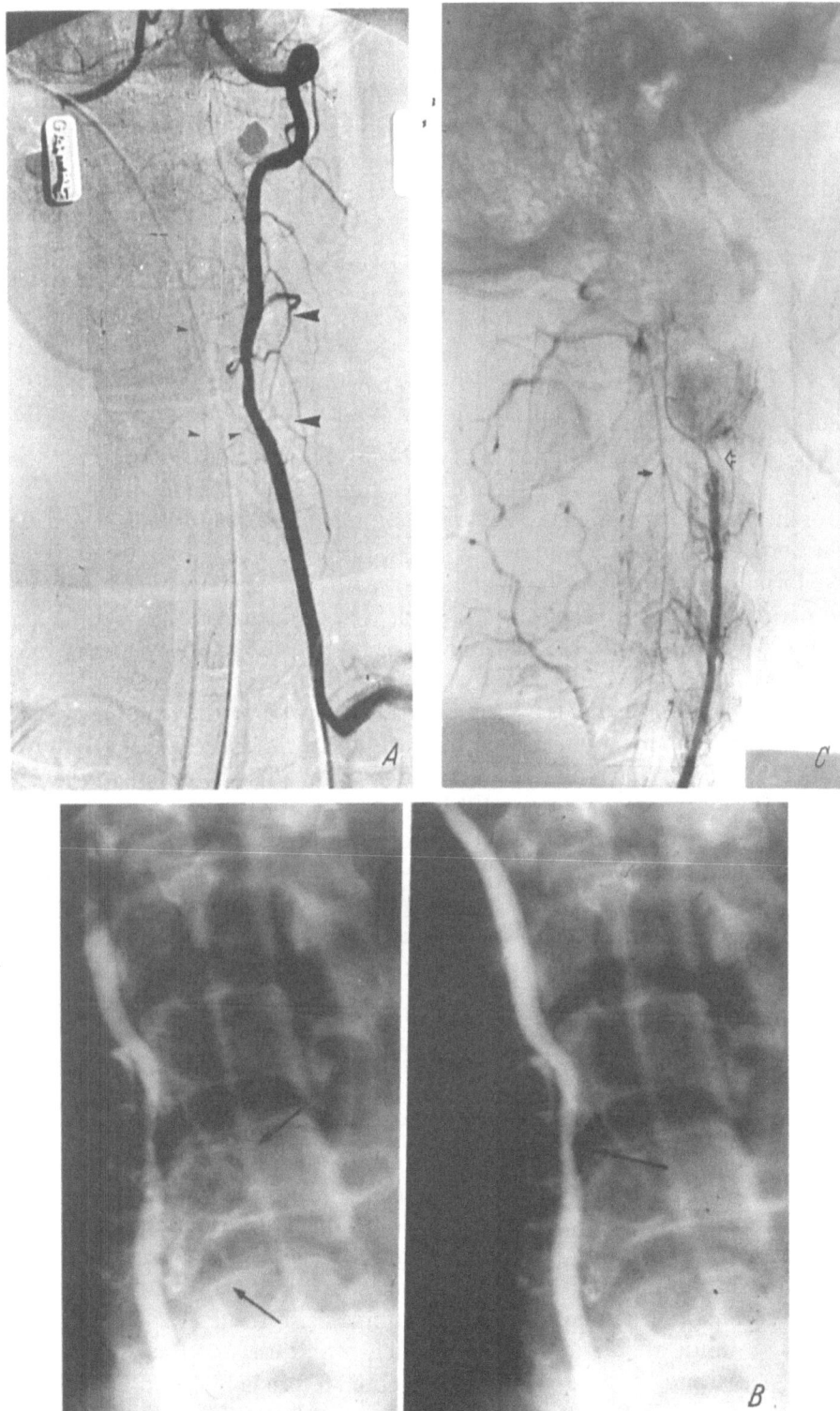

Fig. 31. Tumoral compression of the V. A. **A)** Mild stenosis. Sarcoma. **B)** Marked stenosis with hypervascularization. Neurinoma. **C)** Occlusion. Fibrous dysplasia. Notice the anterior radiculo-medullary branch

6.5 Histology of Tumors Involving the V. A.

Tumors that may be related to the V. A. are of many different histologic types and may be benign or malignant. These tumors can be classified according to the structure from which they originate: neuromeningeal structure, paravertebral soft tissues, bony vertebrae.

6.5.1 Neuromeningeal Structures

6.5.1.1 Neurinoma

Neurinoma is the most frequent histologic type encountered in relation to the V. A. In our experience, 25% (13 out of 52) of the tumors involving the V. A. are neurinomas (**Figs. 28, 29, and 30**).

Two forms can be observed: hour-glass and paraspinal tumors.

In all large series, cervical localization of neurinoma is observed in about 25% of the cases, and the hour-glass form is mainly reported at the cervical level. In Kernohan's series (1952) of 226 neurinomas, 17% are extradural and 17% have an hour-glass form. Fields *et al.* (1972) underlined the relative frequency of neurinomas at the level of the second cervical nerve. From a series of 40 reported cases of neurinomas involving the V. A., 10 are located above C 2, 5 below C 6, and 25 between C 6 and C 2 (Kriss and Schneider, 1968, Verbiest, 1970, Geissinger *et al.*, 1972, Rinaldi, 1972, Fields *et al.*, 1972, Rougerie, 1973, Avman *et al.*, 1975, Kamano *et al.*, 1984, George *et al.*, 1982–1985).

Particular mention must be made of intra and extracranial hour-glass neurinoma passing through the foramen jugulare. This rare tumor develops along the ninth, tenth, or eleventh cranial nerve and may extend in the neck down to the V. A.

a) Macroscopic and Microscopic Aspect

Neurinomas include in fact three types of tumor: schwannoma, neurofibroma and malignant neurinoma.

— *Schwannoma*: this tumor is a smooth, encapsulated, generally ovoid or sausage-shaped mass with elastic consistency. Cysts are frequently found on section. It grows slowly, displacing but not invading the nerve fibers since it is a benign tumor taking origin from Schwann cells. Schwannomas are on rare occasions multiple and can be observed in neurofibromatosis.

— *Neurofibroma*: neurofibromas may be either single or multiple. In the latter case, they are a manifestation of Von Recklinghausen's disease or neurofibromatosis, which is inherited as a Mendelian dominant. Unlike schwannomas, neurofibromas arise centrally in the nerve root, which becomes fusiform or globular due to infiltration of the nerve bundles by neoplasia.

— *Malignant Neurofibroma*: sarcomatous change is a well recognized complication observed mainly in neurofibromatosis. Its true incidence is difficult to assess, but the commonly accepted figure is 10% (Robb-Smith and Pennybacker, 1952). It may present as a diffusely infiltrative or a falsely encapsulated mass.

b) Site of Origin and Extension

Neurinomas develop preferentially on the posterior, and to a far less extent on the anterior nerve root.

They may originate from any part of the nerve root, outside or inside the spinal canal. In the latter case, origin may be intra or extra-dural. Therefore, in its most extensive form, an hour-glass neurinoma with intra-dural origin can be divided into three parts: intraspinal and intradural, intraspinal and extradural, and extraspinal.

Tumor development follows the longitudinal axis of the nerve root. Hence, whatever its origin on the nerve root, the tumor displaces the V. A. anteriorly, since the root crosses the V. A. posteriorly. Intraspinal origin may lead to simultaneous lateral displacement; but usually intraspinal, like extraspinal, neurinomas shift the V. A. medially.

Neurinomas originating from intracranial nerves may also take an hour-glass form when they extend through the jugular foramen (George and Laurian, 1986).

The anterior aspect of the capsule is adherent to the periosteal sheath of the V. A. but never invades it. A plane of cleavage is therefore always present between the arterial adventitia and the tumor capsule.

c) Age and Sex

Neurinoma is mainly observed in adult life, with a peak in the second and third decades, but may occasionally be encountered in infancy. In Rougerie's report (1973), among 66 cases in infants, localization was cervical in 17 cases, of which 3 were extradural and 6 had an hour-glass form. No sex predominance is known.

d) Vascularization

Neurinomas are usually weakly vascularized tumors but they may occasionally present with high vascularity, even suggesting malignancy (Moscow and Newton, 1975).

6.5.1.2 Meningioma

This tumor originating from the dura is the second cause, after neurinoma, of spinal cord compression. V. A. involvement is observed in the rare occurrence of an hour-glass extension.

The dumb-bell form of meningioma is frequent for intracranial localizations (falx, tentorium) but rare in spinal locations. A meningioma of the skull base may grow through the jugulare foramen in similar fashion to a neurinoma, or through the atloïdo-occipital interspace. In this type of extension, the tumor may come into contact with the V. A. and also take part of its vascular supply from the V. A. (George and Laurian, 1986).

An extraspinal location of a meningioma is an exceptional possibility reported by Ibrahim et al. (1986). In this case, the tumor received most of its blood supply from the V. A. At surgery, the tumor encircled the artery, which was sacrified. In fact, this meningioma had an hour-glass form, with its main bulk almost totally outside the spinal canal.

Meningiomas present as firm, tough masses with unevenly nodular surfaces, firmly attached to the dura at their implantation site.

These tumors are predominantly seen after the age of forty and have a marked female predominance.

High vascularity is a common feature, the vessels radiating from the tumor's dural attachment.

Malignant forms with metastases in the lungs, bones and liver are exceptional and have only been reported from intracranial localizations. According to Rubinstein (1972), the criteria for malignancy are:

— rapid recurrence after removal,
— local invasiveness,
— atypical histologic features, and
— high mitotic index and remote metastases.

Angioblastic tumors are generally considered potentially more malignant.

Histologic differentiation of this type of meningioma with hemangiopericytoma is a longstanding subject of debate (Bailey and Cushing, 1928).

6.5.1.3 Paraganglioma (Figs. 32, 33 and 34)

This is a rare tumor originating from a paraganglion of the autonomus nervous system. Principal localizations are the carotid body and the jugular dome. On rare occasions, it may develop on the autonomic nerve fibers of the spinal roots. Hence like neurinomas, paragangliomas may be extradural and extravertebral, or have an hour-glass form. Paraganglioma developing in the petrous bone, better known under the name of glomus jugulare tumor, is the most frequent intracranial tumor involving the V. A.

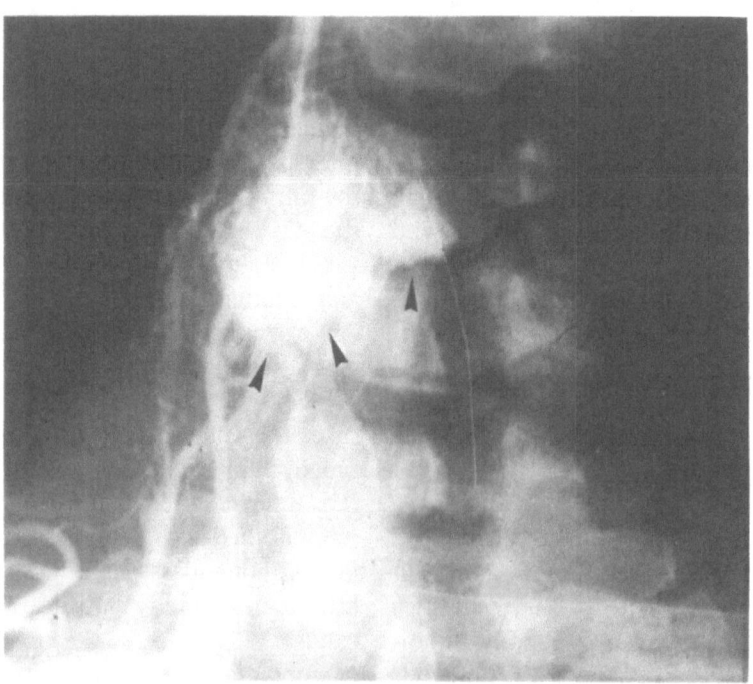

Fig. 32. Hypervascularization in a hour-glass paraganglioma at C 5–C 6

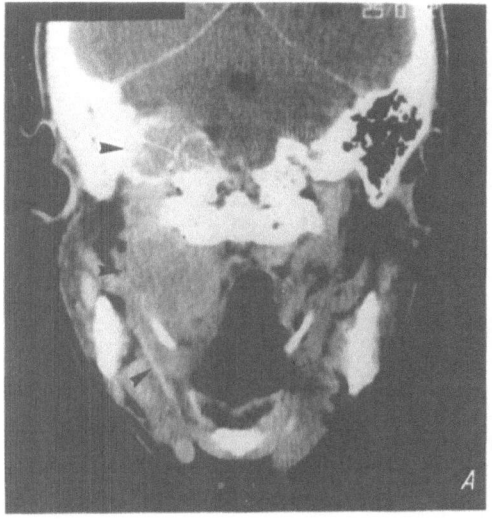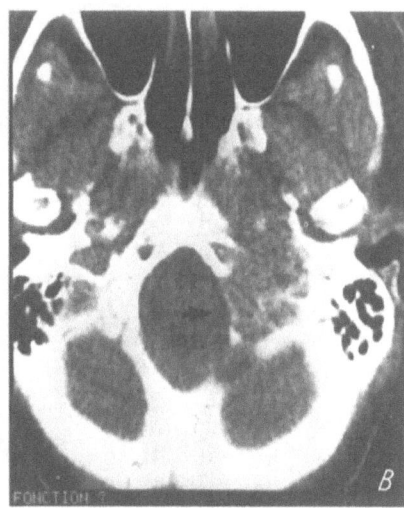

Fig. 33. Intra-extracranial hour-glass paraganglioma. **A)** Frontal view. **B)** Erosion of the foramen magnum margin

Paragangliomas are very highly vascularized tumors with large venous channels. Because of this vascular nature, and the possibility of familial and multiple forms, similarity may be found with hemangioblastomas or meningiomas.

6.5.2 Paravertebral Soft Tissues

Extravertebral tumor may originate not only from extravertebral neuromeningeal structures but also from paravertebral soft tissues. In this case, the V. A. is either shifted anteriorly, or posteriorly and medially, or surrounded by the tumor, depending primarily on the benign or malignant character of the tumor.

6.5.2.1 Haemangiopericytoma

This is a vascular neoplasm associated with numerous capillaries. Tumor cells develop outside the basal membrane from the pericytes. This tumor is often unencapsulated and lacks the neural component found in glomus tumors. It has been found in various soft tissues but has rarely been shown to involve the paravertebral area or the spinal canal (Harris *et al.*, 1978). Among the few cases reported, more than half occurred in the cervical area and developed extradurally, either inside or outside the spinal canal (Kruse, 1961, Pitlyk *et al.*, 1965, George and Laurian, 1986).

Histologically, this tumor can be categorized as either benign or malignant, but there is poor clinical correlation (recurrence and metastases in histologically benign tumors) (Enziger and Smith, 1976). Because of the well-recognized high but unpredictible risk

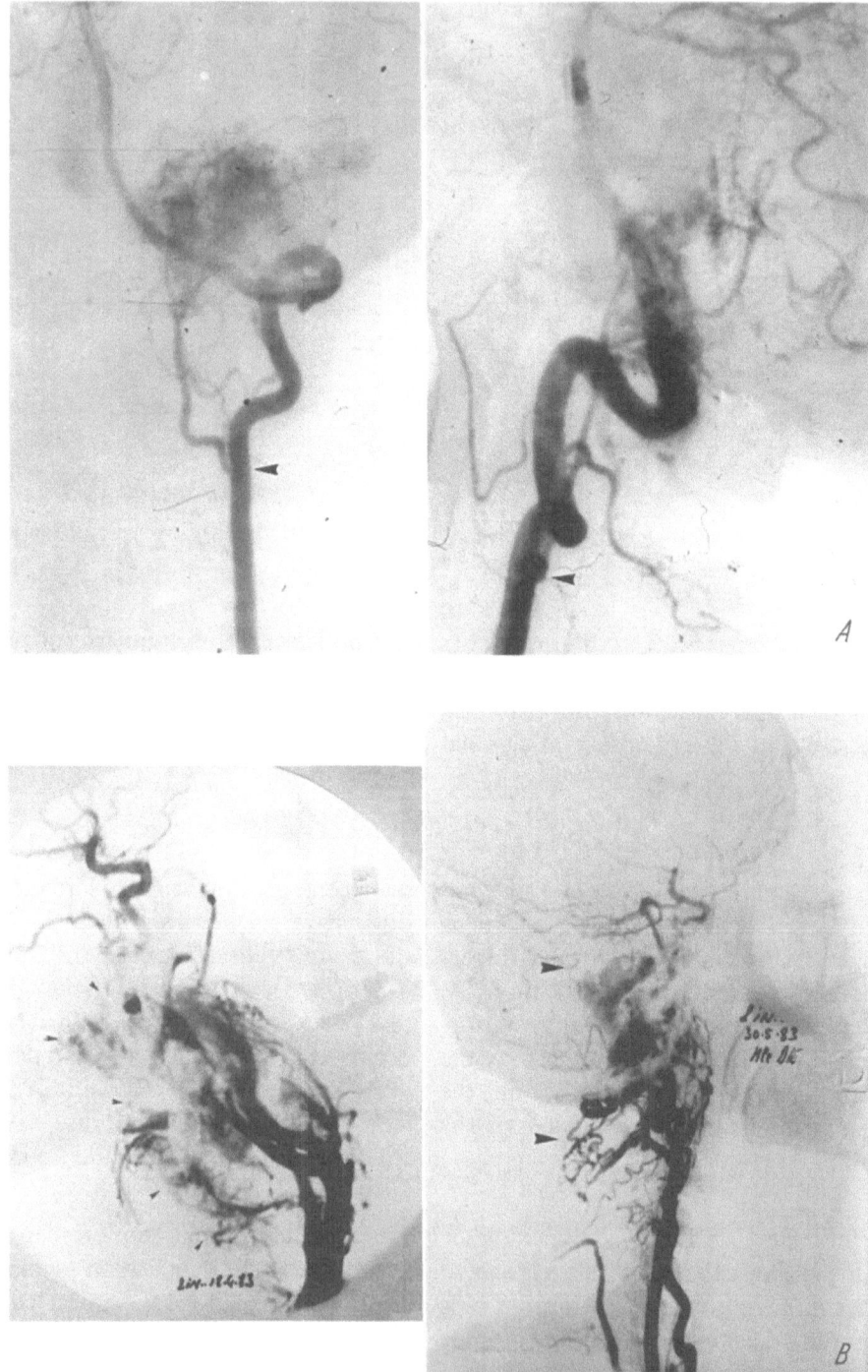

Fig. 34. Vascular supply of paragangliomas **A)** from a branch at C 3, **B)** from several branches in a case with large cervical prolongement

of recurrence, a combination of surgery with radiation therapy is recommended in all cases (O'Brien and Brasfield, 1965, Harris *et al.*, 1978).

6.5.2.2 Sarcoma

Any type of sarcoma, whatever its origin, may involve the V.A.: rhabdomyosarcoma, neurosarcoma, osteosarcoma and undifferentiated sarcoma.

These tumors occur most frequently in the first decades of life. Vascularization has no characteristic feature, as a sarcoma may be weakly or highly vascularized. Usually, a sarcoma presents as an infiltrative lesion, but on occasion, it may appear as a falsely encapsulated mass (**Fig. 31 A**).

6.5.2.3 Carcinoma

Carcinomas involving the V.A. are neoplasms arising in the apex of the lungs and extending to the supraclavicular area: Pancoast-Tobias syndrome (Dartevelle *et al.*, 1984).

6.5.2.4 Lymphangioma and Hemolymphangioma

This is a vascular lesion presenting as multilobulated cysts containing brownish fluid. The capsule of the cysts is poorly vascularized. It is a benign and slowly growing lesion which can progressively erode the vertebrae (George and Laurian, 1986).

6.5.2.5 Other Non-tumoral Processes

Non-tumoral lesions developing in the paravertebral space may also involve the V.A. These lesions include infections and parasitic lesions, such as actinomycosis (George and Laurian, 1986) or tuberculosis (**Fig. 35**).

6.5.3 Osseous Lesions

Any type of osseous lesion involving the cervical spine may come into contact with the V.A. This may be tumor, dystrophy or osseous localization of general disease. **Table 6** mentions the types of tumor already reported with V.A. involvement.

Tumor may be benign or malignant, hypervascularized or not. Obviously, surgical control of the V.A. is far more important in the case of hypervascularized and benign lesions. Whatever the type, if complete cure is the goal of the procedure, removal of abnormal bone should not be limited by the degree of proximity of the V.A. or by the degree of vascularity.

6.5.3.1 Benign Tumors

Benign tumors are usually encountered in young patients, with a peak frequency in the second and third decades of life. Benign tumors of the spine account for 9% of all osseous tumors, among which 20 to 30% are located at the cervical level.

Benign tumors are usually classified according to the cell type of origin into five major groups: osteogenic tumor,

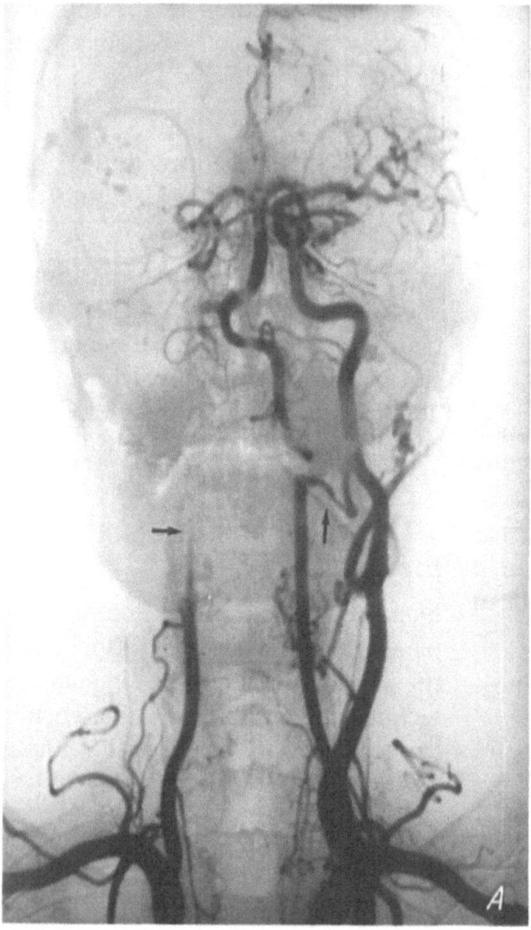

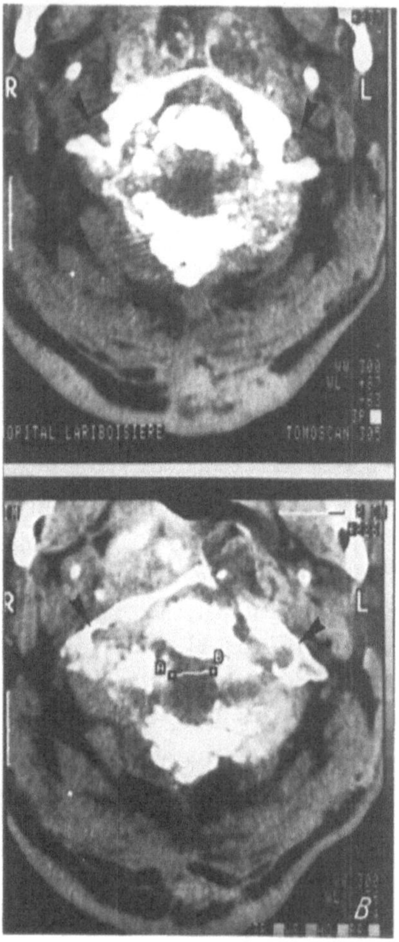

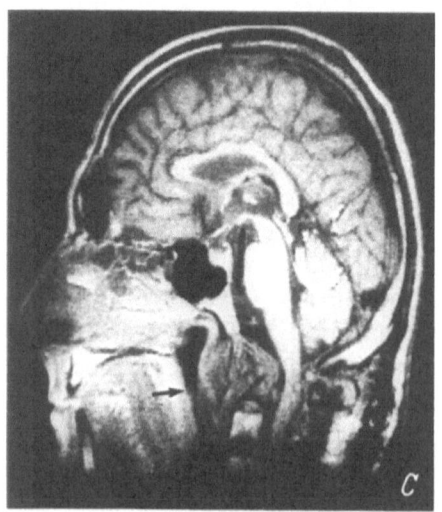

Fig. 35. Tubercular abscess at C1–C2. **A)** Angiography: left V. A.: occlusion; right V. A.: shift and stenosis. **B)** C. T. scan: bone destruction of the anterior arch of C1 and C2, extending laterally towards the transverse foramina. **C)** NMRI: tubercular abscess extending from the lower clivus down to C2 with posterior displacement of the medulla oblongata

Table 6. Osseous tumor and V. A. involvement

	Benign		Malignant	
Osteogenic tumor	osteoid osteoma osteoblastoma	+	osteosarcoma	−
Chondrogenic tumor	osteochondroma chondroma	+	chondrosarcoma	−
Giant cell tumor	giant cell tumor	+	malignant G. C. T.	−
Spindle cell tumor	fibroma	−	fibrosarcoma	−
Embryogenic tumor	chordoma	+		
Dystrophy	aneurysmal cyst	+		
	fibrous dysplasia	+		
General disease	hystiocytosis-X	−	metastasis	+
	paget's disease	+	myeloma	−
			hemopathy	+

+ Indicates reported cases with V. A. involvement.

chondrogenic tumor, giant cell tumor, spindle cell tumor and vascular tumor (**Table 6**).

Extensive and highly vascular lesions are the most likely to require surgical control of the V. A. Osteoblastoma is the best example and the most frequent benign tumor.

a) Osteogenic Tumor

The two main types of osteogenic tumor are osteoid osteoma and osteoblastoma. They are histologically similar but differ in biological behavior; osteoid osteoma is confined and self-limiting in its growth pattern, while osteoblastoma is more extensive and increases in size. Therefore, they are generally differentiated by size: greater or smaller than 2 centimeters. Male predominance is common to both. Preferential localization is on the lamina and spinous process. Soft tissue infiltration is frequently observed in osteoblastoma as the result of cortical rupture. Sarcomatous change is a rare possibility that should not be confused with a primary osteosarcoma.

Involvement of the V. A. by osteoblastomas has been observed by George and Laurian (1983–1986) and Chirossel et al. (1985).

b) Chondrogenic Tumor

Osteochondroma and chondroma are the two main types of chondrogenic tumors. Their growth is due to the proliferation of cartilagenous cells of the posterior spinal arch. Sarcomatous change is frequent, as it accounts for 20 to 50% of the multiple forms. Involvement of the transverse canal has been reported by Nubourgh et al. (1979) but the V. A. artery was atretic on the tumoral side. Tumoral resection after V. A. control was achieved by Chirossel

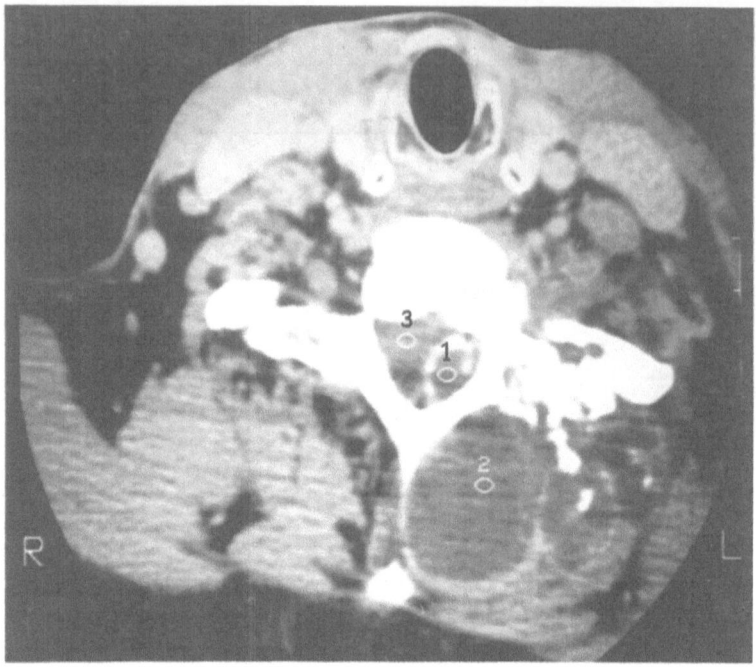

Fig. 36. Hour-glass chondroma with intrathoracic prolongement

et al. (1985) in a case of osteochondroma at C 5. In our series, there are two cases of chondroma, one with hour-glass intraspinal and intrathoracic extension, and the other, an osteogenic chondroma originating from the second transverse process (**Fig. 36**).

c) Giant Cell Tumor

This tumor is rare at the cervical level, since it preferentially occurs in the sacrum. It has a female predominance, and the vertebral body is the usual site. Sarcomatous transformation may occur, especially after roentgenotherapy.

Giant cell tumors are always hypervascularized and may even contain areas similar to aneurysmal bone cysts. No case of giant cell tumor involving the V. A. has yet been reported.

d) Vascular Tumor

Angiomas and hemangiomas are exceptional tumors with female predominance. The vertebral body is the usual localization. These tumors are dramatically hypervascularized and are frequently compared to a "vascular sponge". This fact explains the importance of V. A. control in their treatment.

e) Chordoma

This is a rare embryonic tumor derived from persistant portions of the notochord and usually located in the sacrum, but any part of the spine may be involved (Wellinger, 1975). It is a weakly vascularized but very infiltrative tumor, which explains its frequent reccurrence. Moreover, some chordomas present with metastases and must be considered malignant.

Jeanmart et al. (1967) reported one case with V. A. displacement, and Bach (1970) reported one case at the C 2 level with death from subdural hemorrhage after V. A. wall invasion. One case at the C 2–C 3 level with intra and extraspinal extension is reported in the series of George and Laurian (1986).

f) Other Benign Osseous Lesions

Spindle cell tumors are exceptionally located on the cervical spine.

6.5.3.2 Osseous Dystrophy

— Aneurysmal bone cyst.

The usual spinal localization of aneurysmal bone cysts is at the lumbar and cervical level. C 1–C 2 is the most frequent site. Vascular lacunae are the main histologic characteristic. Extension is usually rapid, with body lysis and involvement of paravertebral soft tissues (Paillas et al., 1963). Unproven symptomatic compression of the V. A. by a cervical aneurysmal cyst at C 3 with transient ischemic attacks has been reported by Iraci et al. (1981).

— Fibrous dysplasia.

This is a bony dystrophy which may involve any part of the skeleton. Spinal localization occurs in about 5%. Hypervascularization is a common feature. Asymptomatic occlusion of the V. A. in a case at the C 2 level was observed by George et al. (1982).

6.5.3.3 Osseous Localization of General Disease

Histiocytosis-X or Paget's disease may present with a cervical spine localization and lead to V. A. occlusion, as in the case reported by George et al. (1982).

6.5.3.4 Malignant Tumor

Malignant tumors of the cervical spine are of three different types: primary tumors, metastases and localization of malignant diseases.

a) Primary Malignant Tumor

Every type of primary malignant skeletal tumor may be observed at the cervical level: osteosarcoma, chondrosarcoma, fibrosarcoma. These are rare and present as hypervascularized, extensive and poorly limited tumors.

b) Metastases

These are the most frequent type of spinal tumor. They are predominantly

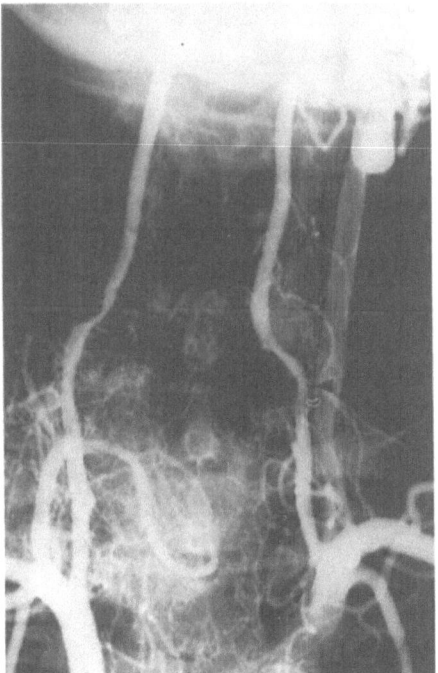

Fig. 37. Bilateral shift and stenosis; thyroid carcinoma metastasis

observed after the fourth decade of life, which explains why the frequency of malignant tumors of the spine increases progressively with age. Cervical localization of metastases is less common than thoracolumbar sites and accounts for only about 10% of all spinal metastases. V. A. involvement is mainly seen with hypervascular metastases from thyroïd or kidney carcinomas (**Fig. 37**).

c) Localization of Malignant Disease

— Myeloma.

Either solitary or multiple myeloma is rarely located at the cervical level (8% of all osseous localizations). Although a high degree of vascularization is commonly observed, no case of resection with V. A. control has yet been reported.

— Hemopathy.

Spinal localization of hemopathy has a very uncommon incidence at the cervical level. V. A. occlusion in the context of Hodgkin's disease has been observed by George and Laurian (1982).

7. EXTERNAL COMPRESSION

External compression of the cervical V.A. is certainly not as common as stenotic or occlusive disease due to atherosclerosis, but the number of patients affected by various causes of V.A. compression is probably underestimated. In fact, except for osteophytic spurs, other causes of V.A. compression are not widely known. Moreover, most clinicians are unaware of the pathophysiology, symptomatology, methods of diagnosis and efficient forms of treatment. At the same time, cervical arthritis is frequently evoked as an easy way to explain vertigo, dizziness or other subjective symptoms; this attitude generally leads to symptomatic medical therapy with variable results. Moreover, as symptoms are essentially subjective and the neurologic exam usually normal, a diagnosis of functional or psychosomatic origin is not uncommon.

External compression of the V.A. in its second portion is predominant and will therefore be discussed first.

7.1 Second Portion

7.1.1 Pathophysiology

Two main mechanisms producing vertebro-basilar symptoms from external compression of the V.A. have been proposed: sympathetic irritation and intermittent occlusion of the V.A.

7.1.1.1 Sympathetic Irritation

Barré (1926) and Liéou (1926) first referred to symptoms caused by irritation of the V.A. from cervical arthritis and described these symptoms as "the posterior cervical sympathetic syndrome". It includes vertigo, dizziness, tinnitus, visual symptoms, hoarseness and occipital headaches following rotation of the neck; the presence of arthritis irritates the sympathetic vertebral nerve at the fourth, fifth and sixth cervical vertebrae level and explains the symptoms.

The Barré and Liéou concepts were largely followed in France, and hypertonicity of the vertebral nerve due to cervical arthritis is still considered by many as the primary factor producing symptoms.

7.1.1.2 V.A. Intermittent Compression

In 1961, Powers first described the syndrome of intermittent V.A. compression. It is characterized by symptoms very similar to those attributed by Barré and Liéou to vertebral nerve irritation; namely vertigo, syncope, tinnitus, visual disturbances and positive Adson's sign. The same dynamic factor, rotation or extension of the neck, is also frequently observed.

At the same time, Bauer *et al.* (1960) reported the first series of V. A. compression by osteophytic spurs, and angiographic demonstration of intermittent V. A. compression on living patients was performed by Meyer *et al.* (1960) ans Sheehan *et al.* (1964).

Consequently, treatment directed toward relieving V. A. compression was developed (Hardin, 1960–1965, Gortvai, 1964, Keggi *et al.*, 1966, Verbiest, 1968).

The positive results of decompressive surgery confirmed in their position those who thought that the Barré-Liéou syndrome did not exist, but other authors are still not convinced. The pathophysiology of intermittent vertebro-basilar symptoms associated with cervical arthritis thus remains controversial.

7.1.1.3 Sympathetic Irritation plus V. A. Compression

Following Nagashima's reports on electrical stimulation of the vertebral nerve and on effects of temporary V. A. occlusion during V. A. surgery under local anaesthesia, the two concepts can be reconciled. Both experiments provoke symptoms similar to those observed in intermittent V. A. compression by osteophytic spurs. Nagashima and Iwana (1972) consequently recommended not only removing the osteophytic spurs (the V. A.

compressing agent) but also removing the connective scar tissue which surrounds the V. A., since it is presumed to be the cause of the sympathetic nerve irritation. This technique has also been applied by Gortvai (1964), Hardin (1963), Verbiest (1968) and Sullivan *et al.* (1975).

In fact, no series has yet been reported comparing with the same methodology the results of surgery aimed at both the compressing and irritating factors and at each separately. Therefore, there is still no agreement on which of these is principally responsible for symptoms in cervical arthritis.

7.1.1.4 Collateral Flow

Furthermore, interruption of the flow in one V. A. is not systematically accompanied by symptoms. The size of the controlateral V. A. and the configuration of the circle of Willis influence to a large degree the onset of symptoms. This is clearly demonstrated by the consequences of V. A. ligation. On reviewing 100 cases of V. A. ligation in the literature, Shintani (1972) indicates that mortality and morbidity are unlikely to occur as long as there is adequate flow through the opposite V. A. The same finding was established by Nagashima *et al.* (1970) after temporary V. A. occlusion; subjective symptoms were not manifested by patients having a normal configuration of the circle of Willis. Such data indicate that symptoms should be attributed to external compression of the V. A. only if there is a controlateral lesion compromising V. A. flow, or if it is associated with a hypoplastic controlateral V. A., and/or an abnormal circle of Willis.

7.1.1.5 Dynamic Compression

V. A. compression by osteophytic spurs appears or increases clinically as well as angiographically during head and neck movements, principally hyperextension with rotation to the ipsilateral side (**Figs. 38** and **39**).

However, rotation of the neck has long been shown to be responsible for stretching of the controlateral V. A. under normal conditions.

In 1884, from studies on cadavers, Gerlach recognized that excessive rotation at C 1–C 2 resulted in stretching of the V. A. He agreed with Henke (1863) that no true neck rotation occurs but rather a screwlike movement. Subsequently, many reports have confirmed the possibility of V. A. compression during extension and controlateral rotation; most of these studies were performed on cadavers using perfusion techniques: De Kleyn and Versteegh (1933), Holzer (1955), Toole and Tucker (1960), and Lazorthes et al. (1971) or post-mortem angiography: Tatlow et al. (1957), Fielding (1957), Schneider et al. (1972). V. A. stretching was demonstrated by Selecki (1969) to begin at 30° rotation of the neck to the opposite and to become marked at 45° rotation. For the majority of the authors, the site of V. A. obstruction during head rotation is at the C 1–C 2 level, but Bladin and Merory (1975) presented evidence that with excessive rotation of the neck a sheering effect is observed on the V. A. as it penetrates the posterior atlanto-occipital membrane.

Moreover, some authors have demonstrated simultaneous internal carotid artery compression by the lateral process of the atlas (Boldrey et al., 1956, Toole and Tucker, 1960, Lazorthes et al., 1971).

Therefore, during extension and rotation of the head and neck, the V. A. flow may be compromised on the ipsilateral side by external compression from osteophytic spurs and on the controlateral side by mechanical stretching at C 1–C 2.

Hence it may be concluded that unilateral external compression of the V. A., whatever its origin, can be symptomatic if there is a controlateral lesion capable of compromising vertebrobasilar hemodynamics. This controlateral lesion may be:

— an additional agent of external compression,

— an atheromatous stenosis or occlusion,

— a controlateral hypoplastic V. A.,

— a controlateral stretching of the V. A. more or less aggravated by a carotid artery lesion or compression, or a nonfunctional circle of Willis.

7.1.1.6 Embolism

An embolic mechanism of producing symptoms seems unlikely in external compression of the V. A., since no pathologic changes in the internal wall of the kinked V. A. segment, especially no increased tendency of atheroma, were described in autopsy material by Hutchinson and Yates (1956) and Stein et al. (1962). However, one case of embolus to the posterior cerebral artery has already been reported (Sullivan et al., 1975). Nagashima (1970) reported a case of complete obstruction of one V. A. due to probable intimal injury caused by a large uncinate osteophyte. In this case, not clearly proven, no embolic complication was observed. Intimal lesion due to external compression must therefore be considered an exceptional possibility.

7.1.2 Aetiology

7.1.2.1 Cervical Spondylosis

Cervical spondylosis is the most common cause of V. A. compression. The term "cervical spondylosis" describes degenerative lesions of spinal vertebrae with consequent development of osteophytosis. Enlargement of the osteophyte is a slow but progressive phenomenon which may encroach upon soft tissues, causing symptoms. Depending on their site and direction of growth, osteophytes may produce three distinct syndromes:
— nerve root syndrome due to uncinate or facet osteophyte directed towards the intervertebral foramen,
— myelopathic syndrome due to body margin osteophytes directed towards the spinal cord and the anterior spinal artery,
— V. A. syndrome due to uncinate or facet osteophytes directed laterally towards the transverse canal.

a) Uncinate Osteophytes

Arthritic bony spurs may compress the V. A., essentially if the site of formation is on the uncinate portion of the vertebrae (see chapter Anatomy). This part of the vertebrae, which in the embryonic stage is the junction of the centrum and lateral masses, is called the "neurocentral joint", the "uncovertebral joint" or Luschka's joint. There is disagreement of whether or not it is a true joint (Frykolm, 1951, Boreadis, 1956, Hadley, 1957).
Osteophytic spurs compress the V. A. in its second transverse portion mainly at the C4–C5 and C5–C6 levels. At these levels, where arthritis predominates, the V. A. is relatively fixed in the transverse canal, and very close to the uncinate process.

b) Facet Proliferation

Apophyseal facet proliferation is a less common cause of V. A. compression. More often, it plays a role in limiting displacement of the V. A. dorsally when the head is extended. In this way, it worsens the V. A. compression by uncinate osteophytes. In rare cases of large facet proliferation, the V. A. may be displaced ventrally and medially (Nagashima, 1970).
Uncinate osteophytes are unilateral in 75% of cases, bilateral in 25%, and apophyseal osteoarthrosis is noted in about 15% of cases.
In the first stage, the V. A. is shifted and kinked laterally and dorsally, since uncinate osteophytes develop at a level between two transverse processes. In a second step, the V. A. is stenosed because of the arthritic spur growing toward the level of the transverse process. The margins of the transverse process prevent any external displacement of the V. A., whereas the superior

articular facet of the inferior vertebra (which may also be associated with facet proliferation) limits the possibility of posterior shift. This latter fact explains that V. A. stenosis symptoms are elicited not only by head and neck rotation, but often require associated extension.

Another factor which prevents the V. A. from escaping compression is the progressive development of a connective tissue scar reinforcing the periosteal sheath and fixing the V. A.

c) Diagnosis

Clinical symptoms are very similar to those produced by atherosclerotic occlusive disease. The most common complaint is that of dizziness and/or vertigo: 15 out of 20 cases for Nagashima (1970). The next most frequent symptoms are visual disturbances and drop-attack.

The main characteristic that suggests the diagnosis of V. A. external compression is the circumstances in which these symptoms occur: extension and rotation of the head and neck, generally to the ipsilateral side of the involved V. A. Manoeuvers such as turning the head abruptly to look over the shoulder, or looking upward at the ceiling or on backing a car are frequently reported by the patients. As in any other type of vertebro-basilar insufficiency, symptoms appear most often on arising from bed and may be precipitated by orthostatic hypotension.

The dynamic factor of producing symptoms has been noted by a number of authors: Ryan and Cope (1955), Kremer (1958), Tatlow et al. (1957).

Generally, the same type of movement regularly reproduces the symptoms. It may help the physician to observe neurologic signs; but in resting position, the neurologic examination is usually normal. These signs may include nystagmus, positive Romberg, fifth to twelfth cranial nerve involvement, gaze palsy and cerebellar signs. Involvement of motor and sensory systems on one or both sides of the body should not be presumed to be due to V. A. compression alone, since it may also be related to cervical spondylosis with spinal cord compression.

Whatever the symptoms described and observed, a careful history specifically asking the patient about the circumstances producing symptoms is essential: the head and neck position which

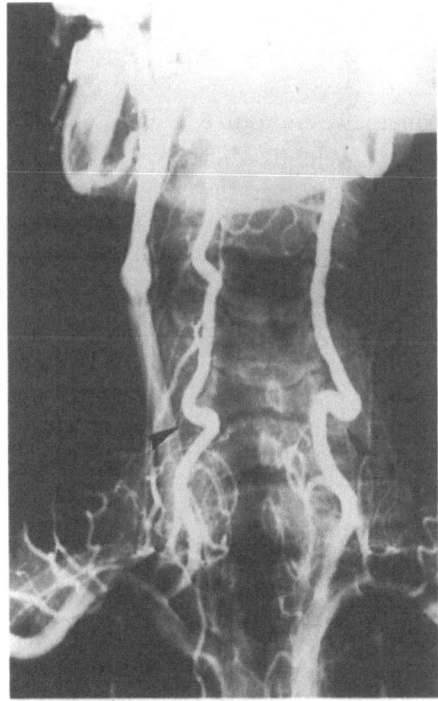

Fig. 38. Bilateral V. A. compression by osteophytic spurs at C 6 but without stenosis

elicites symptoms must be clearly defined. The same manoeuvers must be reproduced before the neurologic exam and during the angiography. It is only in the case of marked V. A. stenosis, demonstrated angiographically by the same movement of the neck as that producing symptoms, that a correlation between osteophytic spurs and symptoms of V. A. compression can be accurately established. Bilateral angiographic study is required to understand the mechanism by which the vertebro-basilar flow is compromised, since it implies insufficient compensation by the controlateral V. A. (**Figs. 38** and **39**).

7.1.2.2 Fibrous Bands

Fibrous bands correspond to a thickening of the periosteal sheath of the V. A. in the transverse canal (Hardin and Poser, 1963, Carney, 1984), which is principally composed of the ligaments of the scalenus muscles at their insertion sites on the transverse processes. Rainer *et al.* (1970) out of 51 patients, mentioned 9 cases of fibromuscular compression of the V. A. Similarly, Herrschaft and Duus (1972) reported 5 such cases among 63 cases of vertebro-basilar insufficiency.

These fibrous bands are mainly observed at three sites: below C 6, above C 2 (see next chapter) and at C 5–C 6 (**Fig. 40**).

Fibrous bands form a fixed and incompressible element, crossing and encroaching upon the anterior aspect of the V. A. Therefore, significant compression of the V. A. is generally demonstrated during hyperextension of the head and necessitates an abnormally high entry of the V. A. into the transverse canal. In resting position, the V. A. exhibits a bayonnet course: it first passes over the transverse process of C 6 (and sometimes C 5) and then under the fibrous band. Hyperextension

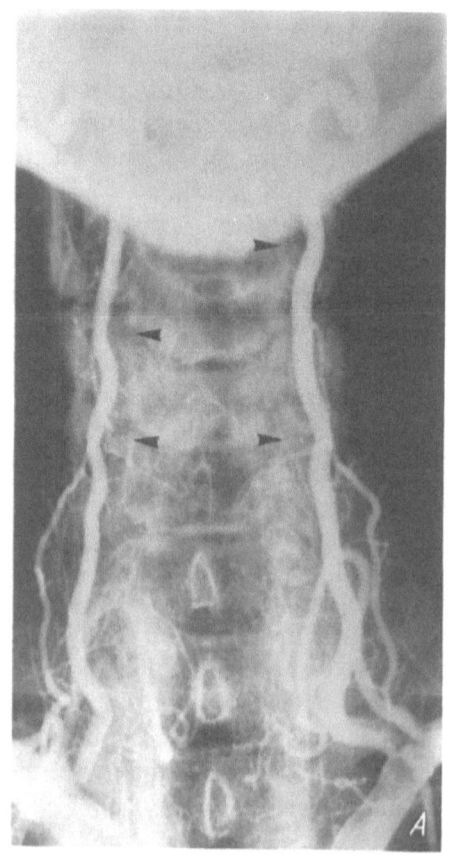

Fig. 39. A) Multiple encroachments upon both V. A.'s by bilateral osteophytes; **B)** right V. A.: on the left, head and neck ipsilateral rotation producing marked stenosis at C 4, C 5, and C 6 levels, on the right, head and neck controlateral rotation producing no V. A. compression, **C)** left V. A.: on the left, ipsilateral rotation with severe stenosis at C 3–C 4 and mild compression at C 5–C 6, on the right, controlateral rotation with moderate V. A. compression

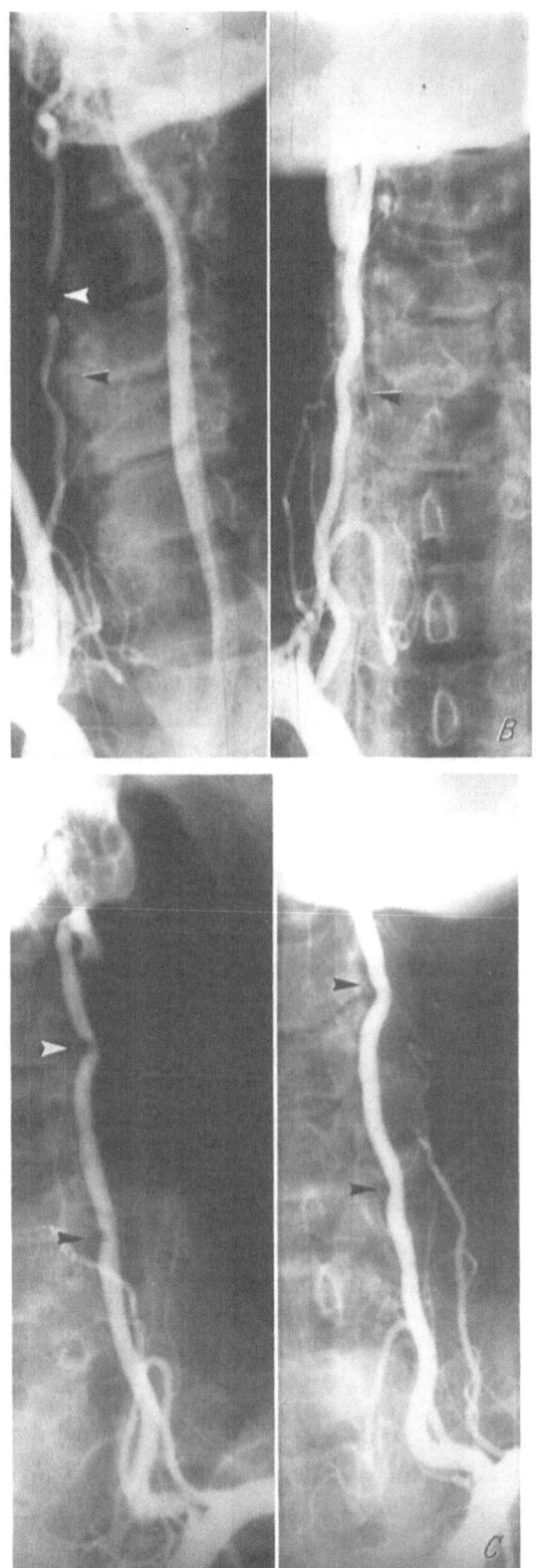

Fig. 39B and C

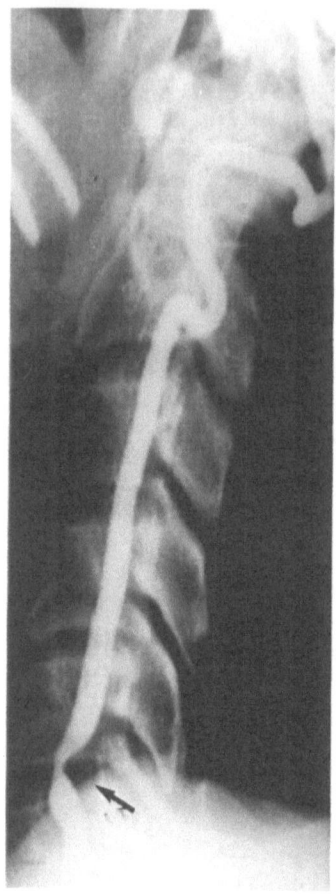

Fig. 40. External compression by fibrous band in the transverse canal at C 5–C 6

exagerates this "cigar-cut" effect and in this way may produce symptoms if the controlateral V. A. flow is insufficient. Fibrous tissue surrounding the V. A. is also associated with osteophytic spurs and plays a role in spondylotic compression of the V. A. by fixing the vessel against the spurs (see chapter 7.1.1.3 and 7.1.2.1).

7.1.2.3 Disc Herniation

Spinal nerve root compression is a common finding in cervical disc herniation, but not much emphasis has been given to possible V. A. compression, as already reported by Gortvai (1964), Verbiest (1970), Brunon and Goutelle (1974). In the same way as an osteophytic spur, a cervical disc may protude in different directions, compressing the spinal cord, the nerve root, and the V. A.; compression of the latter is rarely recognized, probably for multiple reasons:

— posterior or postero-lateral herniation is much more frequent than a strictly lateral one,

— nerve root compression appears before V. A. compression, and patients are referred early for cervico-brachial neuralgia,

— bilateral lateral herniation is very rare, and haemodynamic consequences are unlikely to occur.

7.1.2.4 Cervical Canal Stenosis

Mention must be made of V. A. compression associated with congenital cervical fusion and cervical canal stenosis, as in the case reported by Itoh *et al.* (1978). In this case, occlusion of the V. A. at C 3–C 4 was discovered but no clear demonstration of the main compressive factor was made, while cervical spondylosis was also present. Brunon and Goutelle (1974) mentioned a similar case with vertebro-basilar insufficiency manifestations they thought to be related to external compression of the V. A. at the level of a congenital fusion of cervical vertebrae.

7.1.2.5 Trauma

Among the different mechanisms of V. A. injury (see chapter Trauma), external traumatic compression is the least commonly recognized. It is mainly observed on the second and third portion of the V. A.

Any fracture with dislocation of the spine above the level of V. A. entry into the transverse canal may lead to V. A. compression at the level of the displaced intervertebral foramen (Schneider and Crosby, 1959). As the dislocation is frequently bilateral, both V. A.'s may be compressed, with vertebro-basilar insufficiency as a consequence.

The V. A. injury may not initially be recognized, masked behind the spinal and frequently associated brain injury. Aneurysm and arteriovenous fistula may reveal initial V. A. injury months after trauma. Cervical angiography should be performed more frequently after cervical spine injury, particularly if brain stem or cerebellar signs are present, or if symptoms overtake the level of spinal cord injury.

V. A. compression may also be discovered long after the injury in the case of exhuberant callus following insufficient reduction (Hugues, 1964, Verbiest, 1973).

Also not rare is the late discovery of intermittent V. A. compression related to an unrecognized atloido-occipital dislocation or cervical subluxation or pseudarthrosis (Brunon et al., 1974).

7.1.2.6 Tumor

Displacement of the V. A. by any type of paravertebral or hour-glass tumour is frequent, but hemodynamic consequences are very rare, even in the case of complete occlusion (see chapter Tumor). This fact may easily be explained by the slow and unilateral development of this type of V. A. compression. Only a few symptomatic cases have been reported; all of them were manifested by intermittent symptoms on head and neck movements, suggesting a mechanical factor associated with the tumoral compression.

7.2 First Portion

V. A. displacement and subsequent stenosis are far less common on the first portion than on the second or third. This fact is obviously explained by the differences in anatomic location and course of the V. A.

Case reports are scarce and refer to various causes:

Fibro-muscular elements: the anterior scalenus muscle, deep cervical fascia or longus colli may compress the V. A. if there is an anomaly of the V. A. in its first portion. Powers et al. (1961) stated that the V. A. can be occluded by compression produced by the medial border of the anterior scalenus muscle and the thyro-cervical trunk when the V. A. arises from the posterior surface of the subclavian artery behind this arterial trunk. Hardin and Poser (1963) reported 15 cases of intermittent rotational symptoms due to fascial compression enhanced by kinking of the V. A., but this type of V. A. compression may be present even if the V. A. has a normal course. Kojima et al. (1985) suggested that the V. A. can be obliterated by compression with fi-

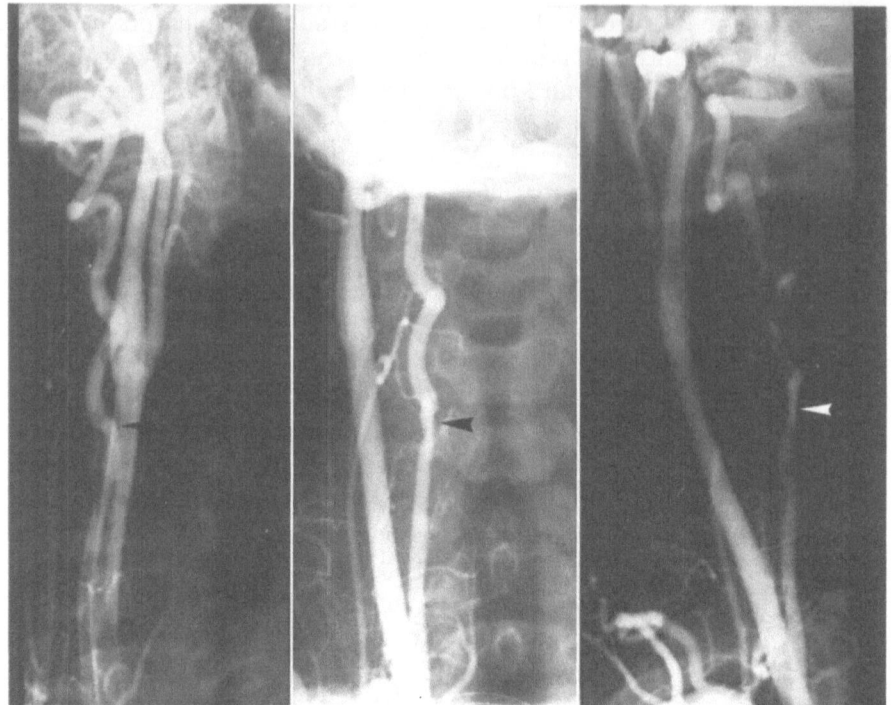

Fig. 41. External compression by a fibro-muscular element at the "scaleno-vertebral angle" corresponding to an abnormally high level of V. A. entry (C 4) into the transverse canal. Center: head in rectitude position and extension, left: ipsilateral rotation, right: controlateral rotation

brous bands of the longus colli and the anterior scalenus muscle during head rotation. Obstruction occurs at the distal part of the first portion, just below its entry into the transverse canal at the C6 level. This dynamic V. A. occlusion at what Kojima called the "scaleno-vertebral angle" is more likely to be symptomatic if there is insufficient controlateral flow due to atretic V. A., as in the case of Husni *et al.* (1966) and Mapstone and Spetzler (1956). On the contrary, in the case of Kojima *et al.*, the opposite V. A. was of normal size (**Fig. 41**).

Scar formation around the proximal V. A. in a hematoma following thy-roidectomy was reported by Wagner *et al.* (1963). One such case after trauma is present in our series.

Sympathetic Nerve: the rami connecting the vertebral nerve and the stellate ganglion or the ansa subclavia may encroach upon the anterior aspect of the V. A. We observed one case with pseudo-occlusive compression which was released surgically.

Thoracic Outlet Compression Syndrome is sometimes suggested to explain symptoms of vertebro-basilar insufficiency, but the osteo-fibrous abnormalities observed in this syndrome (apophysomegaly of C 7 transverse process, scalenus muscle tendon or cervical rib) compress the subclavian artery, usually at a point distal from the V. A. origin. Vertebro-basilar manifestations cannot therefore be explained by direct compression, but may be secondary to retrograde embolism or to subclavian artery thrombosis extending to the V. A. ostium (Symonds, 1927, Blank and Connar, 1974).

Tumor: any type of tumor and especially lung apex carcinoma, may involve the first portion of the V. A. and displace this vessel, but stenosis appears only in the case of very extensive tumors surrounding the V. A. No case of symptomatic involvement of the V. A. at this level has yet been published.

7.3 Third Portion

Many dynamic factors may be involved in producing V. A. compression above C 2. In fact, the third V. A. segment has a particular course which is supposed to be adapted to head and neck movements, especially rotation. However, as described in the previous chapters, demonstration of V. A. mechanical stenosis or even occlusion during head and neck movements has been made by anatomic, perfusion and angiographic studies on patients without pathologic anomalies. For most of the authors, the V. A. is compressed during rotation associated with extension at the level of the atlanto-axial joint. Some others consider that the narrowing of the foramen magnum by the sliding movement of the atlas on the occiput during hyperextension is an important factor of V. A. compression.

Whatever the mechanism applied to the V. A. under normal conditions, some pathologic conditions may increase the phenomenon.

7.3.1 Congenital Abnormality

7.3.1.1 Cervico-occipital Anomalies

Many cervico-occipital anomalies may lead to V. A. external compression: defects of occipital articulation, atlas and axis; basilar invagination; Klippel-Feil malformation.

Moreover, hypoplastic or absent V. A. is more frequently observed in association with these cranio-cervical malformations (Djindjian and Hurth, 1964, Janeway et al., 1966, Recordier, 1966). The role of vertebro-basilar insufficiency in the pathogenesis of basilar impression symptoms was suggested as early as 1940 by Gustafson and Oldberg and then by Ford (1952) and Taylor and Chkravorty (1964).

The first demonstrations were made by Djindjian et al. (1964) on post-mortem angiographies, and then by Janeway et al. in 1966, and Herrschaft and Duus in 1970, on living patients.

7.3.1.2 Atlanto-occipital Subluxation

See below.

7.3.2 Atlanto-occipital Subluxation

Atlanto-occipital subluxation, whatever its cause (congenital, traumatic, rheumatoïd) may stretch the V. A. in the transverse foramen of C 1. Subluxation at the atlanto-occipital joint associated with V. A. compression has been reported from congenital origin by Ford (1952) and Singer et al. (1975), from traumatic origin by Pratt-Thomas and Berger (1947), Ford and Clark (1956), Mant (1972), and Hayes et al. (1980), and from rheumatoid arthritis. Particular mention must be given to odontoid dislocation in rheumatoid arthritis. Sudden death in this disease may occur after complete dislocation at the atlanto-axial joint level (Boyle, 1971). V. A. occlusion is one of the possible causes (Webb et al., 1968). Rheumatoid arthritis with atlanto-occipital subluxation may also manifest as vertebro-basilar insufficiency produced by intermittent V. A. compression secondary to atlas slip during flexion of the head (Robinson, 1966, Jones and Kaufman, 1976).

7.3.3 Infantile Atlanto-occipital Instability

This particular cause of V. A. compression is due to sliding and slipping movements between the vertebral column and the skull such as observed in early infancy. As well desribed by Gilles et al. in 1979, the posterior arch of the atlas may invert through the foramen magnum during extension of the head because of the laxity of the atlanto-occipital joint. This results in a narrowing or even closure of the V. A. over the arch of the atlas, which may explain some sudden infant death syndromes or stillbirth syndromes.

A similar mechanism is advanced by Yates (1959) to explain V. A. dissection causing death at birth.

Table 7. External compression

	1st Portion	2nd Portion	3rd Portion
Osteophytes	−	+	−
Fibrous bands	+	+	+
Disc herniation	−	+	−
Nerve	+	−	+
Trauma	+	+	+
Congenital anomaly	−	±	+
Rheumatoid arthritis	−	−	+
Tumor	+	+	+

+ Indicates already reported cases of V. A. compression.

7.3.4 Other Causes

Other causes, identical to those observed on the second portion of the
V. A., have been reported, but they are
much less frequent on the third segment. Tumors (George, 1985), fibrous
bands, and entrapment by the 2nd
cervical nerve (Carney, 1981) have
occasionally been demonstrated to
cause stenosis or occlusion of the V. A.
above C 2 (**Fig. 42**).

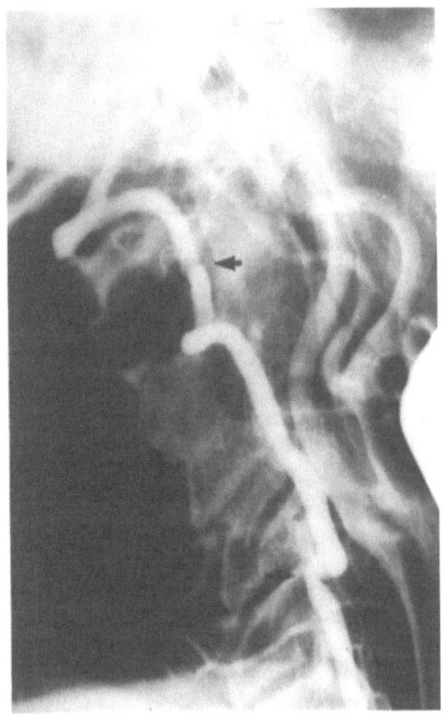

Fig. 42. External compression at two levels: C 4
by a fibrous band, C 1–C 2 by the anterior
branch of the second cervical nerve

8. TRAUMA

The modalities and mechanisms of traumatic lesions of the V. A. may be of many different types. Most have already been reviewed in previous chapters. They are grouped within this separate chapter in an attempt to give a synopsis of the possible V. A. consequences of cranio-cerebral trauma.

8.1 Modality

Both penetrating and non-penetrating trauma may be responsible for V. A. injury **(Table 8)**.

Table 8. V. A. injury

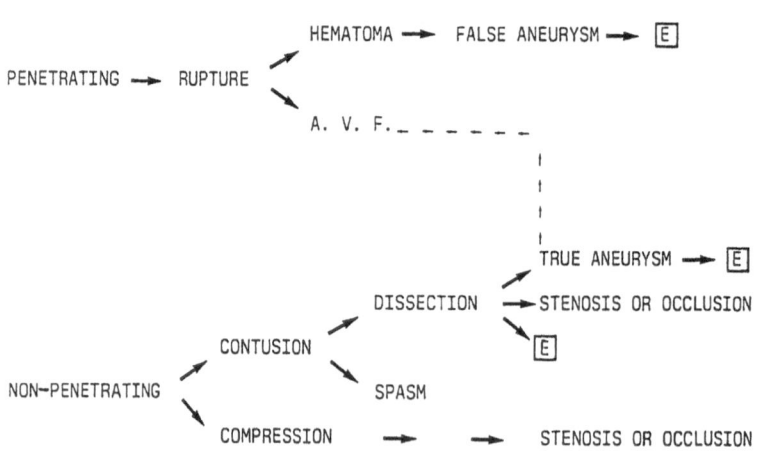

E : EMBOLISM

8.1.1 Penetrating Trauma

This type of trauma is most frequently observed in the military practice, and each war from the American Civil War to the Viet-Nam War contributed to new reports of V. A. injuries.

However, because of the deep location of the V. A., this vessel is far less frequently injured than any other.

For similar reasons, V. A. injury is quite uncommon in civilians, and case reports are scarce (Contostavlos, 1971, Heros, 1979).

In contrast, iatrogenic penetrating injuries of the V. A. were frequent in the past, following direct puncture of the V. A. Until 1970, reports on arteriovenous fistulae (A. V. F.) following puncture for vertebral angiography were numerous (Sugar *et al.*, 1949, Philipson, 1956, Olson *et al.*, 1963,

Garland, 1965, Lester, 1966, Vencken, 1970). Since that time, direct V. A. puncture has been abandoned and V. A. lesions, primarily A. V. F.'s are now an unintentional result of carotid angiography puncture or internal jugular vein catheterization (Reizine *et al.*, 1985).

Iatrogenic lesions of the V. A. have also been described after lateral cervical spinal puncture for myelography, in the case of an abnormal intra-dural course of the V. A. (Rogers, 1983).

Surgical V. A. lesions have also been reported after posterior fossa craniectomy, mastoidectomy, sympathectomy or anterior cervical disc approach (Buscaglia and Crowhurst, 1979, Reizine *et al.*, 1985) and also after radon seed implantation (Early *et al.*, 1966).

8.1.2 Non-penetrating Trauma

8.1.2.1 Hyperextension Injury

Although blunt trauma is a possible cause of V. A. injury (Aronson, 1961, Chou and French, 1965, Avellanosa *et al.*, 1977, Mc Lean *et al.*, 1985), subluxation after severe hyperextension of the cervical spine is a more common finding (Nurick, 1963, Hayes, 1980). Rotation of the neck may be associated with hyperextension in producing these lesions (Sherman *et al.*, 1981). Such injuries have been reported in various circumstances:

— traffic accidents: Simeone and Goldberg (1968), Avellanosa (1977), Six *et al.* (1981),

— sports, including yoga (Hanus *et al.*, 1977), football (Marks, 1973, Schneider *et al.*, 1972), wrestling (Rogers and Sweeney, 1979) and diving (Suetching and French, 1955).

8.1.2.2 Compression Injury

Prolonged abnormal position of the neck may injure the V. A. by a similar mechanism, except that hyperextension and/or rotation is not forced and acute but moderate and sustained (Murray, 1957, Okawara and Nibbelink, 1097). This prolonged compression of the V. A. has even been suggested by Holzer (1955) as the cause

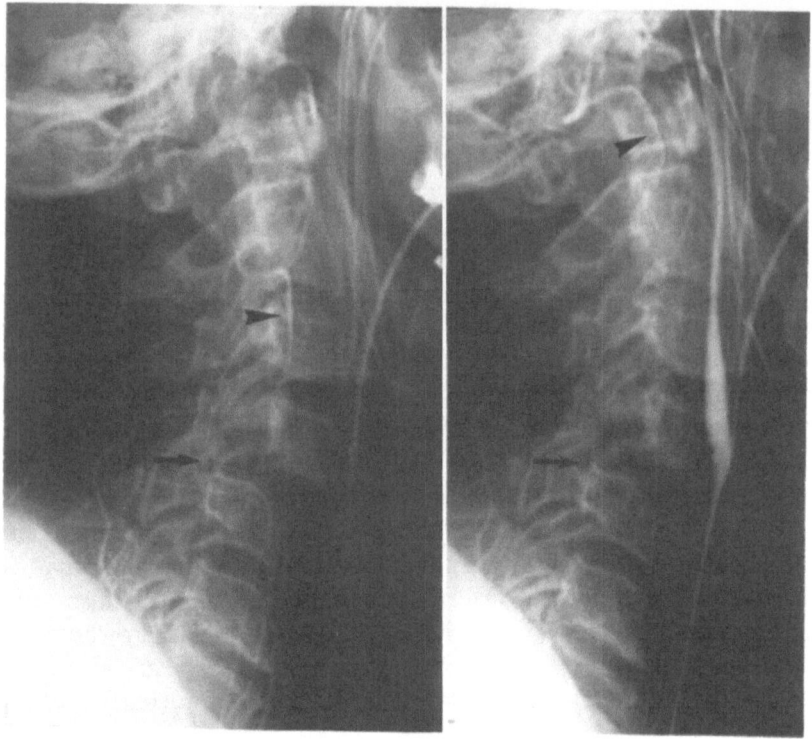

Fig. 43. Luxation of the cervical spine at C 4–C 5 with complete occlusion of both V. A.'s Weak distal reinjection (first post-traumatic day)

of V. A. occlusion at the C 1 level after surgery on the stellate ganglion.

A compression mechanism is far more obvious after severe trauma to the cervical spine with fracture and/or luxation, since the displacement of the vertebrae or of a bony fragment easily explains the V. A. deformity (Fig. 43). Traumatic atloïdo-occipital dislocation is a particular example that may lead to intermittent and sometimes severe V. A. compression (Nurick, 1963, Verbiest, 1970, Brunon et al., 1974).

Lateral exclusion of disc fragments through the intervertebral foramen may also encroach upon the V. A. (Verbiest, 1970, Brunon et al., 1974).

8.1.2.3 Iatrogenic Injury

V. A. compression of iatrogenic origin is fairly well known, as reports of V. A. injury after chiropractic manipulations are numerous. Again, sustained hyperextension and rotation of the head and neck is the most frequent maneuver described (Pratt-Thomas and Berger, 1947, Ford and Clark, 1956, Boudin and Barbizet, 1958, Green and Joint, 1959, Smith and Estridge, 1962, Miller and Burton, 1974, Schmitt, 1976, Sherman et al., 1981).

As previously mentioned, prolonged abnormal position during surgery is another possible iatrogenic cause (Holzer, 1955).

8.2 Mechanism

Three main mechanisms are proposed to explain the various consequences of direct or indirect V. A. injury: contusion, rupture and compression of the V. A. wall (Schneider and Crosby, 1959, Carpenter, 1961, Gurdjian *et al.*, 1963, Dragon *et al.*, 1981, Zimmerman, 1983) **(Table 8)**.

8.2.1 Contusion

Contusion of the arterial wall is due to direct trauma, by either a penetrating injury (bullet, shell fragment, knife . . .) or blunt trauma or tearing of the intima after V. A. stretching (hyperextension injury).

The contusion may subsequently evolve into a dissecting hematoma within the arterial wall, between inner or outer layers (Bostrom and Lillie-quist, 1967, Simeone and Goldberg, 1968, Schmitt, 1976, Stringer and Kelly, 1980). According to the extension and development of the dissection, different consequences may be observed:

— stenosis or even occlusion (Schott *et al.*, 1965, Mantak, 1972, Schmitt, 1976, Sherman *et al.*, 1981). Six *et al.* (1981) reported a case with bilateral

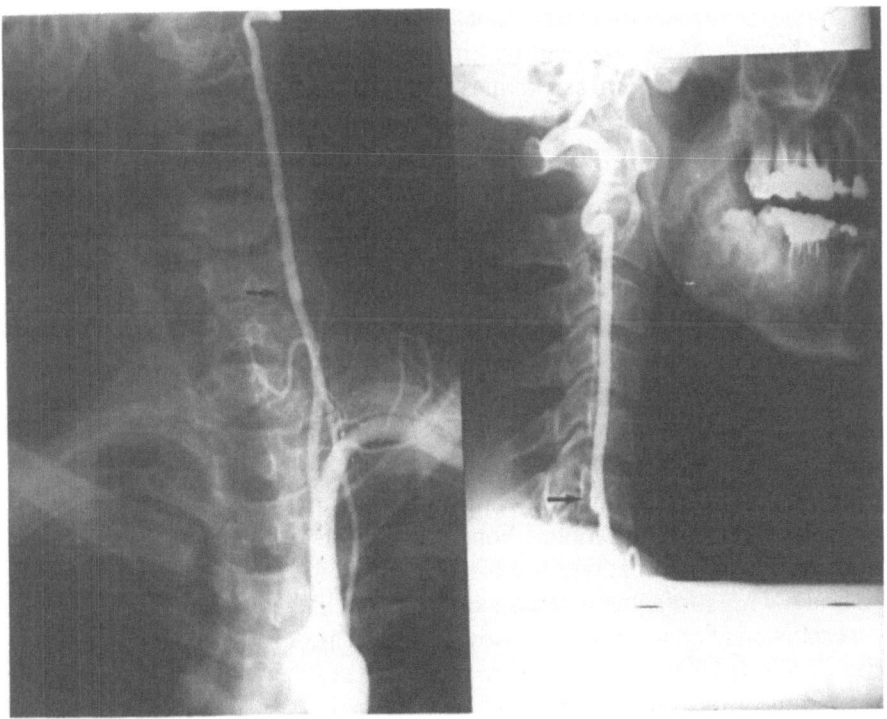

Fig. 44. Dissecting aneurysm at the V. A. entry into the transverse canal (C 6)

occlusion, and Simeone and Goldberg (1968) reported a case treated by endarterectomy,

— embolism from the site of intimal rupture (Murray, 1957, Heilbrun and Ratcheson, 1972, Sherman *et al.*, 1981),

— aneurysm, if the dissection develops between the media and the adventitia (**Fig. 44**).

This form of aneurysm is sometimes called "true" aneurysm and must be differentiated from "false" aneurysm resulting from the organization of a hematoma (Heifetz, 1945, Kister and Rankow, 1966, Adeloye, 1970, Alves and Black, 1972, Davidson *et al.*, 1975, Case *et al.*, 1979, Kempe, 1979, Paul *et al.*, 1980).

Contusion of the arterial wall may also lead to complete rupture of the inner or the outer wall of the vessel. The former gives rise to clot accumulation inside the lumen of the vessel and the latter to aneurysmal dilatation. Both comport the risk of embolism in the vertebro-basilar territory.

8.2.2 Rupture

Direct rupture of the entire wall of the V. A. usually follows a penetrating trauma but may appear secondarily from aneurysm or dissecting hematoma. Complete rupture is associated with blood irruption in various anatomic spaces. Most frequently, it occurs in the paravertebral soft tissues, producing a hematoma which may evolve into a false aneurysm (Matas, 1893, Makins, 1919).

Rupture of an abnormal intradural V. A. or of the V. A. at its point of dural penetration, provokes a subarachnoïd hemorrhage and/or a subdural hematoma (Fraenkel, 1927, Wolff, 1928, Contostavlos, 1971, Rogers, 1983, McLean *et al.*, 1985).

Rupture into an adjacent vein produces an arterio-venous fistula. Reports on this type of V. A. injury are numerous; arteriovenous fistulas may be observed after penetrating or nonpenetrating injuries, after arteriographic puncture, or even after cervical spine surgery (Elkin and Shumacker, 1946, Aronson, 1961, Faith and Ducker, 1961, Tsuji *et al.*, 1968, Deutsch and Hill, 1969, Nagashima *et al.*, 1977, Avellanosa and Glasauer, 1977, Buscaglia and Crowhurst, 1979, George and Laurian, 1982, Reizine, 1985).

8.2.3 Compression

The V. A. may be permanently compressed by a vertebral luxation, a bony fragment, a distal herniation, or a foreign body, with subsequent stenosis or even occlusion (Schneider and Crosby, 1959, Verbiest, 1970, Mantak, 1972).

Intermittent V. A. compression may be due to an unstable fracture or intermittent luxation, as observed in atloïdo-occipital dislocation. Suetching and French (1955) reported on a patient with V. A. compression which disappeared after tong traction and appeared again each time the traction was released.

8.2.4 *Aggravating Factors*

— Osteophytic spurs: these may worsen the V. A. injury in the case of trauma with hyperextension of the neck, as emphasized by Gurdjian *et al.* (1963).

— Embolism, while uncommonly observed in atherosclerotic lesions, occurs frequently after certain traumatic lesions: contusion, dissecting hematoma and aneurysm (Murray, 1957, Heilbrun and Ratcheson, 1972, Sherman *et al.*, 1981).

— Hemodynamic factors: as in any other vertebro-basilar pathology, vertebro-basilar symptoms are better explained if other factors of flow reduction are associated: bilateral V. A. lesions, controlateral atretic V. A., carotid artery lesion, abnormality of the circle of Willis (Simeone and Goldberg, 1968, Heilbrun and Ratcheson, 1972, Six *et al.*, 1981).

In the same way, a V. A. lesion may be asymptomatic if it occurs on a small, non-dominant V. A. (Gurdjian *et al.*, 1963).

— Arterial spasm: arterial spasm has been suggested by some authors (Schneider and Crosby, 1959, Mantak, 1972) to explain the consequences of certain traumatic lesions of the V. A. While presumably the onset of arterial spasm is a possibility in the V. A., just as in any other vessel, its demonstration and its role in producing symptoms is still unclear; moreover, some angiographic aspects interpreted as evidence of spasm may have actually been due to dissection.

8.3 Level of Injury

The V. A. is most frequently injured at three principal sites, and may even be injured at all three simultaneously, according to Schneider and Crosby (1959).

These sites are: above the C 6 intervertebral foramen, at the C 1 intervertebral foramen, and above C 1. These are the most frequent sites of fracture dislocation and correspond to three particular points in the course of the V. A.: entry into the transverse canal, exit from the transverse canal, and dural penetration. They are points of V. A. fixity between segments of relative mobility; around these points, the amplitude of head and neck movements is more important than anywhere else.

8.4 Onset of Symptoms

Symptoms may appear in two different modes following trauma.

8.4.1 Early Onset

Symptoms may be observed either immediately after trauma, or after a short period of time (several minutes to few hours). This delay is assumed to be due to the time required for a contusion to evolve into one of the previously described lesions (Schneider and Schemm, 1961, Vasin *et al.*, 1977, Meier *et al.*, 1981). For some authors (Lyness and Simeone, 1978, Dragon *et al.*, 1981), a latent interval between cervical injury, whatever its severity, and the onset of neurological symptoms should evoke trauma to the V. A.

In the case of early symptoms, diagnosis may be easy after minor trauma or penetrating injury; conversely, a diagnostic problem often results from intercurrence of symptoms which are non-vascular in origin: cerebral concussion or spinal cord lesions. Probably some cases of unexplained aggravation after cranio-cervical trauma, are related to cervical vessel injury; but this needs to be demonstrated in order to recommend more frequent angiographic explorations. The advent of routine C. T. scan for investigation of head injuries has probably led to misdiagnosis of some traumatic lesions. Correct analysis, however, requires vertebral as well as carotid angiography with cranial and cervical films (Heilbrun and Ratcheson, 1972), which is difficult to propose.

8.4.2 Late Onset

Late onset of symptoms, i. e. several days or months following trauma, is related to various causes:
— embolism from an arterial wall lesion (aneurysm),
— intermittent V. A. compression due to unrecognized spinal fracture or subluxation,
— tinnitus more or less associated with vertebro-basilar signs, secondary to an arterio-venous fistula.

In these cases, a diagnostic problem may arise from the fact that the cervical trauma has been forgotten or underestimated. However, when the vascular origin of the symptoms is obvious, vascular investigations are, of course, indicated and the V. A. lesions will not be missed (Marks and Freed, 1973, Avellanosa and Glasauer, 1977, Six *et al.*, 1981).

9. INFANCY AND CHILDHOOD

V. A. lesions in the newborn and child are infrequent and consequently, not well known. However, they are of sufficient importance to warrant a separate chapter, even though the lesions encountered (dissection, arteriovenous fistula) are described in previous chapters as well.

Lesions of traumatic origin and congenital arteriovenous fistulas are the two main types of V. A. lesions observed at this age.

Early recognition should help decrease the mortality and morbidity secondary to the cerebro-vascular consequences of these lesions.

9.1 Traumatic Lesions in the Newborn

Yates' work (1959) underlined the importance of cervical injuries occurring during delivery, whatever its modality. The great manipulative strain, in any method of delivery, imposed on the infant's neck, can explain various traumatic lesions at this level.

According to Yates, three cervical structures may be involved:

— cervical spine: distortional trauma of the cervical spine,

— spinal cord: direct damage of the spinal cord or tearing of the spinal nerve roots is observed in only a few cases,

— vertebral artery: damage to the V. A. is observed in one third of the infants examined after neo-natal death.

9.1.1 V. A. Lesions

In Yates' experience: one or both V. A.'s are usually injured in their course through the transverse canal. The mechanical injury to the V. A. produces a dissection which consistently develops in the subadventitial plane.

It is of particular interest to note that in these cases, the dissecting hematoma arises from tearing of V. A. branches at their junction with the major trunk. In no case, is the V. A. itself torn.

— Associated venous lesions.

In some cases, venous plexus rupture is observed in addition to arterial lesions. This can be related to the severity of the trauma.

— Associated cervical spine injury.

In the V. A. lesions seen by Yates, there was evidence of associated distortional trauma of the cervical spine.

9.1.2 Consequences of V. A. Lesions

There is considerable evidence that stenosis or occlusion secondary to V. A. dissection at the time of birth, is an important factor in the production of ischemic damage to the brainstem, or of hemispheric lesions in many cases of cerebral palsy.

In fact, many of the pathologic changes found in cases of cerebral palsy or epilepsy lie within the V. A. territory. Unfortunately, no corrective treatment is yet available in the aftermath of these traumatic lesions.

9.2 Traumatic Lesions in Childhood

Traumatic lesions of the V. A. in the child present particular, fairly specific features: symptoms of vertebro-basilar insufficiency are very unusual at this age, the V. A. lesion has distinctive characteristics, and a particular mechanism of injury is related to osseous and ligamentous anomalies.

9.2.1 Vertebro-Basilar Insufficiency

Symptoms of vertebro-basilar insufficiency are quite infrequent in children. For a long time, their etiology remained less certain than in adults.

Autopsic (Fowler, 1962) and then angiographic studies (Dooley and Smith, 1968) showed the possible occurrence of embolism to the basilar trunk, but without demonstration of any embolic source.

Ouvrier and Hopkins (1970) published the two first well-documented reports on occlusive lesions of the extracranial V. A. associated with intracranial V. A. occlusion. For these authors, the angiographic appearence of the V. A. was that of "arteritis".

Fraser and Zimbler (1985) were the first to believe that the best explanation for this vertebro-basilar lesion was traumatic.

9.2.2 V. A. Lesion

The particularity of this lesion in the child stems from its localization and angiographic aspect:

9.2.2.1 Localization

The lesion is always located at the C 2 transverse foramen level (Ouvrier and Hopkins, 1970, Devico and Fareil, 1972, Philippe et al., 1974, Singer et al., 1975, Klein et al., 1976, Simmerman et al., 1976, Pascual-Castroviego et al.,

1977, Malik and Chhabra, 1982, Fraser and Zimbler, 1985). In the newborn and the adult, traumatic lesions are never observed at this site. According to the cases reported in the literature, the lesion is most frequently bilateral.

9.2.2.2 Angiography

Three angiographic aspects have been described:

a—Segmentary occlusion, extending for 1 or 2 cm, with distal V. A. reinjection by a muscular network at C 1–C 2.

b—Regular segmentary stenosis.

c—Fusiform ectasy.

From the descriptions, and despite of the lack of pathologic studies and repeat angiographic controls in the follow-up, it can be concluded that these lesions result from V. A. dissection of traumatic origin.

9.2.2.3 Associated Arterial Lesions

Although the dissection usually affects only the V. A.'s, associated internal carotid artery thrombosis was reported by Philippe et al. (1974) and Malik and Chhaba (1982). This association can be explained by the same mechanism as that proposed for the V. A. lesions: C 1–C 2 subluxation (see blow 9.2.3).

9.2.2.4 Basilar Trunk Embolism

Bilaterality and intimal localization of the arterial wall lesion may explain the frequency of distal emboli into the basilar trunk and its collaterals (Ouvrier and Hopkins, 1970, Zimmerman et al., 1976, Fraser and Limbler, 1985).

9.2.3 Pathogenesis. Osteo-ligamentous Anomalies

Several hypotheses have been proposed to explain these lesions, though their pathogenesis has long remained unclear.

— Congenital tortuosity or kinking at the level of the second cervical vertebra favoring intermittent occlusion, has been suggested, but such anomalies are infrequent at this level and at this age.

— Fibromuscular dysplasia has never been demonstrated in children exhibiting these lesions.

— The most acceptable explanation is trauma, due to repeated subluxation at C 1–C 2. This may cause mechanical deformation and occlusion of the V. A. with consequent traumatic dissection. The subluxation at C 1–C 2 may be due to:

— cervical spine anomaly.

A lack of union of the odontoïd with the body of C 2 (os odontoideum) produces chronic and intermittent mechanical trauma with stretching of the V. A.'s due to anterior sliding of C 1 over C 2 when the head is flexed (Singer et al., 1975, Fraser and Zimbler, 1985).

— ligament laxity.

Without any bone defect or anomaly, subluxation may result from laxity of the ligaments connecting the atlas and axis. Radiological changes are, in this case, only apparent on flexion-extension films.

If the suspicion of such anomalies is properly confirmed, surgical cervical spine fusion is indicated.

In children with unexplained repetitive transient brainstem and cerebellar symptoms, increased awareness of this lesion should lead to exploration and diagnosis of this pathology. Diagnosis is important, since this is an extra-cranial occlusive cerebro-vascular disease for which surgical stabilization of the cervical spine provides appropriate therapy and removes further risk of stroke.

9.3 Congenital Arterio-venous Fistula

Congenital A. V. F.'s are often missed in the neonate; they are usually recognized later in childhood. Most of the reported cases were identified and treated between the ages of 5 and 15.

9.3.1 Clinical Symptoms

These fistulas are rarely symptomatic; systematic examination is the most frequent circumstance leading to the discovery of a continuous palpable thrill under the ear or a suboccipital pulsating mass. In only two cases, symptoms of cardiac failure led to the diagnosis (Norman et al., 1950, Bartal and Levy, 1972).

9.3.2 Type and Topography

9.3.2.1 Type

Most of the congenital fistulas develop between the V. A. and the perivertebral venous plexus; only two cases between the V. A. and the internal jugular vein have been reported to date (Bartal and Levy, 1972, Suen et al., 1972).

From an anatomic point of view, the fistula always consists of a single communication between artery and vein, without any supply from neighboring arteries. In several cases with surgical treatment (Mathey and Cormier, 1957, Ehrlich et al., 1968, Cinqualbre et al., 1978), direct arteriovenous communication through a persisting vestigial vessel was described; such vestigal arteries might be persistent intersegmentary arteries (see chapter Embryology).

9.3.2.2 Localization

Arteriovenous fistulas involving the V. A. are most frequently encountered at its extremities (ostial and suboccipital portions). The distal V. A. above C 1 is the most frequent localization (Chou et al., 1967, Ehrlich et al., 1968, Greenberg et al., 1970, Bartal and Levy, 1972, Fabiani et al., 1979, Reizine et al., 1985). Arteriovenous fistulas on the proximal V. A. are mainly observed just below the V. A. entry into the transverse canal (Mathey and Cormier, 1957, Cinqualbre et al., 1978, Reizine et al., 1985).

Localizations on the transverse portion of the V. A. are scarce and may be situated anywhere along the transverse canal (Norman et al., 1950, Shumacker et al., 1966, Suen et al., 1972, Moret et al., 1979).

9.3.3 Therapeutic Approach

The discovery, almost always incidental, of an arteriovenous fistula in an asymptomatic child, raises the difficult problem of deciding whether or not there is an indication for treatment.

For some authors, the technical difficulties of surgical treatment limit therapeutic indications to cases with either cardiac failure, vertebro-basilar insufficiency, or incapacitating murmur.

Others (Norman *et al.*, 1950, Bartal and Levy, 1972, Reizine *et al.*, 1985) consider that such arteriovenous fistulas tend to increase in size and therefore they prefer to propose cure of the fistula even in asymptomatic cases.

Therapeutic indications have recently been modified by the development of embolization techniques. An attempt at fistula occlusion with a detachable balloon is now justified as an initial procedure, whatever the symptoms; in case of failure of endovascular techniques, new surgical approaches to the V.A. can be applied with safety.

10. PATHOPHYSIOLOGY

Surgery on the cervical V. A. may be discussed to treat different pathological states as described in the previous chapters; but there are two principal indications for this surgery:
— to spare the V. A. in case of involvement by any lesion which must be removed,
— to restore V. A. flow which has been compromised and thereby prevent ischemic events in the vertebro-basilar territory.

10.1 V. A. Preservation

When surgery is performed on a lesion involving the V. A., the primary goal of treatment is to remove the lesion as completely as possible. The relation of the lesions to the V. A. raises certain more or less important technical difficulties which are best solved by control and freeing of this vessel. In this way, V. A. flow is maintained and the lesions can be completely removed. This situation occurs mainly with tumors related to the V. A. and with arteriovenous fistulas supplied by the V. A. Today, V. A. ligation or trapping should only be accepted as a last resort, even if V. A. occlusion seems to be well tolerated.

Similarly, incomplete removal of a tumor because of fear of injuring the V. A. is not acceptable "a priori".

In other words, deliberate sacrifice or, on the contrary, too much respect for the V. A. leading to incomplete treatment of a V. A. related lesion are now unacceptable.

10.2 Prevention of Ischemic Events

The purpose of V. A. surgery in this second major indication is to restore V. A. flow and prevent vertebro-basilar ischemia.

10.2.1 Clinical Features

Since the first pathologic confirmation of vertebro-basilar ischemia, reported by Kubik and Adams in 1946, many different clinical features have been recognized as belonging to the same etiology: subclavian steal syndrome, lacunar strokes, transient ischemic attack and vertebro-basilar insufficiency, and infarction of different structures including the brainstem, cerebellum and occipital lobe (Millikan and Siekert, 1955, Alajouanine *et al.*, 1960, Wilson, 1962, Fisher, 1965, Caplan, 1981).

10.2.1.1 Subclavian Steal Syndrome

This syndrome will not be discussed here, since the causative lesion is located on the subclavian artery. Nevertheless, among a variety of possible operations, proximal V. A. to common carotid artery transposition now appears to be the best treatment (Bohmfalk *et al.*, 1979). Recognition of the retrograde flow in one V. A. produced by this syndrome has facilitated determination of the hemodynamic origin of some vertebro-basilar insufficiency syndromes.

10.2.1.2 Lacunar Strokes

In the vertebro-basilar system, these strokes are quite similar to those observed in the carotid territory. They are small, deep infarcts in the territory of penetrating vessels. As demonstrated by Fisher (1975–1978), it is a local disease with lipohyalinotic change in small vessel walls, related to hypertension. These lesions are quite distinct from atherosclerosis of large vessels.

10.2.1.3 Vertebro-basilar Insufficiency and Stroke

These are manifestations of vertebro-basilar ischemia, consisting of transient and repetitive symptoms in vertebro-basilar insufficiency and of permanent, more or less regressive, signs in vertebro-basilar infarctions.

a—The incidence of transient ischemic attacks (T. I. A.) in the posterior circulation is approximately half that of anterior circulation T. I. A.'s (Cartlidge *et al.*, 1977). T. I. A.'s in the vertebro-basilar system must be considered warning signs as important as are those in the carotid system.

The probability of subsequent stroke within one year from the time of the first T. I. A. is 22%, and within five years, 35% (Cartlidge *et al.*, 1977). Strokes in the vertebro-basilar system are preceded by T. I. A.'s in approximately 80% of patients (Fisher, 1975, Naritomi *et al.*, 1979). This provides an opportunity for preventive measures.

b—Before such preventive measures can be taken, the clinical diagnosis of vertebro-basilar ischemia must be correctly assessed. A wide spectrum of symptoms and signs can be referable to the vertebro-basilar circulation. Some are of doubtful origin and, if isolated, should not be retained for clinical diagnosis: dizziness, vertigo, syncope, speech impairment and motor or sensory limb dysfunction. The most helpful criteria indicating vertebro-basilar origin are postural incidence, combination of several symptoms and changing laterality and territory of impairment.

c—Except in cases of T. I. A. due to a small embolus, a vertebro-basilar T. I. A. implies a critical level in vertebro-basilar perfusion, which is intermittently overcome under certain circumstances. In this situation, the tissue perfusion level may be sufficiently reduced to provoke localized cerebral suffering manifested by intermittent clinical symptoms; but duration and level of ischemia are not important enough to induce tissue necrosis with permanent neurologic impairment.

Therefore, infarction occurs only if there is a sufficiently sustained and important reduction of tissue perfusion and oxygen extraction.

10.2.2 Hemodynamic and Metabolic Features

Cerebral blood flow (C. B. F.) reduction is the first parameter modified in cerebral ischemia; but, as is well established by metabolic studies, C. B. F. measurement alone cannot determine the actual presence or degree of ischemia.

According to Ackerman et al. (1981–1984), ischemic brain lesions can be classified intro three stages on the basis of pathophysiologic disturbances:

— Stage 1 reflects an impaired perfusion pressure. The lesions is primarily ischemic and should respond to an increase in perfusion pressure. C. B. F. is more or less reduced, but cerebral metabolic rate of oxygen (CMRO 2) is normal, and cerebral blood volume (C. B. V.) increases progressively due to autoregulation with progressive vascular dilatation. In this stage, the oxygen extraction fraction (O. E. F.), which is CMRO 2 reported to C. B. F., is increased.

— Stage 2 refers to a lesion by dysmetabolism. It corresponds to a marked fall in C. B. F., decreased CMRO 2 and persistent increased C. B. V. Autoregulation by vasodilatation is now maximal in order to compensate the C. B. F. decrease. This hemodynamic compensation is the first to act and also the first to be exhausted.

As long as CMRO 2 remains normal, metabolic compensation occurs as O. E. F. increases in parallel with the progressive fall of C. B. F.. When cellular function is impaired, CMRO 2 decreases, with a consequent decrease in O. E. F., which tends towards normal. At this point, the second, or metabolic, mechanism of compensation is exhausted.

— Stage 3 corresponds to cellular necrosis and is associated with a marked fall in C. B. F., CMRO 2 and O. E. F., while the C. B. V. increase persists.

Division into these three stages is also useful from a therapeutic standpoint. In stage 1, a decrease in C. B. F. is the principal impairment, and its correction by any means is efficient. In stage 2, proportionate depression in C. B. F. and CMRO 2 is related to impaired cellular metabolism, which would respond only to agents able to improve metabolic function. Stage 3 corresponds to complete failure of oxygen metabolism, which can only be managed conservatively.

In fact, hemodynamic and metabolic data vary significantly for a given subject at different times in the clinical course of cerebral ischemia. In the early phase, blood flow in excess of metabolic needs is frequently observed. This mismatch in the flow-metabolism relation has been termed "luxury perfusion"

(Baron *et al.*, 1981). It is observed less than 31 days after stroke whatever the absolute value of C. B. F., which can be increased, decreased or normal. This type of mismatch usually disappears progressively, and after 30 days, C. B. F. usually remains decreased whereas oxygen metabolism returns to normal.

In some cases, there is what is termed "misery perfusion" corresponding to insufficient flow to meet oxygen demands. In this situation, C. B. F. is decreased to a larger extent than CMRO 2, with a compensatory increase in O. E. F.. This phenomenon can be observed in the acute phase, but less frequently than luxury perfusion (Baron *et al.*, 1981–1983, Lenzi *et al.*, 1982). Chronic misery perfusion persisting weeks and months after stroke has also been described and its presence is the best indication for surgical revascularization (Grubb *et al.*, 1979, Baron *et al.*, 1981). Surgical by-pass in this condition suppresses the flow-metabolism mismatch, as demonstrated after extra-intracranial anastomosis in the carotid territory (Samson *et al.*, 1985).

In cases of T. I. A. and lacunar strokes, blood flow and oxygen extraction were found to be normal (Baron *et al.*, 1981, Vorstrup *et al.*, 1983).

10.2.3 Factors Inducing Ischemia

10.2.3.1 Systemic Factors

The level of tissue perfusion depends first on general factors such as cardiac output and variations in systemic pressure (Meyers *et al.*, 1960), as demonstrated by the frequent occurrence of vertebro-basilar symptoms with changing position, especially with orthostatism. Clinical presentation in many patients reveals a very labile neurologic condition during orthostatism unaccompanied by systemic hypotension. Roski *et al.* (1982) classified these patients as having "fluctuating neurological deficit" and attributed it to hypoperfusion. For Caplan and Sergay (1976), postural hypotension is one of the must helpful symptoms, since the majority of patients with major vessel atherosclerotic disease in the vertebro-basilar system exhibit this postural symptom.

Increase in blood viscosity secondary to polycythemia, increased platelet aggregation and adhesiveness, and plasma hypercoagulability are all factors which may induce thrombosis. Cases have been reported in which patients had T. I. A.'s or strokes without atherosclerotic carotid or vertebral disease, verified by angiography, and no arteritis, collagen disease, history of migraine or cardiac source of emboli. However these patients had hemostasis perturbations, which must therefore be considered capable of provoking ischemic events without any associated vascular disease (Kalendovski *et al.*, 1975, Wu and Hoak, 1975, Al Meffy *et al.*, 1979).

10.2.3.2 Structural Lesions

a) Embolism

Structural lesions, primarily atherosclerotic stenosis or occlusion, appear to be the most common cause of vertebro-basilar ischemia. However this does not mean that decreased flow in the vertebro-basilar system is the main factor. On the contrary, it is generally accepted that ischemic events are most often embolic in the territory of the upper basilar trunk or the posterior cerebral arteries. This fact is explained by the diameter of the basilar trunk, widest at its origin at the junction of the V. A.'s, and tapering distally (Caplan, 1980); emboli cannot be trapped until they reach narrow lumen vessels. According to Castaigne *et al.* (1973), emboli usually arise from atherosclerotic lesions located in the proximal portions of the V. A. or from the heart.

Conversely, deficits referable to the lower brainstem, especially lateral medullary infarcts, are more often attributed to hemodynamic insufficiency following unilateral V. A. occlusion. In fact, post-mortem studies of patients who died after vertebro-basilar vessel occlusion have documented the frequent presence of small distal emboli. Angiographic evidence of emboli from an occlusion or a stenosis of the cervical V. A. has also been given by several authors (Meyer *et al.*, 1960, Fischer *et al.*, 1961, Sundt *et al.*, 1978, George and Laurian, 1980–1981) **(Fig. 45)**.

In the carotid system, embolus from an atheromatous plaque is a widely admitted phenomenon. Ulceration within the plaque is the major structural lesions involved in producing embolism in these vessels. On the V. A., ulcerated plaques are usually considered uncommon. Schwartz and Mitchell (1961) have observed ulcerated atherosclerotic

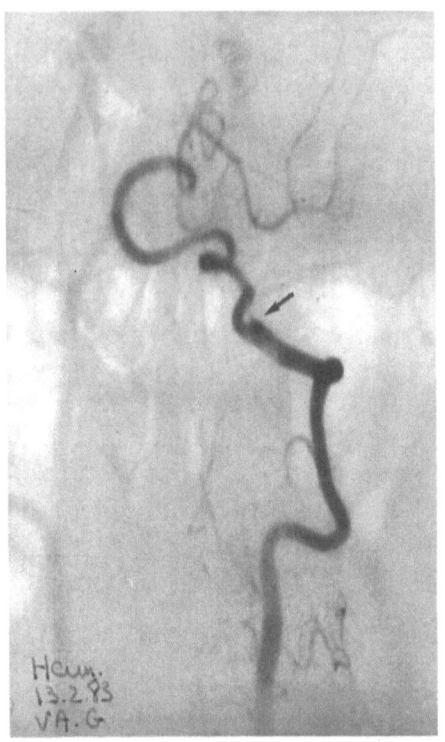

Fig. 45. V. A. occlusion just distal to the PICA origin, probably secondary to embolism from an ostial stenosis

lesions on the subclavian artery and not on the V. A. On the contrary, Hutchinson and Yates (1957), Duffy and Jacobs (1958) observed intraparietal hemorrhage on atheromatous V. A.'s. The exact frequency of ischemic events of embolic origin in the vertebro-basilar system is therefore still controversial. Caplan (1981) speculated whether "ulcerated plaques in the V. A. have the same angiographic appearance as in the carotid artery or if the smaller size and tortuosity of the V. A. alter their appearance".

In certain conditions, embolism seems to be the only way to explain the clinical manifestations; this is the case in unilateral occlusion of a small V. A. with a controlateral dominant V. A. and sometimes even collateral reinjection of the distal V. A. Here, insufficient flow, however abruptly installed, appears quite unlikely as the cause of ischemia (Fisher, 1970, George and Laurian, 1981).

It must not be forgotten that, besides atherosclerosis, many other diseases may be responsible for embolism in the vertebro-basilar system.

Dissection and aneurysm, whatever their cause (trauma, fibro-muscular dysplasia, congenital origin . . .) are frequently revealed after an embolic event.

Emboli may be also of cardiac origin from arrhythmia or valvulopathy. Exceptional occurrence of emboli from V. A. wall irritation by spondylotic spurs has also been reported (Sullivan et al., 1975).

Finally, there is the possibility of embolus migration into the occipital lobe, from an ulcerated internal carotid plaque through a persistent trigeminal artery (Heeney and Koo, 1980).

b) Flow Insufficiency

Insufficient flow in the vertebro-basilar system is frequently suggested but, in fact, rarely documented. Many factors intervene that may protect the vertebro-basilar system against a fall in blood flow:

— Controlateral V. A.: as the two V. A.'s join intracranially to form the basilar trunk, stenosis or occlusion of one V. A. is not likely to produce significant flow reduction if the controlateral V. A. is of good caliber. However, a controlateral hypoplastic or atretic V. A. is an aggravating factor.

Ischemic complications following V. A. ligation have only been observed in those cases where compensation by the controlateral V. A. does not exist or is weak (French and Haines, 1950, Webb and Burford, 1952, Thomas et al., 1959, Jones et al., 1960, Shumacker et al., 1966, Tsuji, 1968, Shintani and Zervas, 1972) (Fig. 46).

— Circle of Willis: suppletory flow from the carotid system through a normal-sized posterior communicating artery is not a constant feature (Alpers et al., 1959–1963). A normal circle of Willis with both posterior communicating arteries of good caliber is observed in 18% of cases; in 19% bilateral hypoplastic posterior communicating arteries or posterior cerebral arteries connect the carotid and vertebral systems (Hodes et al., 1953). Bilateral complete absence of posterior communicating arteries is noted in 1% (Wollschlaeger and Wollschlaeger, 1974).

— Carotid artery: even where there is at least one large posterior communicating artery, flow from the carotid system may be insufficient to maintain correct pressure in the vertebro-basilar system if there is an associated atherosclerotic lesion on the cervical or intracranial internal carotid artery. Castaigne et al. (1973) reported a 40% incidence of associated anterior and posterior circulation atherosclerotic disease in an autopsy series. This percentage is quite similar to that observed by angiography in our surgical series (see chapter Personal Experience) (Fig. 47).

A significant decrease in cerebral blood flow is observed mainly in cases of

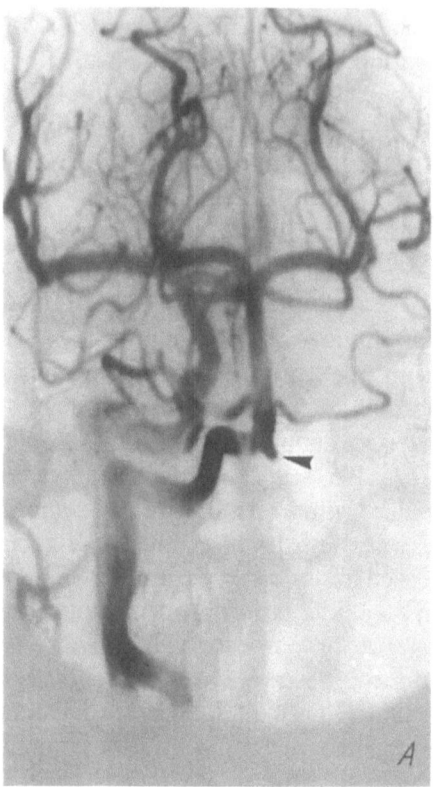

Fig. 46. A) Distal V. A. occlusion on the left side. Good filling of the vertebro-basilar system by the controlateral dominant V. A. B) Ostial stenosis with slow proximal filling of the left V. A.; double localization of atherosclerotic lesions or embole from the proximal one?

associated carotid and vertebral atherosclerotic lesions, whereas in cases with lesions limited to the vertebral artery, cerebral blood flow remains in the normal range. A good correlation was also found between the direction of flow in the posterior communicating arteries and the mean value of cerebral blood flow. If flow is anterograde, mean cerebral flow values are lower than in retrograde flow (Koga and Austin, 1982). This fact demonstrates the predominance of carotid flow in the

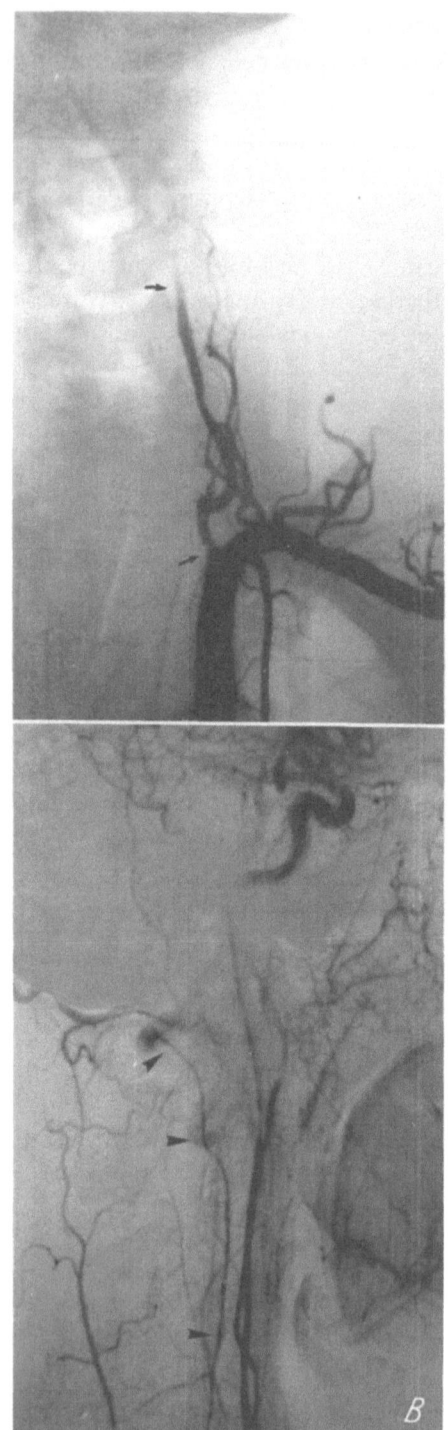

Fig. 46 B

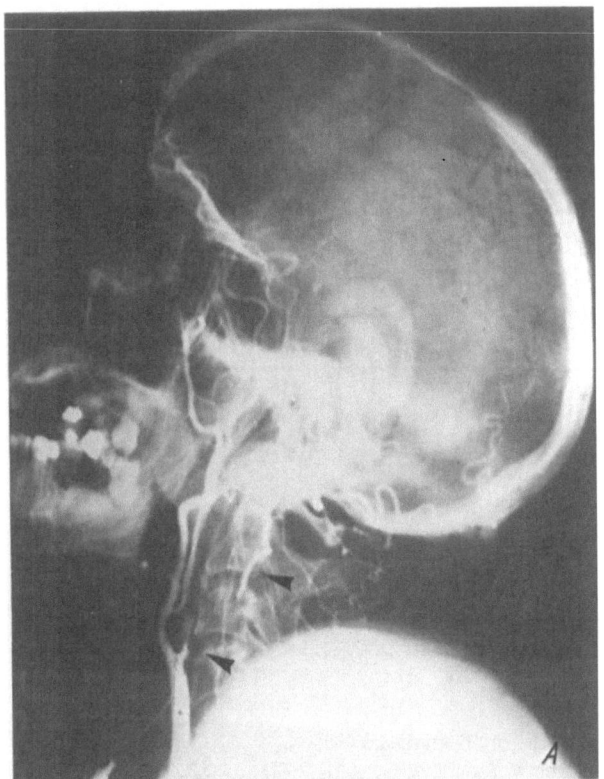

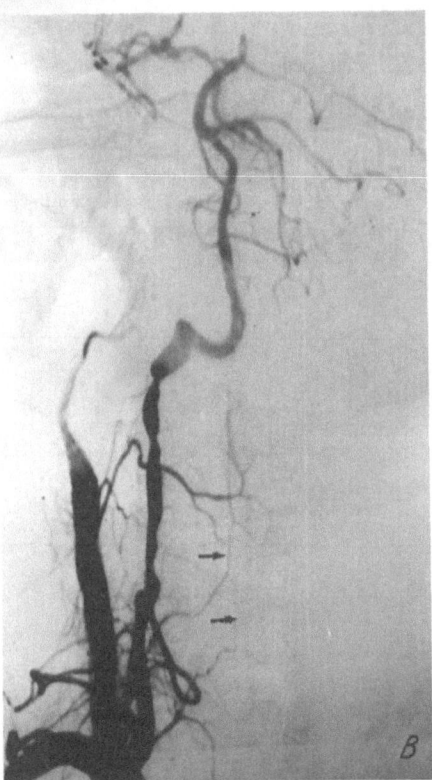

Fig. 47. A) Associated occlusion of the internal carotid artery and the V. A. on the same side.
B) Associated extensive stenosis of the carotid artery and V. A. after radiation therapy

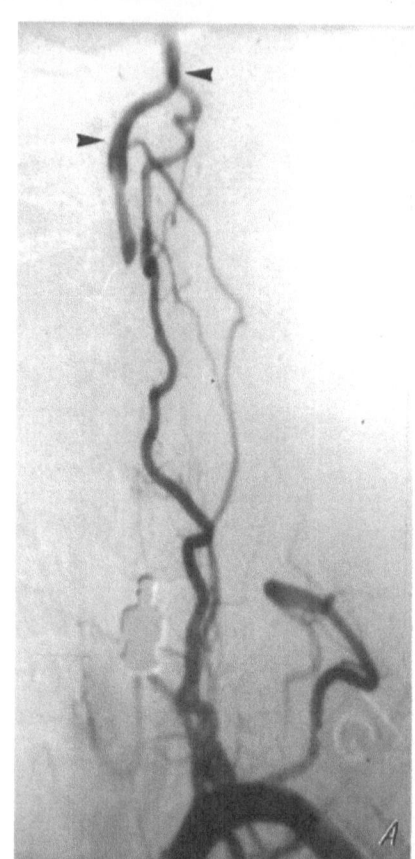

Fig. 48. A) Muscular network from the cervical arteries reinjecting the V. A. above C 3 (atherosclerotic lesion). **B)** Muscular network from the occipital artery reinjecting only on selective injection the V. A. above C 2 (tumoral occlusion)

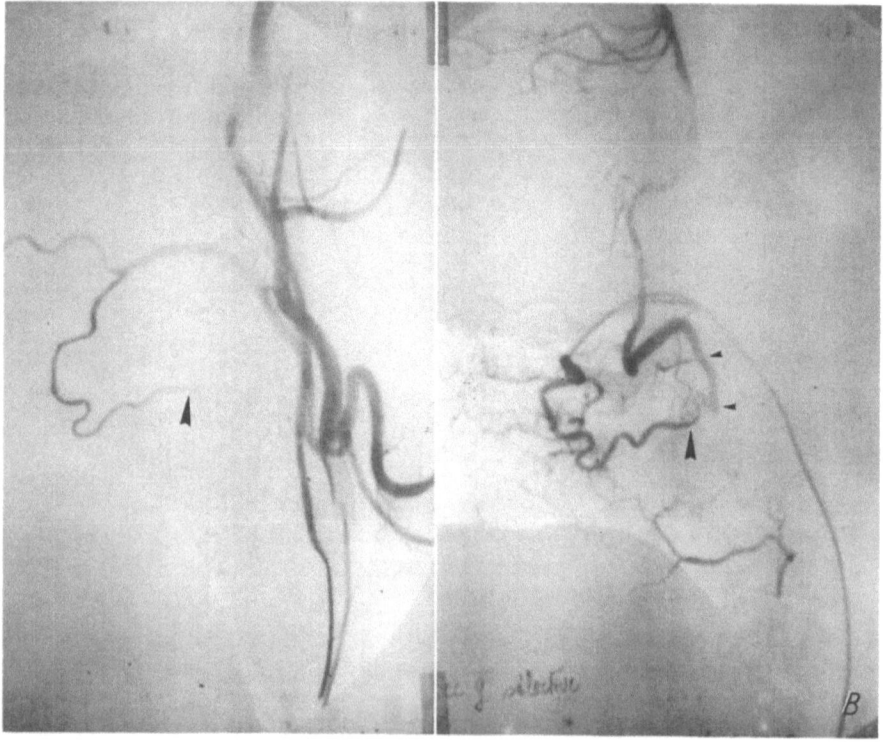

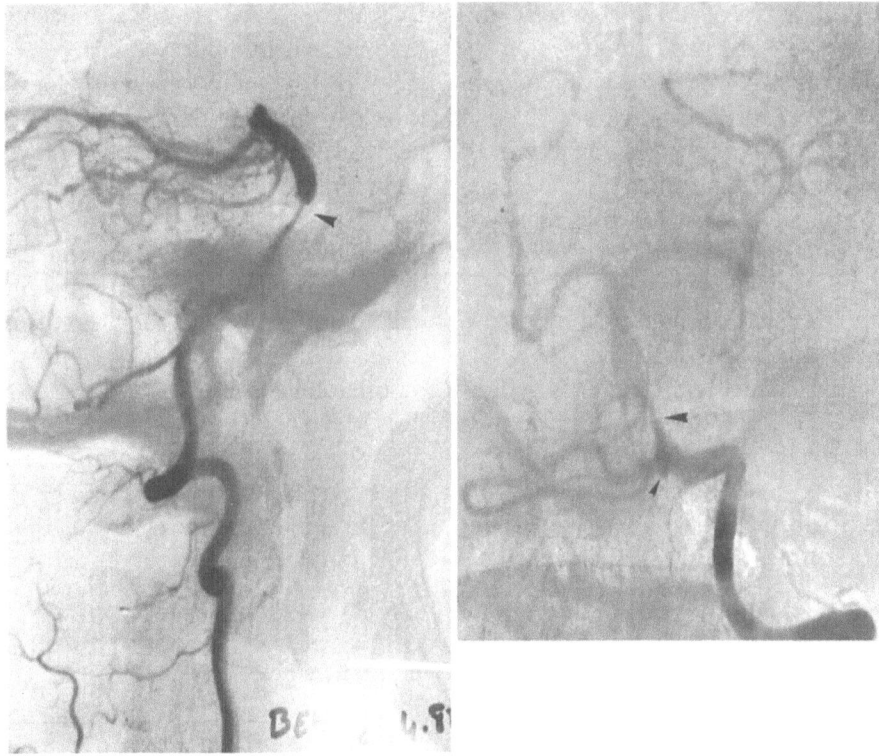

Fig. 49. Severe stenosis of the basilar trunk in its middle part with controlateral V. A. occlusion

cerebral blood supply. The mean ratio of carotid to vertebral artery flow was estimated to be about 70 : 30 (Dumke and Schmidt, 1943, Lee *et al.*, 1965), with a normal V. A. flow in the range of 45 to 90 ml/mn (Bohmfalk *et al.*, 1979). A good example of the importance of the carotid collateral contribution to the vertebro-basilar system is given by the subclavian steal syndrome, in which completed stroke is very rarely observed unless carotid artery atherosclerotic disease is associated (Caplan, 1981). Many reports have also demonstrated that some patients presenting with signs of vertebro-basilar insufficiency and associated internal carotid artery disease could benefit from carotid surgery (Meyer *et al.*, 1960, Humphries *et al.*, 1965, Ford *et al.*, 1975, Correll *et al.*, 1979). Benefits are predictable if a posterior communicating artery of good caliber is visualized on carotid angiography.

— Collateral circulation: vascular territories are usually interconnected in such a way that collateral networks can develop after occlusion or severe stenosis of one feeding vessel.

This collateral network take minutes to weeks to appear on angiography, depending on the rapidity and severity of onset of the flow reduction, and also on local possibilities. It must be noted that vascular occlusions of tumoral origin are almost always well-tolerated, probably because of their slow and progressive installation.

Vascular networks connecting two different territories distally, are observed extracranially and intracranially in the vertebro-basilar system.

In the neck, muscular branches from the occipital, ascending cervical and deep cervical arteries are frequently demonstrated on angiography distally reinjecting a proximally occluded V. A. (Bosniak and Morton, 1964, Fredy *et al.*, 1978). However, it cannot be determined whether such collateral circulation is sufficient to permanently assure normal flow under normal pressure in the vertebro-basilar system. In the acute phase after V. A. occlusion and related infarction, it can be stated that this vascular network does not prevent embolus migration and either is insufficient or develops too slowly to compensate flow reduction (George and Laurian, 1981) (**Fig. 48**).

Intracranially, there are connections between occipital lobe and sylvian vessels and between branches of each cerebellar artery. However, this intracranial collateral circulation is usually less developed than the extracranial, and the protection it may offer is presumably limited

— Dynamic factors: as already discussed in the chapter External Com-

Table 9. Vertebro-basilar ischemia from cervical V. A.

Flow insufficiency		
Suppletive flow	Local factors	General factors
Controlateral V. A.	dynamic factor	cardiac output
Circle of Willis	external compression	hypertension
Collateral flow	intracranial lesion	postural hypotension
Carotid arteries		blood viscosity platelet aggregation hypercoagulability

Embolism	
Atherosclerotic lesion	Stenosis: ulcerated plaque Occlusion: tail of thrombus
Dissection. aneurysm	trauma fibromuscular dysplasia congenital
Cardiac origin	arrhythmia valvulopathy
External compression	spondylotic spurs

pression, head and neck rotation and hyperextension may induce a reduction in, or even an arrest of V. A. flow. Details from the patient on the circumstances of onset of symptoms are thus highly important.

— Other factors: external compression from any origin, especially when slowly progressive, cannot, if isolated, explain vertebro-basilar insufficiency. An aggravating dynamic factor or atherosclerotic lesion must be associated. Conversely, spondylotic V. A. compression may help to explain a reduction in the vertebro-basilar flow caused by a unilateral atherosclerotic lesion.

— Site of lesion: intracranial atherosclerotic disease is far less common than extracranial disease, but far more likely to be symptomatic. Concerning cervical V. A. lesions, it must be remembered that many are pauci or asymptomatic. If an embolic mechanism cannot be imputed, it is difficult to consider a cervical lesion, even an occlusive one, as being sufficient to produce ischemic events without any other associated factors (**Fig. 49**).

11. PRE-OPERATIVE INVESTIGATIONS

Pre-operative investigations must be directed to answer three questions before contemplating surgery on the V. A. (**Table 10**).

— What is the lesion in relation with the V. A.?

— What are the type and importance of the relation between the lesion and the V. A.?

— What are the consequences of the relation between the lesion and the V. A.?

Obviously, the same examination may give a total or partial answer to more than one of the above questions. For instance, computerized tomography is useful to recognize a tumor and its type, but also to demonstrate any infarcted area in the posterior fossa. Hence, according to the type of lesion to investigate, the importance and the goals of each examination are different (**Tables 11** and **12**).

According to the informations they provide, pre-operative investigations can be classified into two categories: morphologic and functional.

Table 10. Pre-operative investigations

Cause	standard X-ray	tomography
	C. T. scan	NMRI
	B. mode echography	
	angiography	
Relation to V. A.	ultrasonic imaging	
	C. T. scan	NMRI
	angiography	
Consequences	Doppler ultrasound	
	angiography	
	evoked potentials	
	C. T. scan	NMRI
	C. B. F.	CMRO2

11.1 Morphologic Exams
11.1.1 Ultrasonography (Echography)

Real time B mode ultrasound is now a well established tool to visualize the lumen of a vessel and is routinely used to explore carotid artery lesions, usually in combination with pulsed Doppler scanning.

Table 11

Angiography	
Size of both V. A.'s Basilar trunk and V. B. system Radiculo-medullary branch Congenital anomaly	any lesion
Carotid artery Distal reinjection of V. A. Circle of Willis (Occlusion test)	ischemia revascularization
Vascularization V. A. displacement V. A. compression	tumor
Distal V. A. filling Venous drainage Selective injection (balloon)	A. V. M.
Dynamic study (flexion-extension)	external compression

Table 12

Ischemia	Tumor
X-ray tomography Cochleo-vestibular invest.	X-ray tomography
C. T. scan NMRI	C. T. scan NMRI
Ultrasonic imaging Angiography	angiography
Evoked potentials C. B. F. CMRO2 (Occlusion test)	(occlusion test)

Echography is more sensitive than Doppler scanning to detect stenotic lesions, but less accurate in the diagnosis of occlusion (Comerota *et al.*, 1984). Moreover, echography appears more reliable than angiography for demonstrating ulcerated plaques and plaque hemorrhage (Callow, 1985). However, the results of ultrasound are mainly related to the quality of the scan; this is why its application to the V. A. is far less useful than for the carotid artery, except at its ostium. The main problem raised by ultrasound on the V. A. are the depth, small size and bony environment of this vessel.

This technique is very useful per and post-operatively, as already reported for carotid endarterectomy (Sigel *et al.*, 1982); it may help choose the best site for grafting or reimplantation techniques and control the adequacy of V. A. revascularization.

11.1.2 Standard X-Ray and Tomography

Plain X-rays and tomography of the cervical spine may be demonstrative in many ways, revealing:
— anomalies in the course of the V. A., such as calcifications of the retro-glenoidal ligament or bony canal over the arch of atlas,
— bony erosion of the vertebral body or pedicle, with enlargement of the intervertebral foramen by V. A. looping,
— tumoral signs: enlargement of the intervertebral foramen by an hour-glass tumor; enlargement of the jugulare foramen, lysis of the petrous bone or the clivus by a skull base tumor; lysis, calcification or densification of any vertebral part involved by an osseous tumor,

— external compression factors: osteophytic spurs, traumatic lesion of the cervical spine (fracture, luxation or atloido-occipital dislocation which may necessitate dynamic studies with flexion-extension films); foreign body more or less close to the transverse canal; cranio-cervical junction abnormalities such as a basilar impression, dens aplasia or Klippel-Feil syndrome; apophysomegaly or cervical rib.

Therefore, a great deal of information can be obtained from an examination as simple as standard radiography. It should be performed routinely as the first step of investigations in any suspected case of vertebro-basilar insufficiency.

11.1.3 Computerized Tomography Scan

C. T. scan has now become a routine examination, but in V. A. surgery, it can only really be helpful if every question is correctly asked and answered. This assumes that clinical data have previously delineated the areas to explore. There are two main areas which can be explored by C. T. scan: the cervical area to investigate the V. A. lesion, and the cranial area to seek eventual consequences in the vertebrobasilar territory. The examination must be performed with and without intravenous contrast injection; the C. T.

scan study must also be directed to visualize soft tissues as well as bony elements.
— Cervical area.
C. T. scan in this area can demonstrate the transverse canal. Any abnormality of this canal raises a suspicion of V. A. involvement. Tumors and most causes of external compression of the V. A., can be demonstrated. Correct analysis should give information on extension of a tumor or any other lesion, particularly towards the transverse canal. After contrast injection, the V. A. itself can be

visualized and its displacement frequently demonstrated.

Others extensions that are mandatory to know before defining the surgical approach, can also be seen on C.T. scan: extension to the paravertebral soft tissues, the lung apex, the posterior fossa or towards the spinal canal and the spinal cord. In the latter case, C.T. scan after intrathecal injection of Metrizamid may be necessary. However, this mode of investigation and, similarly, myelography are now supplanted by nuclear magnetic resonance imaging (N.M.R.I.).

— Cranial area.

Areas of infarction in the cerebellum, brainstem, occipital lobe and spinal cord may be delineated on C.T. scan. However, this study is frequently normal in the first hours and days following onset of infarction, and it must be repeated. Another limitation of the visualization of an infarcted area in the vertebro-basilar system is the small size of these infarcts, especially in the brainstem and spinal cord (Welch *et al.*, 1975) **(Fig. 50)**.

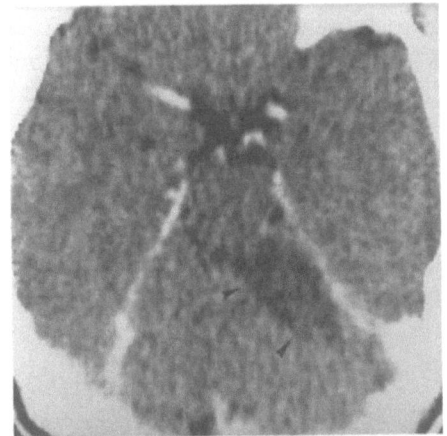
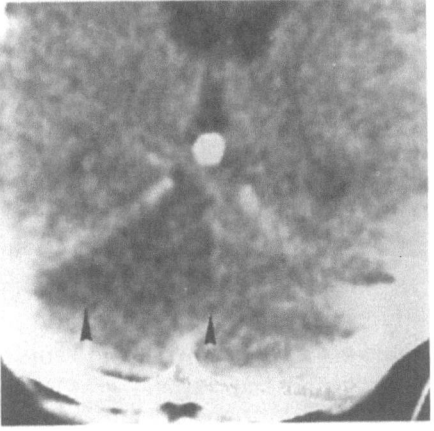

Fig. 50. Cerebellar softenings visualized on C.T. scan

11.1.4 Nuclear Magnetic Resonance Imaging

N.M.R.I. is a new imaging instrument of higher sensitivity than C.T. scan in most pathologic fields and especially in the central nervous system. It is not yet available in many centers, but its use will undoubtedly increase and rapidly replace other forms of investigations. N.M.R.I. exploits the physical and chemical properties of hydrogen nuclei to produce an image in the three spatial planes. Thus, N.M.R.I. can easily detect a variation in the water content of any structure. This explains its high sensitivity in detection of ischemic areas, since cerebral ischemia increases the water content of brain tissue. In the same way, N.M.R.I. gives much more detailed anatomic information than C.T. scan, and can even visualize large vessels and atherosclerotic plaque (Weinstein *et al.*, 1985).

In the investigation of lesion related to the V.A., N.M.R.I. affords clear demonstration of any tumor or bony anomaly and perfect delineation of extension to adjacent structures, including nerve roots and spinal cord. Infarcted areas and surrounding edema are well demonstrated, even in the brainstem or spinal cord. From experimental data, it appears that N. M. R. I. is able to detect edema at a reversible stage, before ischemic necrosis occurs (Buonanno *et al.*, 1983, Spetzler *et al.*, 1983, Weinstein *et al.*, 1985).

Progress in the understanding of V. A. pathology will undoubtedly follow utilization and development of N. M. R. I. Cerebral blood flow measurements using N. M. R. I. techniques is currently being investigated (Millis *et al.*, 1983).

11.1.5 Angiography

Angiography is still the conventional method for visualizing a vessel and its branches. Angiographic exam can now be performed in standard conditions and by digital subtraction analysis (**Fig. 51**).

— Digital subtraction angiography following intravenous injection of contrast media gives a rough picture of the extracranial arterial axes; therefore, it should not be performed if one wants to obtain details on parietal arterial lesions. Superposition and weakly constrated pictures make this mode of angiography usually insufficient for a well-founded surgical decision. Indications for intravenous digital studies are therefore limited to the elderly and patients in poor clinical condition, to confirm severe lesions such as occlusion.

— Angiography by arterial injection is the only examination which accurately demonstrates the cervical vessels, especially the V. A. Digital techniques present some advantages over standard angiography:

— smaller amount of injected contrast, under lower pressure, allowing repeat injections,

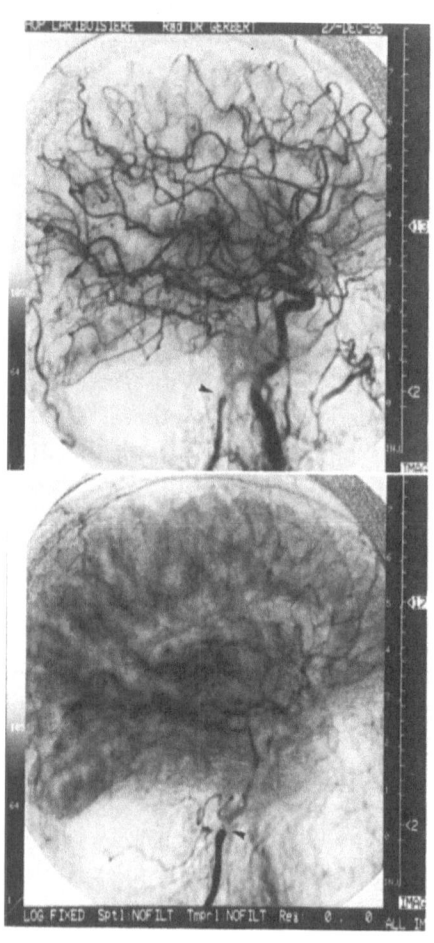

Fig. 51. Digital angiography: early and late arterial phase in a case with distal V. A. occlusion and slow retrograde filling of the basilar trunk and the PICA

— instantaneous subtraction, which is important for the V. A. since it runs beside and within bony elements,

— enlargement of desired portions of the image, enabling magnification of any abnormality,

— selection of sequences and film reproduction, with low volume storage of information,

— stored films can be reutilized at any time.

Digital angiography of the V. A. can be done by the brachial route as frequently used in standard technique, or by transfemoral catheterization. This latter route allows exploration of all the supra-aortic vessels via aortic arch injection as a first step, followed by selective injection of any desired vessels.

A complete study of the entire vascular supply to the cervicocephalic area is therefore possible in one stage and in a simpler way than by standard angiography, which requires bilateral brachial and left carotid angiography.

Whatever the technique, information on five points must be obtained:

1. V. A. lesion: its type, parietal or external; the degree of stenosis or occlusion; degree and direction of displacement.

2. Vertebrobasilar perfusion beyond the lesion.

3. Dominance of the involved V. A. and the controlateral V. A. size.

4. Condition of the internal carotid arteries and of the circle of Willis.

5. Presence of collaterals and their importance, particularly anterior radiculo-medullary branches.

The ability to assess these five points requires a complete study of not only the involved V. A., but of the controlateral V. A. and the carotid arteries as well at both cervical and cranial levels on at least anteroposterior and lateral views.

In marked stenosis or occlusion, collateral flow development must be evaluated: condition of the controlateral V. A., carotid arteries and circle of Willis as well as evaluation of the reinjection of the homolateral V. A. above the lesion by a vascular network from branches of the occipital and cervical arteries. This last study requires injection of the external or common carotid artery and of the subclavian artery.

External compression of the V. A. often requires angiographic study with head and neck rotation to the ipsilateral and controlateral sides.

Such studies, necessitating several injections, are best performed by digital subtraction arterial angiography.

11.2 Functional Examinations

11.2.1 Cochleo-vestibular Investigations

Since the peripheral and central pathways of the cochlear and vestibular systems are supplied by the vertebrobasilar system, their exploration may be of interest. As well demonstrated, the vestibular system is particularly sensitive to ischemia, but there is no pattern of vestibular dysfunction, specific to an ischemic origin (Matsunaga *et al.*, 1979, Nagashima, 1972–1985). It is common knowledge that vestibular disorders may have multiple possible causes, including ischemia, sympathetic irritation, or even psychiatric disorders (Hozawa, 1979, Jacob, 1985, Gauthier, 1985).

Nevertheless, cochleo-vestibular studies are helpful in the following ways:
— to confirm the authenticity of subjective symptoms, such as vertigo or dizziness. The examination must be performed in different head and neck positions, especially those producing symptoms,
— to determine the central or peripheral location of a vestibular disorder,
— to orient investigations in direction other than vertebro-basilar ischemia: cerebello-pontine angle tumor, Meniere's disease,
— for follow up with or without treatment.

Cochleo-vestibular investigations with caloric tests and electro-nystagmography may be completed by auditory evoked potentials.

11.2.2 Evoked Potentials

1—Auditory evoked potentials (A. E. P.); this technique was expected by many authors to give information on brainstem dysfunction at an early stage. In the presence of vertebro-basilar ischemia, it appears that A. E. P. are abnormal essentially in case of infarct, where clinical data are usually sufficient to establish the diagnosis. A. E. P. may even be normal in the case of brainstem infarct if the ischemic area does not involve the auditory pathways (Lynn and Gilroy, 1984). In the case of T. I. A. or vertebro-basilar insufficiency, A. E. P. are rarely perturbed (Fischer *et al.*, 1981, Lynn and Gilroy, 1984, Nau *et al.*, 1985). Therefore, A. E. P. is not a useful examination to demonstrate hemodynamic insufficiency in the vertebro-basilar system and consequently should not be used to test the efficiency of revascularization techniques.

2—Visual and somatosensory evoked potentials: these evoked potentials have been reported to have the same limitations as A. E. P. (Noel and Desmedt, 1975, Koa and Gilroy, 1984). Moreover, they are less accurate at the brainstem level, since here they only relay nuclei at both extremities.

In A. E. P., the first five components are generated from the auditory nerve and auditory pathways in the brainstem (Starr and Hamilton, 1976). Therefore, in the field of vertebrobasilar ischemia, A. E. P. is the most interesting evoked potential, but its interest is limited to determining the level and severity of brainstem infarcts (Uziel and Benezech, 1978).

11.2.3 Sleep Recordings

Structures involved in night sleep organization (R. E. M. and slow wave sleep) are mainly located in the brainstem.

Night sleep recording is a non-invasive method which can give information on these structures, but it is a long and rather difficult procedure. In our experience, significant modification of sleep organization is observed only in the case of severe brainstem suffering of traumatic or ischemic origin (George et al., 1986).

11.2.4 Doppler Scanning

Doppler spectrum analysis imaging is more a functional than a morphologic exam, since it is by means of blood velocity modifications that vascular lesions are demonstrated. In addition, with pulsed Doppler imaging, the actual diameter of the vessel can be measured and a reliable value of the arterial flow can be obtained.

The examination therefore has the great advantage of being non invasive and of rapidly giving a good estimation of the flow in each V. A. Unfortunately, the V. A. is a small caliber vessel, located deeply in the neck, against and partly behind bony structures; V. A. exploration by Doppler imaging, as with any ultrasound technique, thus requires a well-trained examiner performing a patient and complete study. A complete V. A. study should include the first portion including the ostium and the third portion, in neutral position and in different positions of the head and neck. Recordings in the position described by the patient as that producing symptoms is of particular importance.

Recordings should also be performed during flow interruption of each cervical trunk by digital compression (Franceschi, 1981). Conducted in this way, Doppler scanning is usually able to demonstrate:

— quality of flow in each V. A. so as to ascertain the presence of stenosis or occlusion and determine its location,

— any modification of flow after various head and neck movements, suggesting external compression,

— compensatory flow in other vessels, particularly in the controlateral V. A.,

— the possibility of supply to the V. A. by other vessels and the functional quality of the circle of Willis.

Obviously, Doppler scanning is not sufficient for correct and precise diagnosis of all lesions on the cervical and intracranial vessels, but it may simplify the angiographic study by avoiding injection of vessels which appear normal on Doppler imaging.

However, the reliability of the examiner must again be emphasized, particularly in V. A. explorations.

Furthermore, even correctly performed, results of doppler imaging may be equivocal. Pre-occlusive and occlusive lesions may not always be differentiated, and assessement of complete occlusion can only be done on angiography. Doppler study is also unable to give information on the small intracranial branches of the carotid and vertebro-basilar system.

However, transcranial Doppler investigations are currently being developed and appear able to demonstrate the main branches of the internal carotid arteries and the circle of Willis.

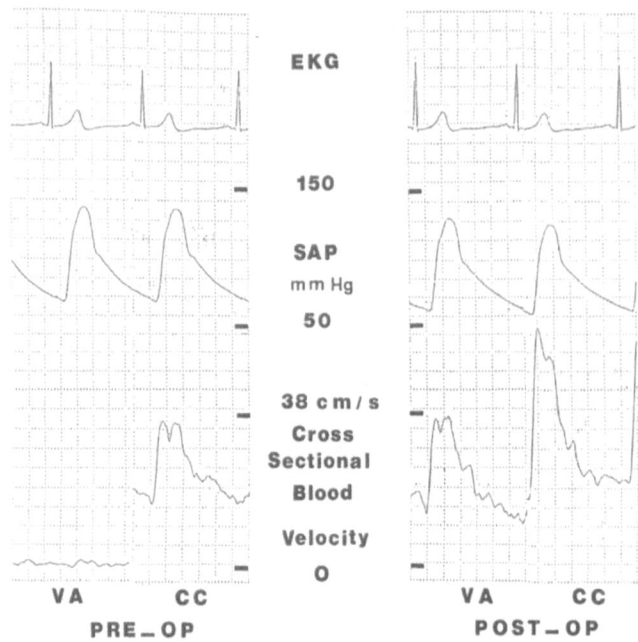

Fig. 52. Intra-operative blood velocity recordings (pulsed Doppler effect). Left: before common carotid to V. A. venous graft by-pass. Mean blood flow value: V. A.: 0 ml/mn (thrombosis), C. C. A.: 266.5 ml/mn, right: after C. C. A. to V. A. anastomosis. Mean blood flow value: V. A. 68.5 ml/mn, C. C. A.: 344 ml/mn

Dynamic studies with digital compression of the cervical trunks can show whether the communicating arteries are functional and determine the direction of flow through these arteries (Aaslid et al., 1982, Aaslid, 1986).

Doppler imaging is of great value in detecting arterial anomalies on cervical vessels, thus removing doubts as to whether to pursue arterial investigations in the case of limited symptoms; it also helps to limit the number of vessels to investigate by angiography and to evaluate the possibilities for supply of the brain by the other cervical vessels and the circle of Willis.

Like B. mode ultrasound, Doppler scanning may be used per-operatively to assess the efficiency of V. A. revascularizations (**Fig. 52**).

11.2.5 Hemodynamic and Metabolic Investigations

Advances in technology have led to the development of several techniques that monitor physiological disturbances in blood flow and brain metabolism:

— Intravenous injection or inhalation of Xe-133 with collimators, which simultaneously gives information on the carotid and vertebro-basilar territories, is non invasive but includes problems such as crosstalk phenomenon or contamination of extracranial flow (Juge et al., 1979).

— Xe-133 intravertebral injection allows selective exploration of the

vertebro-basilar territory but requires catheterization of the V. A. (Skinhoj et al., 1964, Brown et al., 1971, Nagawara et al., 1982).
— Cold Xenon computerized tomography, single photon emission computerized tomography and positron emission tomography (Kuhl et al., 1980, Baron et al., 1981, Bonte and Stokely, 1981, Gur et al., 1982, Hill et al., 1982) give more accurate information on regional blood flow by looking directly at cross section. These methods are excellent because of their non-invasiveness and the possibility of three dimensional imaging of the C. B. F., but unfortunately, they require very expensive facilities.

Furthermore, it is now recognized that complete physiological information on the severity of brain hypoperfusion requires measurements of cerebral blood flow (C. B. F.), cerebral blood volume (C. B. V.) and oxygen consumption (CMRO 2). This data can only be provided by positron emission tomography (P. E. T.). To date, these metabolic investigations have mainly been directed to the carotid territory.

The efficiency of V. A. revascularization should be tested by these advanced techniques in the same way that extra-intracranial anastomoses have (Grubbs et al., 1979, Baron et al., 1981, Meyer et al., 1982).

11.3 Interventional Radiology

This term covers all radiological techniques which are performed for other than purely diagnostic purposes. It includes primarily embolization, balloon techniques and angioplasty.

11.3.1 Embolization

Embolization is now a highly perfected procedure. Numerous techniques using various catheters and embolus materials have been developed and are widely used.

The main indications for embolization are arteriovenous malformations (A. V. M.) and tumors. This procedure reduces vascularity and makes surgical treatment easier. In some cases, even complete cure can be obtained by embolization alone.

Embolization is routinely performed on branches of the external carotid and subclavian arteries. Embolization into small cervical branches of the V. A. are much more rarely undertaken because of the risk of cerebral embolism. Nervetheless, it can be performed under the protection of a balloon occluding the vessel distally (Merland et al., 1979) (**Fig. 53**).

Embolization can be used preoperatively in two ways:

1. to attempt to reach the center (or the nidus) of vascular lesions; this is necessary if the subsequent surgery will necessitate piecemeal removal,

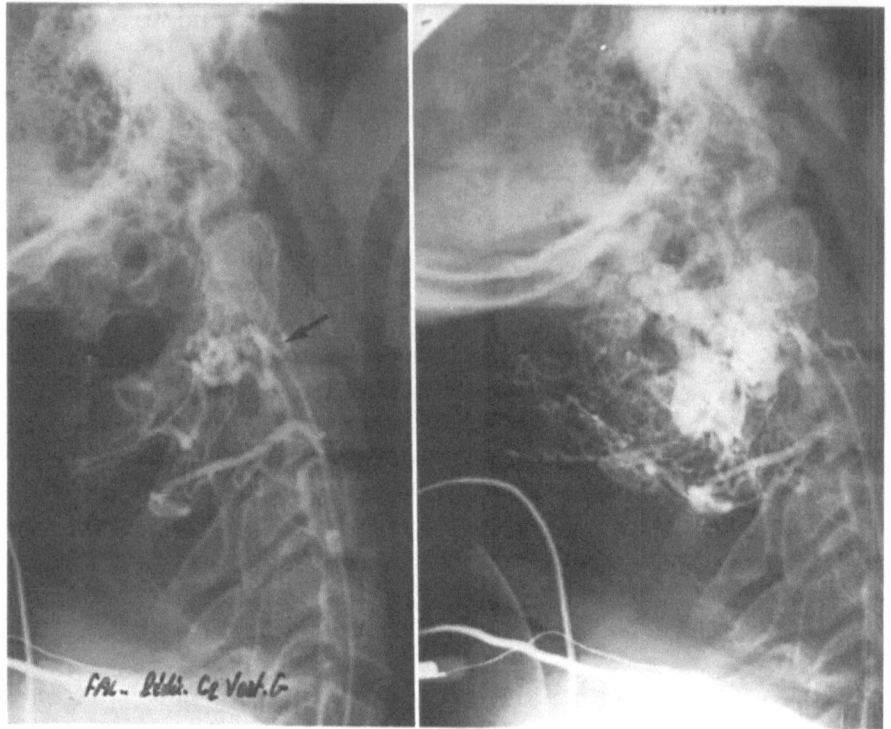

Fig. 53. Selective injection of one V. A. branch at C2 supplying a hemangiopericytoma

2. to occlude vascular branches close to the lesion if "en bloc" removal is expected; in this case, surgery must follow embolization as soon as possible, before collateral vascular channels develop.

11.3.2 Balloon Techniques

Use of a balloon placed at the tip of a catheter has three main interests:

11.3.2.1 Diagnostic Interest

It allows better definition of highly vascular lesions, especially A. V. M. In this lesion, venous drainage is often highly developed and this may give the false impression of a complex or multiple fistula. Repetitive injections above an occluding balloon progressively moved up in the V. A., can determine if there is one or several fistula, their location and their importance (**Fig. 54**).

11.3.2.2 Therapeutic Interest

Arteriovenous fistulas are now initially treated by balloon techniques. A detachable balloon can occlude the fistula while preserving V. A. flow (Debrun et al., 1978, Reizine et al., 1985). Surgery is considered only if the balloon technique has failed to completely occlude the fistula or if it cannot be

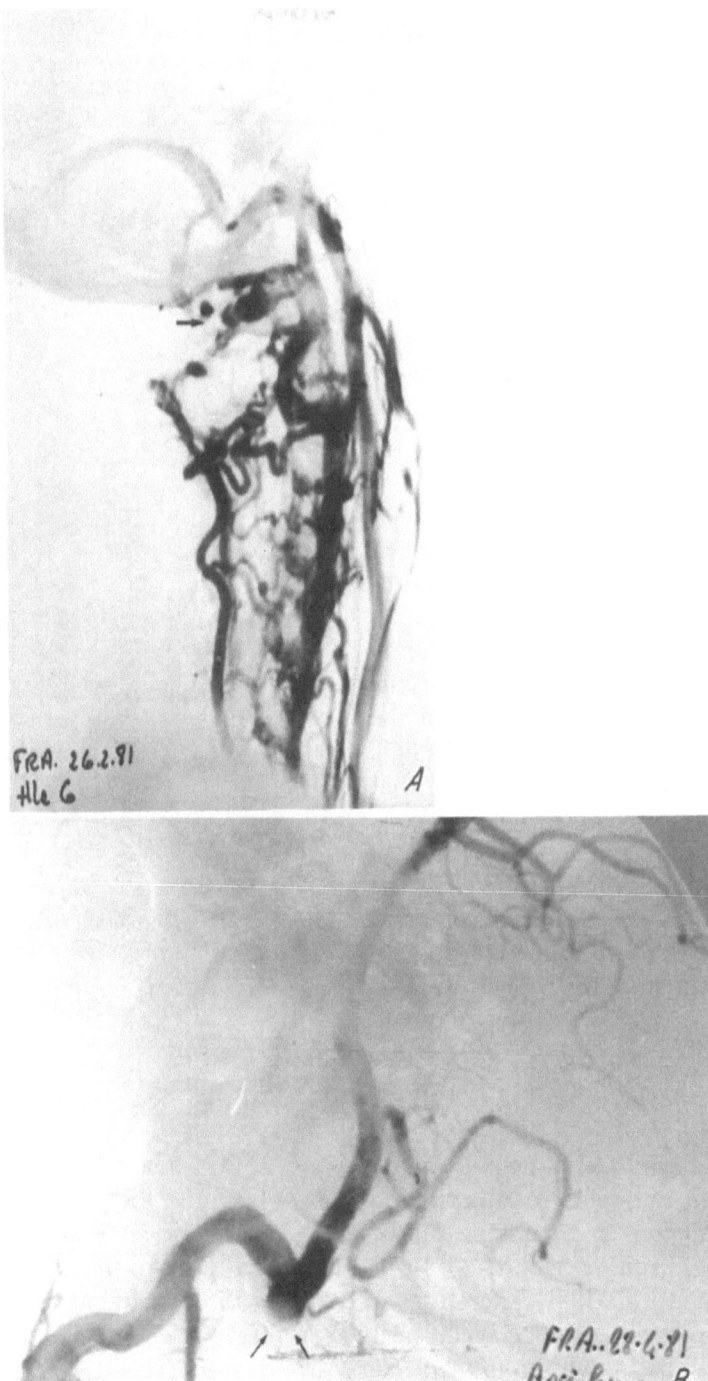

Fig. 54. A) Arteriovenous fistula appearing falsely complex. **B)** Balloon occlusion demonstrating a single fistula at C 1 achieving a correct treatment

performed without encroaching upon the lumen of the V. A.

Balloons may also be used for internal carotid or vertebral artery occlusion during embolization. At the end of embolization, the balloon may be left in place, definitively occluding the vessel, or removed after washing out any residual clot or embolus (Merland *et al.*, 1979). Tolerance of these occlusions must obviously be controlled prior to the procedure.

11.3.2.3 Pre-operative Interest

Whenever temporary or permanent occlusion of the V.A. is expected during surgery or embolization, a previous test of occlusion tolerance must be performed. Under local anaesthesia, a balloon is led to the chosen site in the V. A. and inflated to occlusion of the vessel for 15 minutes. If no neurologic sign is observed, it is considered that prolonged or even permanent V. A. occlusion can be tolerated (**Fig. 55**). This technique can be sensitized by the adjunct of Xe-133 intravenous or intra-arterial C. B. F. measurement before and after inflating the balloon.

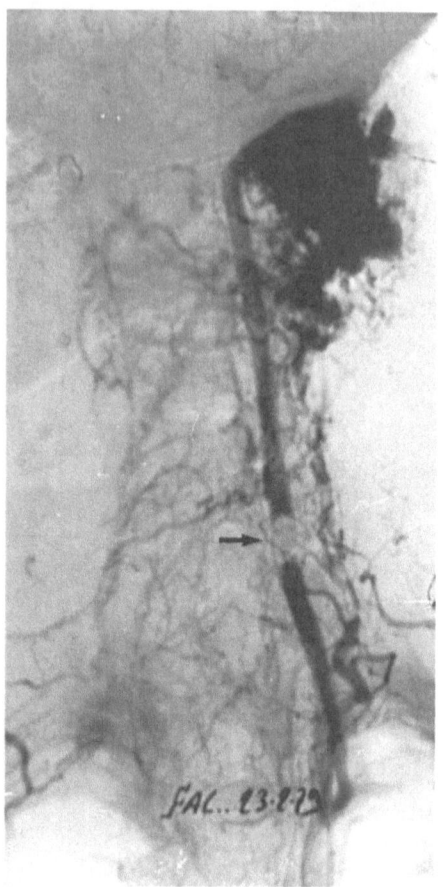

Fig. 55. Balloon occlusion test in a case of hemangiopericytoma

11.3.2 Angioplasty

This is a recently developed technique which is now applied to supra-aortic arteries (Dotter and Judkins, 1964, Gruntzig and Hopff, 1974, Motarjemme *et al.*, 1981, Theron *et al.*, 1984). Treatment of subclavian steal syndromes has been attempted by several authors (Mathias *et al.*, 1980, Bachman and Kim, 1980, Motarjemme *et al.*, 1982, Ritter *et al.*, 1982, Moore *et al.*, 1982, Garrido and Garofola, 1983).

Atherosclerotic stenosis or fibromuscular dysplasia of the external carotid artery (Viteck and Morawetz, 1982, Yagamata *et al.*, 1985), the internal carotid artery (Hasso *et al.*, 1981, Belan *et al.*, 1982) or even the basilar artery (Sundt *et al.*, 1980) treated by endoluminal dilatation, have also been reported with more or less successful results. To date, angioplasty on a vertebral artery stenosis has not yet been published. However, techniques for this vessel, allowing efficient correction of stenosis without risk of distal embolization, has now been developed.

11.4 Management of Pre-operative Investigations

Patients with lesions related to the V. A. are referred for symptoms of two main etiologies: vertebro-basilar ischemia and tumor (**Table 12**).

As previously indicated, each examination will not be of the equal interest in demonstrating the various causes and consequence of V. A. lesions (**Table 10**).

11.4.1 Vertebro-basilar Ischemia

Transient or permanent vertebro-basilar symptoms (vertebro-basilar insufficiency and T. I. A. or stroke) may be due to parietal lesions (atherosclerosis, dissection, dysplasia …), external compression, or more rarely, A. V. M. or tumor.

11.4.1.1 Vertebro-basilar Insufficiency

Initially, plain X-rays of the cervical spine (with flexion-extension films), cochleo-vestibular investigations and non invasive vascular imaging (Doppler and B mode ultrasound) are performed. C. T. scan or N. M. R. I. are not useful in this case except in the exceptional vertebro-basilar insufficiency of tumoral origin.

If the former examinations are conclusive, then angiography is performed to demonstrate the compromise in V. A. flow.

11.4.1.2 Vertebro-basilar Infarct

C. T. scan or N. M. R. I. is usually performed initially to image the ischemic area and the eventual consequences of surrounding edema (brainstem compression and hydrocephalus). Conservative management is usual but, operative treatment (resection of edematous and infarcted cerebellar tissue or ventricular shunting) may be required in severe cases.

During this acute period, cervical X-rays and non invasive vascular imaging may be performed to start the etiologic inquiry. Functional investigations (A. E. P. and metabolic measurements) may help to evaluate the severity of cerebral ischemia.

After recovery from this acute phase, which may take several weeks, angiography can be performed with safety and practical interest. A. E. P. and metabolic studies are repeated, especially if V. A. revascularization is intended in order to establish a pre-operative reference.

During the acute phase of a vertebro-basilar stroke, angiography may have deleterious effects on patients in critical condition. Furthermore, no surgery is usually indicated at this time, except in the rare occurrence of pre-occlusive stenosis with progressive neurologic worsening. In fact, progressive neurologic deterioration is far more often due to development of edema surrounding the infarcted zone, as demonstrated on C.T. scan or N.M.R.I., which must be repeated in such cases.

11.4.1.3 Pre and Post-operative Examinations

Information required from angiography varies, not with the clinical symptoms and the severity of ischemia, but according to the lesion involving the V.A. as indicated in **Table 11**.

Each time any compromise of V.A. flow is demonstrated, functional investigations must be performed to assess as accurately as possible its hemodynamic and metabolic consequences on the brain. This provides a rational basis for subsequent therapeutic decisions.

A balloon occlusion test under local anesthesia may be necessary if temporary or definitive clamping of any vessel (carotid or vertebral artery) is necessary and appears hazardous.

Post-operatively, treatment adequacy must be verified by non-invasive imaging and angiography. Demonstration of therapeutic efficacy in correction of hemodynamic and metabolic impairment requires repeat functional investigations.

11.4.2 Tumor

Tumors related to the V.A. exceptionally have hemodynamic consequences, even if V.A. stenosis or occlusion is present. Investigations may therefore be less extensive than in vertebrobasilar ischemia (**Table 12**).

Standard X-rays and tomography, C.T. scan or N.M.R.I. are sufficient to show the tumor and its extension. Vascular data are given by angiography: caliber of both V.A.'s, V.A. displacement, V.A. compression, hypervascularization and existence of a radiculo-medullary branch in the vicinity.

If there is a risk of V.A. injury during surgery, or if revascularization is proposed, a V.A. balloon occlusion test is a safe pre-operative measure.

12. APPROACH TO THE CERVICAL V. A.

12.1 Historical Background

The first approach to, although not for surgery on, the V. A. seems to have been performed by Boudot in 1864, who mentioned the possibility of transverse process resection through a retromastoid route. This is actually the first technical note on the technique of V. A. surgery. Following reports were essentially devoted to treatment of V. A. injuries, such as Matas' report. Although V. A. surgery did not further develop at this time, these papers indicated that the V. A. could be approached, particularly on its first portion where V. A. ligations were performed.

Then, during World War I, German surgeons studied how to expose the transverse processes (Kuttner, 1917, Oljenick, 1917). However, Henry's work is the masterpiece in the story of cervical V. A. surgery. He described in great detail the technique of surgical exposure of the V. A. in the transverse canal. He underlined that the elective level for control of the distal V. A. is between C1 and C2, which has now been widely confirmed. Henry's conclusion, however, was that this anatomic description was quite theoretical and had no surgical application, since he thought to have proposed "a cure for which there was no disease". In fact, we can now say that there is a need to expose the V. A. in many pathologic states, and any surgeon who has attempted to expose the V. A. since the time of Henry has used, more or less consciously, the surgical principles he established in 1917.

Elkin and Harris (1946) were the first to propose a standardized technique to treat arterio-venous malformations of the V. A. Since 1960, external compression by osteophytic spurs has been released through an approach primarily directed at the V. A. Hardin (1960) was the first to use this approach and was soon followed by many others (Jung et al., 1964, Gortvai, 1964, Verbiest, 1968). Verbiest (1970) was the first in the modern era to give particular attention to the V. A. while working on the cervical spine. He controlled the V. A. to release external compression of spondylotic, discal and traumatic origin. He was also the first to propose V. A. control during tumor removal.

In spite of the work of these pioneers, it was not before the eighties that much interest was devoted to the distal V. A.; even now, surgical approach to the second and third portion of the V. A. is considered a real challenge by most surgeons.

The ostial portion of the V. A. did not

suffer from this lack of surgical aggressiveness. This is probably due to its proximity with the subclavian artery and to its anatomic location outside the transverse canal. Endarterectomy of the V. A. ostium followed the first end-arterectomy of the internal carotid artery by only few years (Cate and Scott, 1957, Eascott *et al.*, 1954). Now, V. A. surgery at the base of the neck is routinely performed by many surgeons.

12.2 General Principles

Various surgical approaches may be used to expose and control the different portions of the cervical V. A. The necessary, of its whole length, including the intracranial part (**Figs. 56** and **57**).

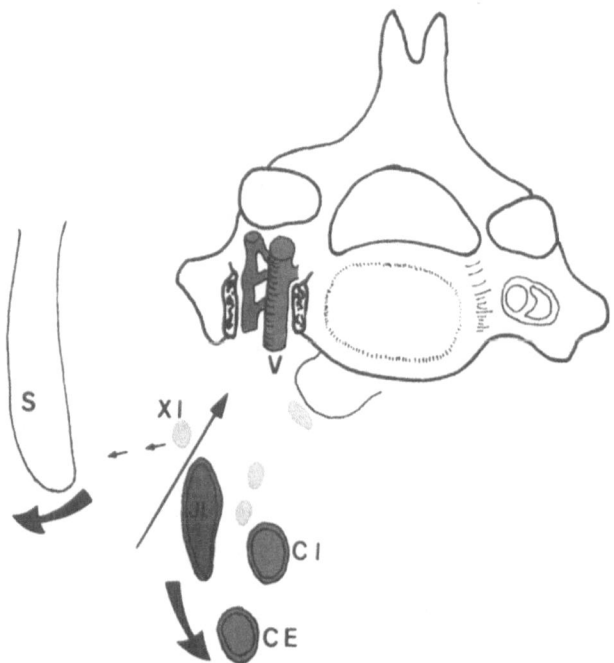

Fig. 56. Lateral-anterior approach between the sternocleidomastoid muscle (*S*) and the internal jugular vein (*JI*); internal carotid artery (*CI*) and external carotid artery (*CE*) are left medially. The accessory spinal nerve (*XI*) is the only one element to control in the approach above C3. *V* vertebral artery

lateral anterior approach which we have developed is the only route to allow exposure of any part of the V. A., or if Whatever the surgical route chosen, principles of exposure and control of the V. A. are similar.

12.2.1 Periosteal Sheath

Except in the first (ostial) portion, the V. A. is surrounded by its venous plexus and enclosed inside the periosteal sheath.

Initially, this periosteal sheath must be respected, thus avoiding any troublesome bleeding from the venous plexus before complete exposure of the desired length of the V. A. Resection of the muscles (inter-transversary muscles) and bone overlying the V. A. must therefore be performed very carefully.

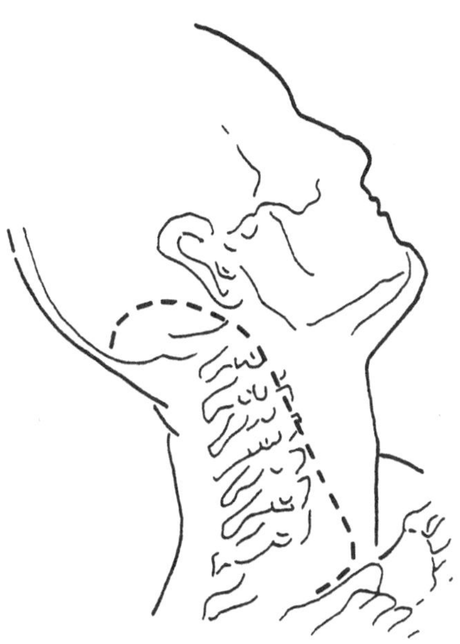

Fig. 57. Skin incision in its whole extent allowing V. A. exposure from the ostium to its intracranial part

12.2.2 Venous Plexus

Thereafter, the periosteal sheath may be opened in a correctly and bloodlessly prepared field. At this time, hemorrhage from the venous plexus may occur. This venous plexus is more or less developed according to the level exposed, the pathology involved, and the individual patient. Bipolar coagulation and/or packing with Oxycel usually results in fairly easy control of this venous bleeding. More precise control of the venous plexus may be achieved with the help of the microscope. The V. A. can then be controlled on its whole circumference and mobilized.

12.2.3 Collateral Branches

Care must be taken to avoid injury to collateral branches, which must have been identified on pre-operative angiography. Particularly, the exact location of any anterior medullary branch must be determined. If not, dividing of any branch with an internal course towards the intervertebral foramen carries the great risk of spinal cord ischemia.

12.2.4 Use of Magnification (Microscope)

Control of the V. A. can be performed under normal view, but any type of magnification, especially the surgical microscope, is a very useful tool. Under the microscope, the venous plexus appears as individualized veins which can be spared during opening of the periosteal sheath and then coagulated separately one by one. Collateral branches of the V. A. are also better identified. Finally, any repair or sutures for by-pass performance is more accurately realized under magnification.

12.2.5 V. A. Wall

The second and third portions of the V. A. are more comparable in thickness to the intracranial part than to the first portion or to the other cervical vessels. On the first portion, V. A. surgery, except for the diameter of this artery, is very similar to general cervical surgery as performed on the subclavian or carotid arteries. The vertebral veins at this level are quite separate venous channels which can be ligated. The use of the microscope is of no benefit on this first portion.

12.2.6 V. A. Clamping

Clamping of the V. A. is easily and atraumatically performed with Heifetz aneurysmal clips. Usual vascular clamps could be used on the first portion of the V. A., but are certainly too agressive for the two upper portions. In fact, even on the first portion, Heifetz clips are quite sufficient to clamp the V. A. Moreover, because of their small size, they are a very useful adjunct in a fairly narrow field. Different shapes and length of blades exist, and one may choose the most appropriate type in each case, i. e. the one causing the least hindrance to working on the V. A.

12.2.7 Suturing

Polypropylene monofilament is used in the same way as for the carotid artery. At the ostium, 6-0 or 7-0 polypropylene is suitable; in the second and third portions, 7-0 is generally used, but under magnification, 8-0 is prefered.

12.2.8 Retractor

A self-retaining retractor with smooth blades, such as a Cloward retractor, is a useful tool, mainly in exposure of the second portion of the V. A. One is applied on the jugulo-carotid track and the other on the deep aspect of the S. C. M. muscle. Care must be taken not to angulate the carotid artery behind the retractor blade, in order to prevent ischemic complications. At the third portion of the V. A., retraction must not be excessive, to avoid stretching of the accessory spinal nerve. The best prevention of elongation of this nerve is to dissect out the nerve on the greatest length possible from the S. C. M. muscle to the skull base. Protection of this nerve is realized by rolling the lymphatic sheath covering the deep muscles over it.

12.2.9 Mortality and Morbidity

No mortality is to be feared with a well conducted approach and control of the cervical V. A.

Morbidity should be very limited:

— Horner's syndrome is frequently observed, even if the sympathetic nerve has been spared. Recovery is constant, but takes several weeks to months.

— Accessory spinal nerve palsy or paresis should not occur if care is taken in preparing the field and in retractor placement.

— Spinal nerve roots: if the V. A. is controlled inside its periosteal sheath, no injury to the spinal nerve roots can occur.

— The anterior branch of the second cervical nerve, which frequently has to be divided for exposure of the V. A. between C 1 and C 2, produces hypo or anesthesia in the area of the jaw angle. In general this effect greatly diminishes in the weeks following surgery and has no effect on patient confort, except for shaving.

— Lymphatic oozing may be present after approach to the first portion of the V. A. Ligation of all lymphatic vessels, particularly the thoracic duct, is the best prevention. If oozing occurs, drainage until closure is dry, is generally sufficient. If not, it may be necessary to reopen the wound, find the lymphatic vessel responsible, and ligate it.

12.2.10 Anesthesia and Post-operative Care

V. A. surgery must be managed from the anesthesiologic point of view in the same way as carotid artery surgery. The brain must be protected if V. A. clamping is likely to be done. Obviously, this concern is maximal with V. A. revascularization techniques, where vessel clamping is a necessity (in every case for the V. A., in most cases for the carotid artery). Use of barbiturate drugs and particular attention to maintaining stable systemic blood pressure before, during and, most importantly after surgery are the two main points. These are part of the general measures in any neurovascular surgery, which also include pre-operative control of cardiac and respiratory functions and of any general vascular risk factors (hypertension, diabetes mellitus, hyperlipemia, coagulopathy ...).

Anticoagulants

Anticoagulants must be used during surgery when vessels are clamped. They are continued in low dose for the following eight days after revascularization procedures. Particular attention is therefore made to obtain perfect hemostasis of the operative field before closure. After the first post-operative week, no particular treatment is given, except that which may be required by another vascular lesion. Revascularization alone does not justify prolonged anticoagulant treatment or replacement by antiplatelet agents.

12.3 Surgical Routes

12.3.1 First Portion (Ostium)

The surgical route to the first portion of the V. A. is the most well known, since approach to the V. A. ostium is now performed routinely by many surgeons. The same route, with only a few variations, is generally used. It passes between the internal jugular vein and the common carotid artery.

12.3.1.1 Position

The patient is in supine position with the head and neck mildly extended and controlaterally rotated. A cushion is placed between the shoulders to elevate the lower cervical area.

12.3.1.2 Skin Incision

Three different incisions in the supra-clavicular area may be utilized to approach the proximal V. A.

a) An angular reverse "L"-shaped incision is preferable in our opinion, since it allows prolongation, either horizontally to expose the distal subclavian artery, or vertically to control the V. A. up to the transverse portion and carotid artery. The usual incision starts at the lower fourth of the anterior border of the sternocleidomastoid muscle and curves laterally to continue parallel with the upper border of the clavicle for four centimeters.

b) Horizontal supra-clavicular incision.

c) Vertical pre-sternocleidomastoid incision.

These two incisions utilize only one of the branches of the "L" shaped incision.

12.3.1.3 Surgical Approach (Figs. 58 and 59)

The platysma muscle is divided, as are the clavicular and sternal insertions of the sternocleidomastoid muscle.

The internal jugular vein is then controlled and secured with a loop. To permit its retraction, this often requires division of the omohyoideus muscle.

The scalenus fat pad, like the phrenic nerve, is never dissected free.

The common carotid artery is then dissected out, down to its mediastinal segment after partial incision of the infrathyroidian muscles flush with the clavicle.

The vagus nerve (X) is mobilized in its cervical portion, and in its mediastinal portion if the prevertebral subclavian artery needs to be exposed.

The V. A. can now be approached be-

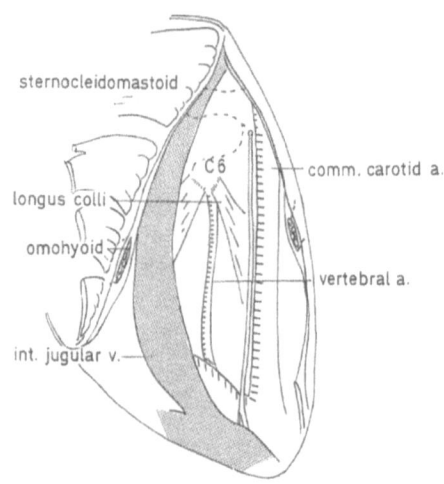

Fig. 58. Lateral-anterior approach to the V. A. first portion passing between the internal jugular vein and the common carotid artery

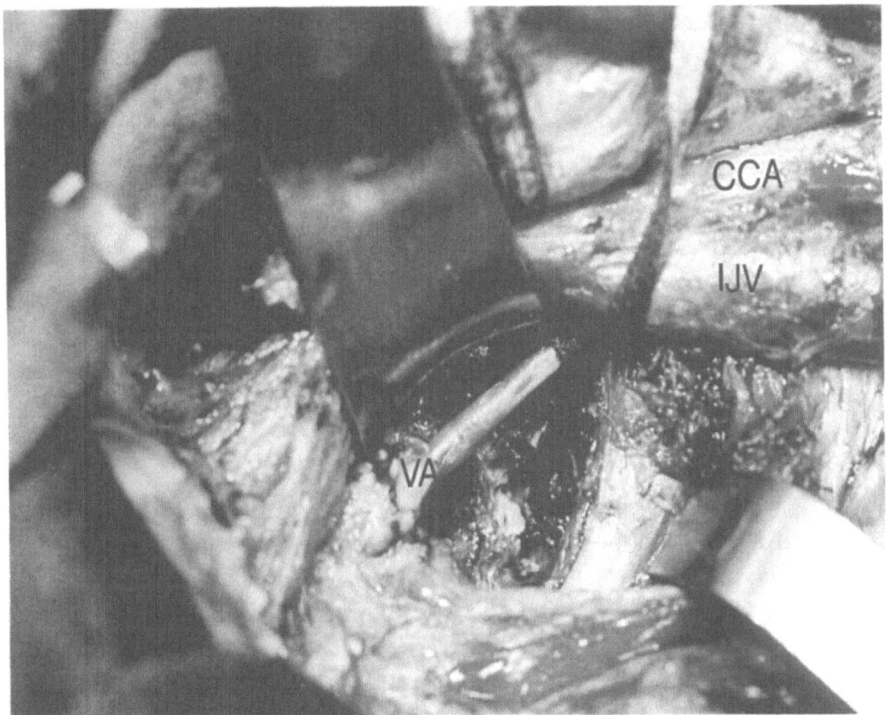

Fig. 59. Operative view of the V. A. first portion (after removal of an hour-glass neurinoma)

tween the internal jugular vein and the common carotid artery (the carotid-jugular interspace).

When the carotid jugular interspace is opened with a smooth bladed retractor placed on the carotid artery, the lymphatic vessels and, importantly, the thoracic duct appears in the field. They must be carrefully dissected and ligated to avoid post-operative lymph accumulation and oozing.

On the deep aspect of the lymphatic sheath, the vertebral vein courses parallel and superficial to the first portion of the V. A. The vertebral vein ends at the posterior edge of the internal jugular vein, where its dissection is started. The vertebral vein should be carefully dissected out and its branches isolated.

It is then resected on 2 to 3 cm before cutting, to avoid dividing it several times along the exposed V. A. The V. A. can then be controlled.

12.3.1.4 V. A. Control

V. A. exposure is generally easier on the right side, since the artery is higher and more superficial than on the left. The first step in control of the V. A. is the control of the subclavian artery dome so as to identify the V. A. origin. Depending on the particular technique which is to be performed, the pre- and post-vertebral segments of the subclavian artery are mobilized or not.

Subsequently, V. A. control starts from its origin and progresses upwards to the C 6 transverse process.

During this, several elements may be troublesome:

a) Nervous Elements

The vertebral nerve passes medially along the course of the V. A. and joins the inferior cervical ganglion which lies behind the V. A.

The intermediate cervical ganglion is lateral to the V. A., but the horizontal anastomoses connect it to the vertebral nerve and inferior cervical ganglion.

Section of the small nerve branches which cross the anterior aspect of the V. A. has no consequences. Subsequent V. A. control inside its periadventitial sheath avoids any risk of sympathetic element injury.

However, in some cases, the intermediate ganglion lies directly on the anterior aspect of the V. A., or large rami from the ganglion pass anterior to the V. A. This requires external mobilization of the intermediate ganglion after division of a few rami, in order to preserve continuity of the sympathetic chain. Sometimes the V. A. can be freed beneath these structures without section of any nervous elements; it is then transposed anteriorly after division at its origin.

b) Inferior Thyroid Artery

The horizontal segment of the inferior thyroid artery must be cut to expose the upper part of the proximal V. A.

c) Muscular Tendons Inserted on the C6 Transverse Process

The uppermost portion of the proximal segment of the V. A. sometimes needs to be exposed. This requires division of the insertions of the longus colli and anterior scalenus muscles on the transverse process of C6. The transverse process itself must also be opened. Prior to this, the anterior vertebral vein must have been ligated at its exit from the transverse canal.

12.3.2 Second Portion (Transverse Portion)

12.3.2.1 Lateral Anterior Approach

a) Position

The patient is in supine position with the head extended and slightly rotated to the opposite side.

b) Incision

The skin incision follows the anterior edge of the sternocleidomastoid muscle (S. C. M.). It is extended upwards to the mastoid tip if the V. A. must be exposed up to C2, and downwards to the clavicle if exposure of the V. A. at its entry into the transverse canal is required.

c) Approach

Approach passes between the medial aspect of the S. C. M. and the lateral edge of the internal jugular vein (I. J. V.).

The I. J. V. and the carotid artery are displaced medially, but they do not need to be dissected out.

This approach leads directly to the lateral aspect of the vertebral bodies and transverse processes. There is no vascular or nervous element to dissect or to divide on the way, except at the upper level (C 3). The accessory spinal nerve (XI) reaches the medial aspect of the S. C. M. at approximately the level of C 3. Therefore, its junction with the S. C. M. must be identified.

The prevertebral fascia covers the prevertebral muscles (longus colli and anterior rectus muscles). Laterally, the sympathetic nerve courses anterior to the prevertebral fascia over the transverse processes. After the prevertebral fascia has been incised, it is retracted laterally with the sympathetic nerve, this avoids dissection of the sympathetic nerve and prevents any damage to it with subsequent Horner's syndrome. Prevertebral muscles are then divided and resected on the required length. Their resection is usually preferred to retraction, as this gives better access to the transverse processes, previously identified with the finger. One must be aware at this time of any abnormality in the course of the V. A., especially of a high entry (C 5 or above) into the transverse canal. In this latter case, the V. A. courses just anterior to transverse processes and behind the muscles.

The periosteum of the anterior branches of the transverse processes is then ruginated so as to be able to pass behind them. This is performed on the required number of vertebrae.

Small intertransversarii muscles are subsequently removed. They are not adherent to the periosteal sheath of the V. A., which can therefore be respected during this procedure.

The anterior branches of the transverse processes are then resected with a small rongeur. If the periosteum of the transverse processes has been well elevated, no injury of the periosteal sheath is to be feared.

If necessary, the periosteal sheath is opened and the venous plexus is progressively coagulated using bipolar coagulation.

If the tip of the transverse processes is respected, the cervical nerve roots remain hidden behind it and the anterior scalenus muscle insertions. Their exposure, if desired, requires separation of these muscle insertions. The nerve roots cross the posterior aspect of the V. A. between two transverse processes and then pass behind the tip of these processes. Complete control of the V. A. performed while the artery remains in its 'periosteal sheath prevents any damage to the nerve roots. These can be exposed behind the V. A. and laterally after resection of the tip of the transverse processes.

12.3.2.2 Anterior Approach

a) Position and Incision

Position and incision are quite similar to those used in the Lateral-Anterior approach.

b) Approach

Approach passes between the aero-digestive track, retracted medially, and the vasculo-nervous elements (I. J. V., carotid artery and vagus nerve).

This leads first to the anterior aspect of the vertebral bodies. Subsequent steps to approach and control the V. A. are identical with the lateral-anterior approach.

12.3.2.3. Lateral Approach

a) Position

The patient is in supine or lateral decubitus position with the head extended and rotated controlaterally.

b) Incision

Incision follows the posterior edge of the S. C. M. muscles.

c) Approach

This is the route primarily described for exposition of the brachial plexus between the scalenus muscles. It passes behind the deep aspect of the S. C. M.

muscle, which is retracted anteriorly and medially.

The V. A. is approached by following the cervical nerve roots until the transverse processes are reached. The transverse canal is thereby exposed on its lateral aspect between the scalenus muscles. The anterior scalene muscle is separated at its insertion level on the anterior tubercules of the transverse processes. It is retracted only after control and freeing of the phrenic nerve, which runs under its anterior aponevrosis. The tip of the transverse processes and the intertransversarii muscles are then resected, giving access to the V. A.

12.3.3 Third Portion (Sub-Occipital)

12.3.3.1 Lateral-anterior Approach

a) Position

The patient is in supine position with the head extended slightly and rotated towards the controlateral side. In the approach to the V. A. between C 1 and C 2, head rotation can be very limited. A 20° to 30° head rotation offers, however, a more comfortable operating field. On the contrary, in the approach over C 1, a marked rotation of at least 45° is necessary, to enable exposure of the posterior arch of the atlas up to the midline and, if required, half of the C 2 lamina and posterior fossa.

b) Skin Incision

Incision follows the anterior edge of the S. C. M. muscle from a point located in front of the mandibular angle up to the mastoid tip.

Depending on what part of the third portion of the V. A. is to be exposed and on the patient's morphology, the skin incision is prolonged inferiorly along the anterior edge of the S. C. M. muscle or superiorly along the mastoid and the superior occipital crest.

Exposure of the V. A. above C 1 requires prolongation of the incision along the mastoid process. Half of the posterior fossa and the intracranial V. A. are approached through an incision running along the occipital crest up to the occipital protuberance on the midline.

c) V. A. Approach Between C 1 and C 2 (Figs. 60 and 61)

This is the easiest part of the V. A. to approach, as it is the most superficial if the head is rotated. At this level, about 2 cm of the vessel can be exposed with-

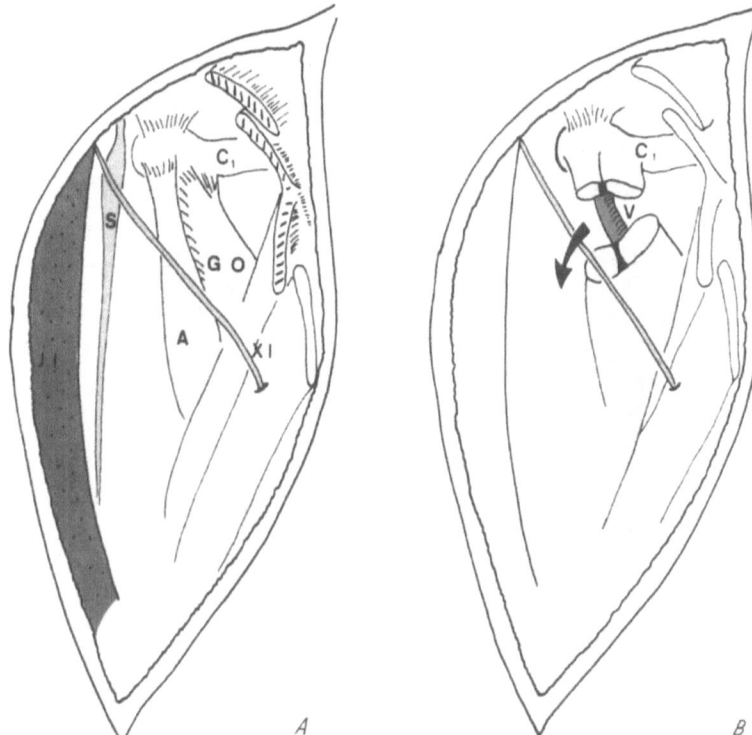

Fig. 60. Lateral-anterior approach to the V. A. segment between C 1 and C 2 (left side). **A)** The space between the sternocleidomastoid muscle and the internal jugular vein (*JI*) is opened. The accessory spinal nerve is freed out and retracted medially. The sympathetic nerve (*S*) is left medially. **B)** The two muscles levator scapulae (*A*) and inferior oblique (*GO*) insertions on the transverse process of C1 are divided. The V. A. appeared just behind these two muscles (*V*). *XI* accessory spinal nerve

out any bone resection. Therefore, it is the preferred site for distal control of the V. A.

Just as for the second portion, approach by the lateral-anterior route passes lateral to the I. J. V.; the carotid artery and the aerodigestive track are left in position and not exposed. This route passes between the medial border of the S. C. M. muscle and the lateral aspect of the I. J. V.

The first and only element to dissect out is the accessory spinal nerve which enters the S. C. M. muscle on the deep portion of its medial aspect, approximately at the level of C 3. It is freed out

from the S. C. M. muscle up to the skull base. It runs superiorly and internally, nearing the I. J. V. over the transverse process of the atlas; then it crosses the vein, usually on its posterior aspect. However, it may cross anteriorly or even be divided in two roots, one passing anterior, the other posterior to the I. J. V. Control of the accessory spinal nerve must be done with care, as its course varies greatly with each patient. It may be very short, so that the nerve crosses the field over the C 1–C 2 interspace, leading to certain difficulties in approach to the V. A.; or it may be long, lying medial and inferior to the field

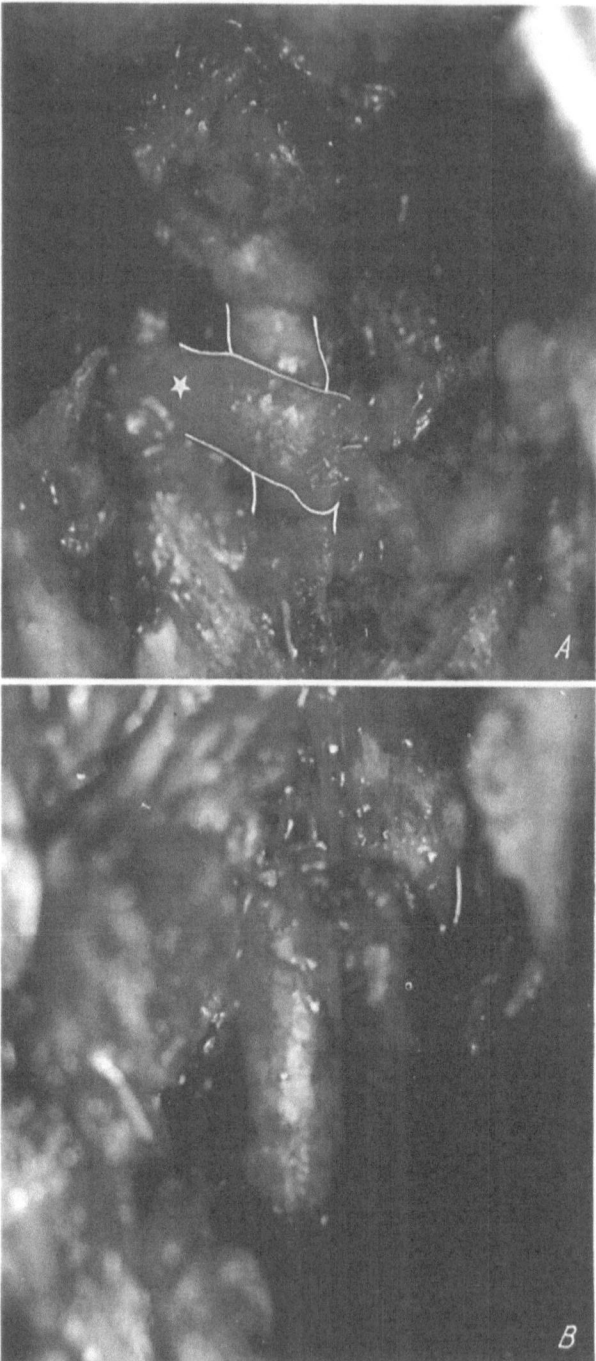

Fig. 61. A) V. A. exposure between C 1 and C 2. The V. A. is still inside its periosteal sheath and behind the anterior branch of the second cervical nerve ☆. **B)** The V. A. is exposed after opening of the periosteal sheath and coagulation of the perivertebral veins

and thus require no particular attention after its isolation. Whatever the case, freeing of the accessory spinal nerve must be extended as high as possible towards the skull base. In most cases, this allows gentle mobilization of the nerve out of the field.

In a second step, the tip of the C 1 transverse process is exposed. This is a very good landmark; even before the skin is incised, it can be identified by palpation, 1 cm inferior and anterior to the tip of the mastoid process.

In a short-necked patient, the anterior part of the digastric muscle may have to be resected to correctly expose the transverse process of C 1. In this case, the hypoglossal nerve (XII) must first be controlled.

Similarly, where necessary, the mastoid head of the S. C. M. may be divided to enlarge the field and afford a better view of the C 1–C 2 interspace.

Usually the field is covered with a more or less extensive lymphatic fascia which must be removed or divided externally and rolled over the accessory spinal nerve. In this way, the nerve can be retracted medially under the protection of the lymphatic fascia.

The C 1–C 2 intertransverse space is now clearly exposed. Two muscles have insertions on the tip of the C 1 transverse process: the levator scapulae and superior oblique muscles. They are divided on the transverse process and retracted downwards and outwards or resected.

The V. A. lies just behind these muscles, so they must be cut with precaution. Care must be taken to divide these muscle insertions as close as possible to the transverse process so as not to leave any muscle remnants overlying the field.

The sympathetic nerve and superior ganglion are usually just medial to these muscles. They do not need to be retracted.

At this point, the V. A. is well visualized, but still surrounded by its venous plexus inside the periosteal sheath and crossed by the anterior branch of the second cervical nerve. This nerve lies in contact with the periosteal sheath on the lateral aspect of the V. A. With the head rotated controlaterally, this nerve covers the anterior surface of the V. A. in its upper or middle third. Recognition of this landmark can thus protect the V. A. from injury during exposure. The next step of V. A. control is division of this anterior branch of the second cervical nerve, which is without significant consequences. Sparing this nerve by retraction has no interest. The periosteal sheath is then opened and the venous plexus suppressed by bipolar coagulation. At this level, the plexus is not highly developed. It predominates on the anterior and medial aspect of the V. A. V. A. control progresses step by step, upwards and downwards from its mid-portion to the transverse foramina of C 1 and C 2.

During V. A. control, it must be remembered that a muscular branch frequently originates between C 1 and C 2 from the postero-lateral aspect of the V. A., usually in the middle third of the C 1–C 2 interspace.

d) Above C 1 (Figs. 62 and 63)

The initial steps of approach above C 1 are quite similar to those just described up to exposition of the transverse pro-

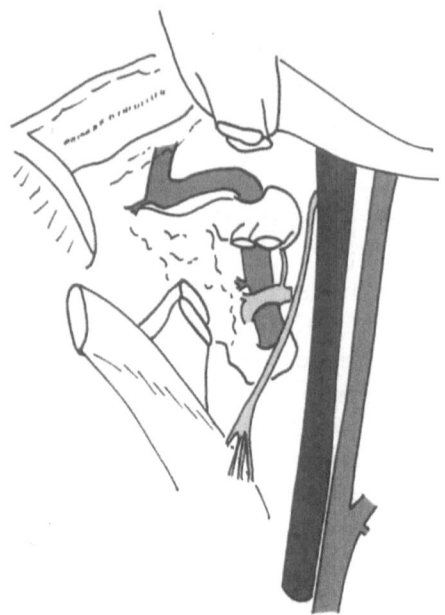

Fig. 62. Lateral-anterior approach to the V. A. between C 1 and C 2 and above C 1

cess of C 1. Here, the mastoid and occipital insertions of the S. C. M. muscles must be divided. The deep cervical muscles (splenius and complexus muscles) are also detached subperiosteally from the occipital bone.

Following this, it is prudent to control the V. A. between C 1 and C 2 before exposure above C 1; but with experience, direct exposure can be realized if one respects careful progression in the surgical approach.

After having controlled the transverse process of C 1, the posterior arch of the atlas is exposed up to the midline. Small muscles are first detached from its inferior margin. The periosteum is then ruginated on the superior margin up to its junction with the periosteal sheath of the V. A. After this, a blunt dissector is

passed between the periosteal sheath and the bony groove of the arch of the atlas. Injury to the V. A. will not occur if permanent contact with the bone is maintained.

The periosteal sheath is then freed from the fatty tissue which covers its posterior and superior surface. This fatty tissue fills the triangular space limited by the arch of the atlas, the occipital bone and the deep aspect of the cervical muscles.

The first cervical nerve crosses the posterior aspect of the V. A. above C 1 to join the cervical muscles. It is usually not seen, since it is injured in retracting the deep muscles. In any case, it is a purely sensitive nerve, which can be divided without consequence.

Near the middle of the posterior arch, the V. A. bends superiorly and anteriorly to join the dura of the foramen magnum. Control of the superior aspect of the V. A. above C 1, as it progresses from the transverse process towards the midline, must therefore proceed cautiously. Again it is safer to control the inferior aspect first, so as to locate this curve of the V. A. Two landmarks help: one is a collateral branch which frequently originates at this level and runs medially; the other is the change in the height of the posterior arch, which increases exactly at this site, so that the medial portion is higher than the lateral one on which the V. A. is lying up to this point of curvature.

Control of the V. A. requires, as for any part of the second and third portions, opening of the periosteal sheath and freeing of the vessel from the venous plexus, which is usually highly developed at this level.

e) Transverse Foramen of C 1

Opening of the transverse foramen of C1 is sometimes necessary to gain more length in V. A. exposure.

It is easier to progress from the C1–C2 interspace than from above C1. However, if complete opening of the transverse foramen is necessary, the V. A. must be exposed on each side of the transverse process. Again it is far more easy and safe to realize this without opening the periosteal sheath.

The loop of the V. A. inside the C1 foramen is rather simple, as it is a single bend in a frontal plane, but it is at an acute angle in the operative position. Actually, with the head rotated controlaterally, the two V. A. segments above C1 and between C1 and C2 run almost parallel, with only the posterior arch of the atlas interposed (**Fig. 63**).

f) Transverse Foramen of C 2

On the contrary, the V. A. loops into the transverse foramen of C2 in a complex fashion, since it exhibits two bends in two different planes (see chapter Anatomy). Opening of this transverse foramen is thus far more difficult. Control of the V. A. on both sides of this foramen must be completed before removing the bone. Progression upwards from C3 is generally the simplest way to open this foramen.

12.3.3.2 Posterior Approach (Fig. 64)

a) Position

Sitting, prone and lateral decubitus positions can be used. The sitting position carries the risk of air embolism, which may be prevented by the use of a G-suit; but it also has the disadvantage of inducing postural hypotension, which, in patients with vertebrobasilar ischemia, may provoke a critical condition and an eventual post-operative stroke (Khodadad, 1981).

The prone position produces more bleeding in the operative field and makes this position unsuitable if the posterior fossa is opened. Moreover, a bloody field is certainly troublesome if a vascular suture has to be made.

The lateral decubitus position is therefore the best choice in most cases. In our experience, the posterior approach has only been used in certain tumor cases and was performed with the patient in sitting position, with protection by a G-suit and a swann-Ganz probe.

b) Incision

There are three posibilities for the skin incision:

— midline incision up to the occipital protuberance and bent laterally along the superior occipital crest.

— paramedian linear incision at equal distance between the midline and the mastoid tip.

— lateral incision vertical to the level of the mastoid tip and bent medially along the superior occipital crest.

Since the posterior approach is mainly used for V. A. exposure above C1 and intracranial hour-glass tumor removal, the midline incision is preferred. However, if the lateral decubitus position has been chosen, the lateral incision is much more convenient.

c) Approach

The occipital muscles are detached and ruginated from the occipital bone and

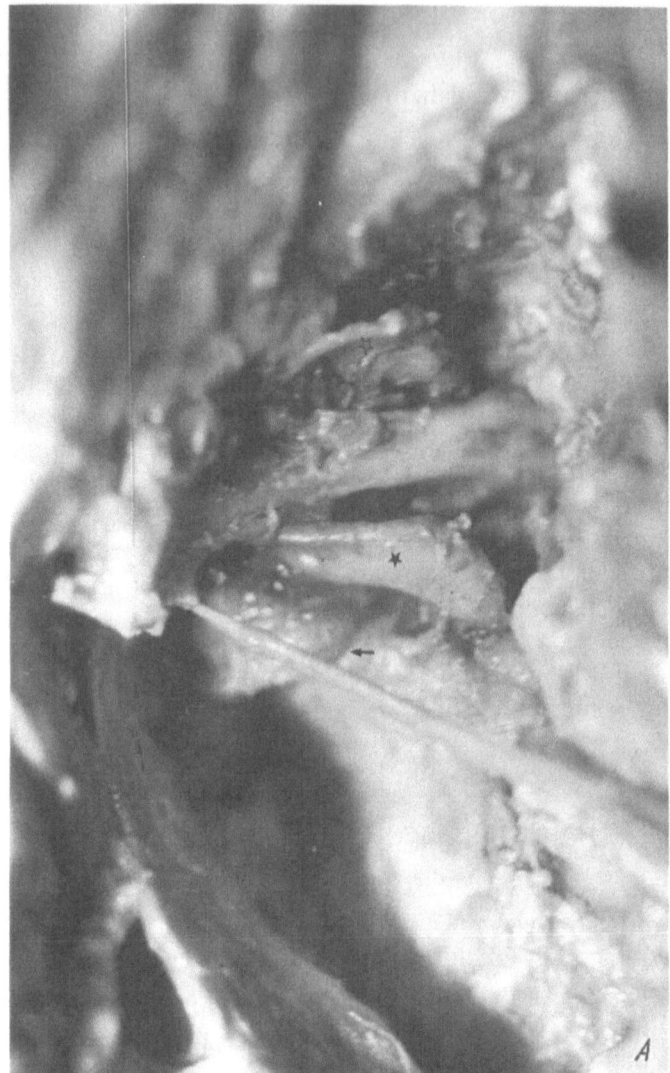

Fig. 63. Anatomical (**A**) and operative (**B**) exposure of the V. A. between C 1 and C 2 ★ and above C 1 ☆. The head is controlaterally rotated. The 2 V. A. segments run parallel with only the arch of atlas interposed between them. Note the proximity of the C 1–C 2 articular facet in **A**) ← . **B**) corresponds to the operative field after removal of an extradural neurinoma

then retracted inferiorly and either laterally or medially depending on the chosen skin incision.

— above C 1: the posterior arch of the atlas is then exposed from the spinous process to the transverse process. The inferior margin is freed out from muscles before the superior one.

Subsequent exposure and control of the V. A. follows the same principles as in the lateral approach.

— between C 1 and C 2: both laminae

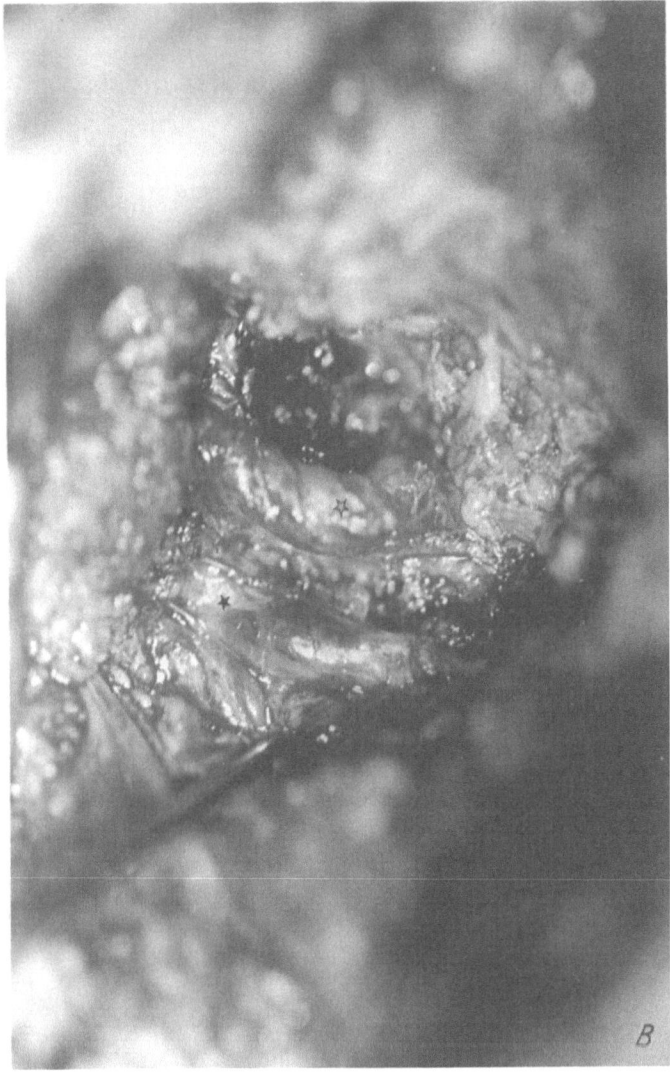

Fig. 63B

of C1 and C2 are exposed from the midline to the transverse processes. The superior oblique muscle is detached from the transverse process of C1, exposing the posterolateral aspect of the V.A. The second cervical nerve is well seen as it emerges from the C1–C2 interspace and crosses the posterior aspect of the V.A. V.A. control then proceeds in the same way as with the lateral anterior approach.

12.4 Discussion of Surgical Approaches (Fig. 65, Table 13)

12.4.1 Lateral Anterior Approach

This approach appears to be the most appropriate surgical route to the V. A. for many reasons:

1—It provides relatively easy access to any part of the V. A., from the ostium up to its intracranial portion. In fact, the skin incision in its fullest extent allows exposition of the whole length of the V. A. Obviously, exposure of only one or two portions can be performed using an adequate part of the skin incision; but any necessity, even appearing during surgery, of V. A. control over a larger distance, does not raise any technical problem. The patient position does not have to be changed, and the skin incision only has to be prolonged.

2—the lateral anterior approach passes through an anatomical plane between the SCM muscle and the IJV without any vessel to dissect out. The lone

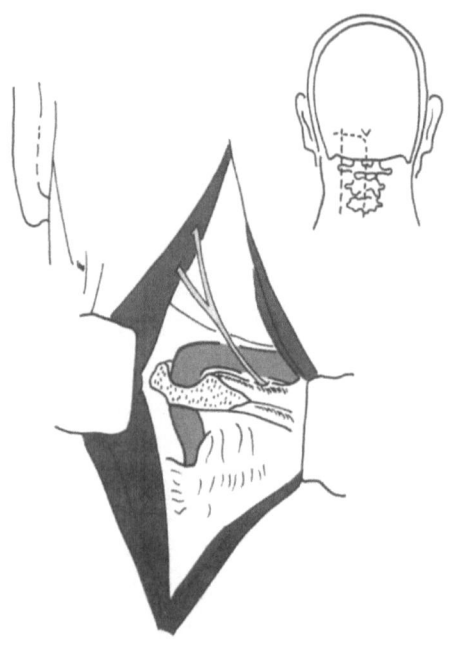

Fig. 64. Posterior approach to the V. A. above C1

Table 13. Surgical approaches

Lateral—anterior	Anterior	Lateral	Posterior
A. V. ostium	ostium	—	—
C6–C1	C6–C3	C6–C3	C1–C2
Intracranial	—	—	intracranial
Vertebral body	vertebral body	—	—
Disc	disc	—	—
Carotid artery	carotid artery	—	—
Nerve roots	—	nerve roots	—
Hemi-laminectomy C1–C2	—	—	laminectomy
Hemi-craniectomy	—	—	craniectomy

Possibilities afforded by the different surgical approaches: control of the V. A., extension to other anatomical structures and complementary techniques.

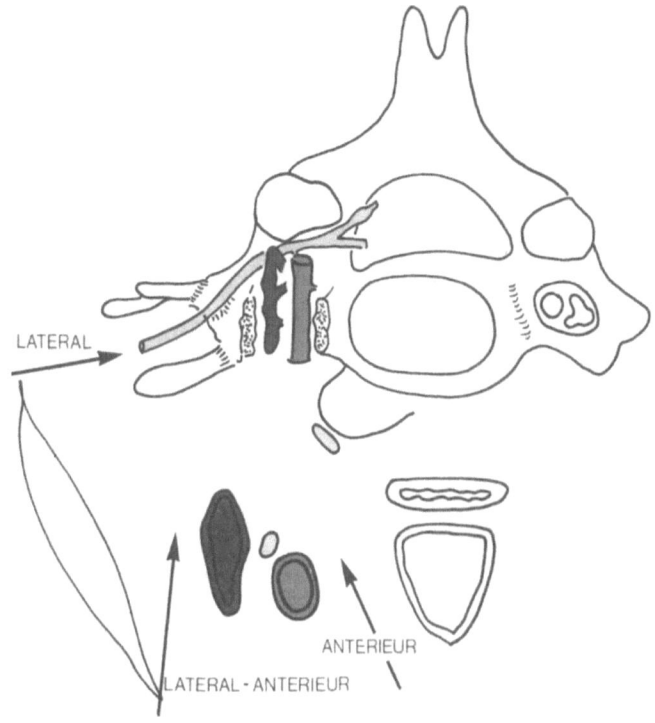

LATERAL

ANTERIEUR

LATERAL - ANTERIEUR

Fig. 65. Surgical routes to the V. A. second portion: lateral, lateral-anterior, and anterior

element crossing the field in the approach to the third portion of the V. A. is the accessory spinal nerve which has to be freed out. Some technical difficulties are shared with the other surgical routes: thoracic duct and lymphatic vessels in the ostial area and perivertebral venous plexus, sympathetic nerve and brachial plexus nerve roots in the second and third portions.

3—More numerous other structures can be controlled by the lateral anterior approach:

— carotid artery, allowing performance of by-pass from any part of it to the V. A. or the simultaneous treatment of a carotid artery lesion.

— cervical nerve roots, of particular interest in hour-glass tumors, especially neurinomas.

— vertebral bodies and discs, permitting resection of bony lesions or repair with bone graft or arthrodesis.

4—The following techniques can be associated in the same procedure using this approach:

— hemilaminectomy of C 1 and even sometimes C 2 for resection by the same route of both intra and extraspinal parts of an hour-glass tumor.

— hemicraniectomy of the posterior fossa in case of intracranial extension or skull base tumor.

— infratemporal approach (Fisch, 1982) to resect petrous bone or clivus lesions.

5—The access to the V. A. afforded by the lateral anterior approach is wide and safe: no vasculo-nervous element crosses the field, with the noticeable exception of the accessory spinal nerve. The SCM muscle can be largely retracted or its insertion severed, giving wider exposure. Surgery is performed outside the carotid-jugular track without any retraction on the oesophagus or trachea.

Other surgical routes are more limited in possibilities for control of the V. A. and other structures. They are also usually less convenient and less appropriate.

12.4.2 Anterior Approach

This is the classical approach described and used for the treatment of osteophytic compression.

This route cannot be extended above C 3, since above this level many vasculo-nervous elements prevent correct exposure.

It gives good access to the vertebral bodies and discs on their lateral aspect as well as on the midline, but it cannot be enlarged laterally towards the nerve roots, since the carotid artery is the outer limit of the field.

The field exposed by the anterior approach is fairly narrow, and is limited laterally and medially by important structures which must be retracted as gently as possible. Moreover the carotid-jugular track laterally and the oesophagus and trachea medially must be protect from accidental injury during surgical manipulations.

12.4.3 Lateral Approach

This is the classical route for surgery on the brachial plexus. Approach to the V. A. is lateral, following the nerve roots up to the tip of the transverse processes. Its interest, which could be important in the removal of paraspinal tumors and especially those originating from the nerve roots, is in fact limited; in these cases, the V. A. is rarely displaced laterally but much more commonly shifted medially and anteriorly. Therefore, with the lateral approach, the V. A. is usually hidden by the tumor and its control as the initial step of the procedure is not possible.

At both extremities of the cervical course of the V. A., the lateral approach is deep and narrow. Correct exposure of the V. A., at these levels requires division of the SCM muscle insertion, on the occipital bone and mastoid process for the third portion, and on the clavicle and manubrium for the first. By doing this, the lateral approach is in fact converted into a lateral anterior approach.

12.4.4 Posterior Approach

This is the common route to the laminae and the posterior fossa. It can be used to expose the third portion of the V. A., but it is not reliable for the other two portions, since this would necessitate lateral extension of the opening so as to remove the apophyseal joints. Furthermore, even if this sacrifice of an important element of spinal stability, were acceptable, the length of V. A. thus exposed, is limited to a very short segment between two nerve roots.

Obviously, the posterior route is quite adequate for exposure of the third portion of the V. A., especially the segment above the arch of the atlas. The field is wide and can be enlarged towards the posterior fossa and down to C 2.

12.4.5 Conclusion

It can be concluded that, as usual in surgery, there is one surgical approach, namely the lateral anterior route, which gives the best access, the widest possibilities and the greatest security for exposure of the cervical V. A.; other possible routes may be proposed, but when used to perform surgery on the V. A., they are deviated from their primary indications and require enlargement which tends to make them similar to the lateral anterior approach. This is the case with the anterior approach, mainly directed to the vertebral bodies and discs, of the lateral approach, devoted to the brachial plexus, and of the posterior approach, classically used to perform laminectomy or posterior fossa craniectomy.

Finally, all these surgical routes must be familiar to any surgeon contemplating surgery on the V. A., so that he is able to choose the most appropriate or to associate technical details of the others as required by the lesion involved. In most cases, the basic surgical technique is the lateral anterior approach to which can be associated elements of the other approaches as required.

12.5 Surgical Competence

In addition to awareness of the different surgical routes, competence in various surgical techniques is necessary if the aim is to be able to treat any type of V. A. lesion.

12.5.1 Vascular Surgery

Performance of V. A. revascularization obviously requires experience of vessel suturing and grafting. However, treatment of external compression of the V. A. carries the risk of V. A. injury and thus should only be performed by a surgeon experienced in vessel repair.

12.5.2 Neurosurgery

Resection of a tumor extending through the intervertebral foramen necessitates minimal training in neuro- surgery to deal with the nerve roots and the dural sac.

12.5.3 Orthopedics

Ability in spinal orthopedics is needed before dealing with a cervical spine fracture or luxation or repairing a bony defect after vertebral tumor removal.

12.5.4 E. N. T.

Lesions at the base of the skull often require competence in E. N. T. sur- gery as well as vascular and neuro-surgery.

12.5.5 Thoracic Surgery

Conversely, at the base of the neck, competence in thoracic surgery, as well as vascular surgery and orthopedics is frequently required.

13. TECHNIQUES OF V. A. SURGERY

13.1 Introduction

Whatever the indication, all V. A. surgery has a common goal: to preserve or to restore V. A. flow.

There are two conditions in which V. A. flow must obviously be protected:
— *Dominant* V. A. with controlateral V. A. of small size or atretic
— *Anterior Radiculo-medullary* branch arising from the V. A., whatever the size of the V. A.

A. In the first condition, the hemodynamic importance of the involved V. A. must be evaluated. If the vessel is occluded, is revascularization necessary?; if it has to be ligated (to treat an embolic lesion) or if it is compressed by an external agent, must it be preserved or can its sacrifice be well tolerated?

In case of occlusion, there is no single paraclinical investigation able to give a correct answer. General agreement is likely to be reached for revascularization of a dominant V. A., or of one V. A. in case of bilateral occlusion of equivalent V. A.'s. In both situations, the entire brain is supplied solely by the carotid arteries and can therefore be considered in nearly critical condition, with little hemodynamic reserve. Any drop in blood pressure can lead to brain ischemia.

In case of external compression or surgical ligation, it must first be stressed that the sacrifice of any vessel supplying the brain, however small, should not be accepted easily. For example, distal revascularization with exclusion of a non dominant V. A. bearing an embolic lesion such as an aneurysm is preferable to ligation or distal balloon embolization on a V. A. filling the basilar trunk in a young patient. Conversely, correct assessment of the risks of surgically controlling a small V. A. completely embedded in a hypervascular tumor may lead to deliberate occlusion before tumor removal. The same treatment is not, however, acceptable on a dominant V. A. without revascularization above the lesion.

External compression with marked stenosis can explain symptoms of vertebrobasilar ischemia, and in this case, release of the compressive agent is indicated. However, in asymptomatic cases of stenosis, numerous factors can compensate the drop in V. A. flow, and in fact obviate the need for surgery except in rare cases. A complete investigation of these factors must be performed before taking any surgical decision.

Finally, the quality of the involved V. A., as well as its importance relative

Table 14

Revascularization	wall lesion
Revascularization + exclusion	embolic wall lesion
	hypervascularized tumor
	complex A. V. M.
Direct control	tumor
	external compression
	A. V. M.
	intraoperative embolization

to the three other major vascular axes supplying the brain (controlateral V. A. and carotid arteries) must be evaluated as accurately as possible before deciding how to solve the V. A. problem. Complete morphologic and functional explorations of the cerebral vascularization are therefore mandatory. Of great help also, is the tolerance test of vessel occlusion performed with a balloon under local anesthesia. This reproduces the clinical condition of a sudden reduction in V. A. or internal carotid artery flow; it may help understand the role of the tested vessel and check the intraoperative possibility of vessel clamping.

B. The second condition, in which there is an anterior radiculo-medullary branch, places limits on what can be done to the V. A. It must be added to the elements cited above in the discussion of V. A. surgical occlusion or

control. Its identification imposes avoidance of V. A. mobilization, as stretching of this branch may induce spinal cord ischemia. A radiculo-medullary branch must therefore be systemically sought on preoperative angiography.

V. A. surgical techniques are of two main types: revascularization and direct control (**Table 14**).

Revascularization by reimplantation or venous grafting is used to restore V. A. flow in the case of a V. A. which is either occluded or is to be occluded in order to allow safe surgical or radiological treatment of an underlying V. A. lesion.

Direct control, whatever the level, exposes the V. A. inside its periosteal sheath after venous plexus coagulation. It is indicated to suppress the vascular supply of a tumor or A. V. M., to alleviate an external compression, or to introduce a catheter for embolization.

13.2 Wall Lesions

13.2.1 Revascularization for Atherosclerotic Lesions

Techniques of revascularization are similar whatever the lesion involving the V. A. However, because, atherosclerotic lesions are markedly predominant, the techniques will be discussed first with reference to these lesions.

These techniques include V. A. reimplantation, grafting, transposition of a donor vessel and direct repair by angioplasty.

The choice of the most adequate is based on several factors, among which the level of the V. A. revascularization is predominant.

13.2.1.1 Reconstructive Techniques for the First Portion of the V. A.

A wide variety of surgical techniques can be utilized on the first portion of the V. A. The particular reconstructive technique to be chosen depends on the extent of the lesions and the distribution of occlusive lesions in other territories.

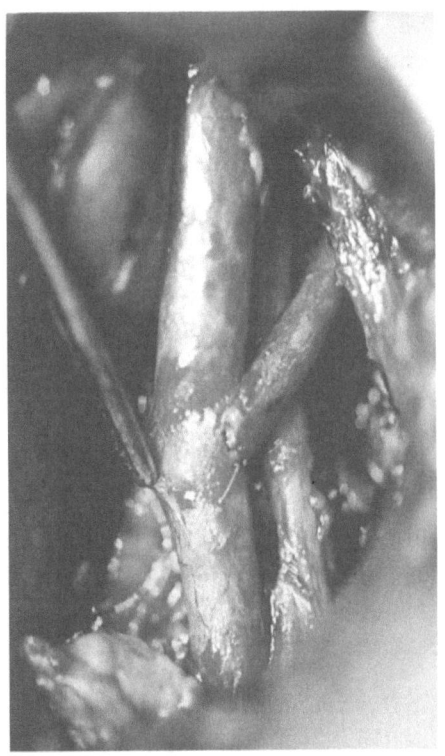

Fig. 66. Operative view of a proximal V. A. reimplantation on the common carotid artery

a) Reimplantation (or Direct Transposition) of the V. A. on to the Common Carotid Artery (Figs. 66 and 67 A)

This is now the procedure of choice (Wylie and Ehrenfeld 1970, Diaz *et al.*, 1984, Feldman, 1984). The V. A. is exposed through a supraclavicular skin incision and approached between the internal jugular vein retracted laterally and the carotid artery and vagus nerve left in place medially. The V. A. is controlled from its origin to its entry into the transverse canal, after resection of the vertebral veins.

The first transverse foramen, at C 6, can be opened to gain some length when the first portion is too short to reach the carotid artery.

The common carotid artery is dissected out down to its upper mediastinal part so as to clamp it behind the clavicle.

Then the V. A. is divided near its origin, flush with the distal extent of the atherosclerotic plaque in order to keep the longest possible segment of V. A.

The V. A. is splayed by a 5 mm incision on its anterior wall.

The chosen site of V. A. implantation on the postero-lateral aspect of the carotid artery can be marked by a stitch. The carotid arteriotomy is performed, with or without a 5 mm arterial punch. The V. A. is implanted directly onto the common carotid artery by anastomosis with continuous suture, completed anteriorly by separated stitches.

The true contra-indications of this technique are:
— parietal carotid lesions with extensive atherosclerosis,
— temporary cerebral ischemia during the carotid artery clamping. The risk can be evaluated pre-operatively by Doppler studies with arterial compression, thus testing the value of the anterior and posterior communicating arteries. The balloon occlusion test is another way to check carotid artery clamping possibilities.

In some patients with controlateral occlusive disease of both the carotid and the V. A., the hazard of clamping can easily be avoided by an alternative technique: grafting.

b) Reimplantation onto the Subclavian Artery or One of Its Branches

This technique requires more V. A. length and is more difficult to realize, in our experience, because of the poor quality of the subclavian artery wall for suturing.

c) Grafting Technique

This technique is performed when re-implantation is not suitable.
The best grafting material is the saphenous vein; the caliber of its ankle segment matches that of the V. A.
The proximal part of the reversed saphenous vein graft is anastomosed end to side to the common carotid artery, low behind the clavicle. As soon as this anastomosis is completed, flow is re-established through the carotid artery and the venous graft is occluded with a microvascular clip.

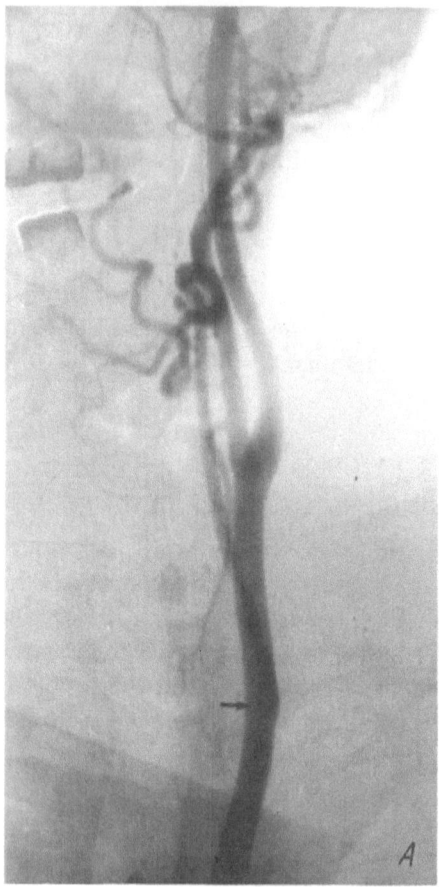

Fig. 67 A

The distal end of the vein graft is then implanted onto the V. A.; this can be achieved by end to side anastomosis, but more frequently, end to end anastomosis is performed after having splayed the V. A. and the graft in complementary fashion.
Proximal implantation of the saphenous vein graft on the subclavian artery requires more extensive dissection (Berguer and Bauer, 1976), therefore, it is rarely used by the present authors.
Indications for grafting techniques on the first portion of the V. A. are generally discussed when reimplantation cannot be realized because of

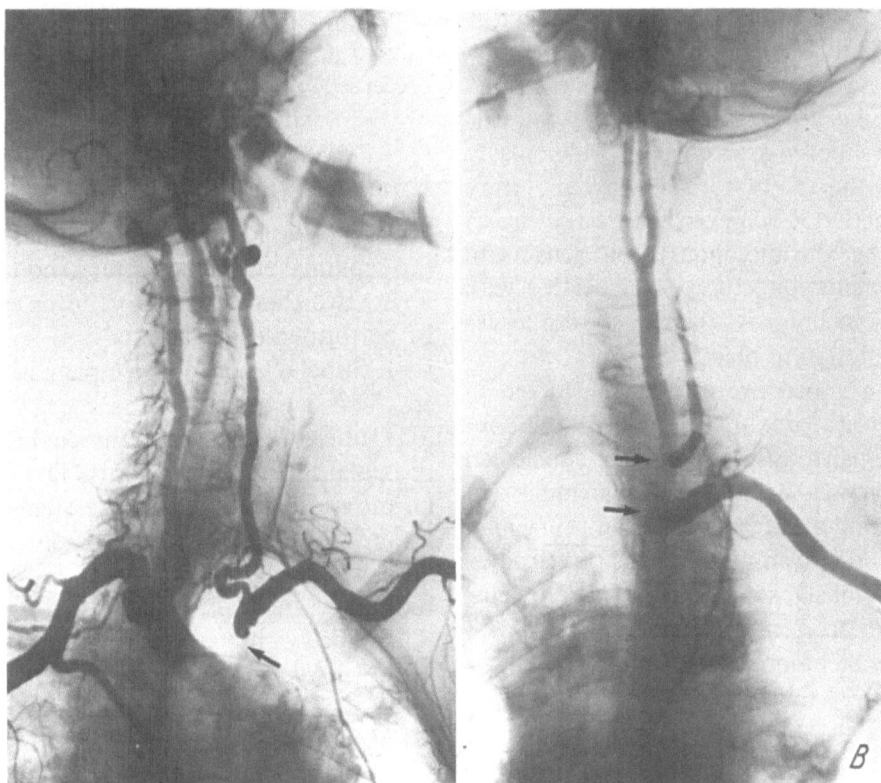

Fig. 67. A) Angiographic control of proximal V. A. reimplantation. B) Angiographic control of a combined V. A. and subclavian artery reimplantation

— too short a segment of V. A. available,

— too great an extent of V. A. atherosclerotic lesions (extensive endarterectomy is in our opinion, an inadequate technique),

— too high a risk of simultaneous carotid and vertebral artery clamping. Consequently, venous graft by-pass, though it achieves very good results, is not frequently utilized.

d) Subclavian and V. A. Angioplasty

Since most lesions involving the proximal V. A. are limited to the ostial region, endarterectomy either via

direct V. A. incision or by transsubclavian approach (Wylie and Ehrenfeld, 1970, Roon et al., 1979, Thevenet and Ruatolo, 1984) could be considered. However, because of the particular friability of the V. A. and subclavian artery, this technique has been abandoned by many authors or substitued by angioplasty (Imparato et al., 1981). In our experience, we have used angioplasty technique in only one case.

A more extensive exposure of the subclavian artery on both sides of the V. A. ostium is necessary. If the V. A. originates very proximally, exposure of the mediastinal segment of the subclavian artery is often required, making this procedure more difficult.

In any case, the arteriotomy is extended on the V. A. across its origin towards the subclavian artery. Then angioplasty of the vertebral subclavian artery junction is achieved with a roof patch using an autologous saphenous vein. No endarterectomy is associated with this technique, which therefore leaves the lesion in place.

This procedure can be considered in severe proximal stenosis without occlusive disease on the subclavian artery and in patients with an important hemodynamic risk of ischemia in whom carotid clamping seems hazardous. Obviously, stenosis manifested by embolic accidents must not be treated with this technique.

e) Combined Treatment of Carotid and Vertebral Arteries

This procedure is indicated in patients who are symptomatic in both the carotid and vertebral territories, or who require carotid surgery and have severe stenosis of the homolateral dominant V. A. The V. A. surgery is performed in this second case as a prophylactic measure.

A single incision along the anterior border of the S. C. M. muscle allows treatment of both arteries. This procedure is performed in a systematic fashion, beginning by V. A. reimplantation onto the common carotid artery. Then flow is restored in the V. A. and the carotid artery clamped above the reimplantation. The carotid endarteriectomy follows.

If atherosclerosis involves the proximal carotid artery extensively, a venous graft by-pass between the common carotid and internal carotid arteries is preferred.

f) Combined Subclavian and V. A. Reimplantation (Fig. 67 B)

In cases of associated stenotic lesions of the proximal subclavian artery and the V. A., two therapeutic procedures can be performed simultaneously.

f—1. Subclavian artery reimplantation and V. A. angioplasty.

The subclavian artery is transected just proximal to the V. A. ostium. The arteriotomy is extended to the stenotic lesion of the V. A. and an angioplasty with a saphenous vein patch is performed on the V. A. origin.

The subclavian artery is then directly reimplanted onto the carotid artery.

f—2. Double reimplantation of subclavian and V. A.'s.

If V. A. stenosis is associated with marked tortuosity which requires proximal V. A. resection, the vertebral and subclavian arteries are reimplanted separately onto the carotid artery.

g) Conclusion

There is no single technique available for every pathologic condition. Therefore, one must be familiar with all procedures that may be used to reconstruct the first portion of the V. A. Reimplantation is now the most frequently adequate technique.

13.2.1.2 Reconstructive Techniques for the Second Portion of the V. A.

Atherosclerotic lesions on the second portion are far rarer than on the first, but revascularization at this level may be indicated in certain conditions:

— ostial occlusion with distal reinjection through a muscular collateral network filling the V. A. down to the C 4 or C 5 level,

— focal areas of stenosis in the transverse canal with tandem stenosis at the ostium,

— long and irregular stenosis extending along the first portion up to the C 6 transverse foramen.

Revascularization of the second portion of the V. A. requires exposure and control of the vessel at this level. As in any other type of surgery, existence of a radiculo-medullary artery must have been identified pre-operatively and must be dealt with so as to preserve vascular supply to the spinal cord.

Techniques on the second portion include endarterectomy, reimplantation and venous graft by-pass (Clark and Perry, 1966, Corkill et al., 1979, George and Laurian, 1979, Carney, 1981, Berguer and Feldman, 1983).

a) Endarterectomy

This procedure may be used to resect focal area of stenosis.

Large areas of stenosis beginning in the first portion can be removed by direct incision along the V. A. or with an eversion technique from the origin of the plaque. Reimplantation onto the common carotid artery must complete this procedure (Diaz et al., 1985).

However, in our opinion endarterectomy is not a reliable technique because of the friability and small caliber of the V. A.

b) Reimplantation

Reimplantation of the V. A. distal to the lesion onto the common carotid artery or the internal carotid artery avoids resecting the plaque, but necessitates to freeing up and mobilizing the transverse portion of the V. A. This is a long and rather difficult procedure.

c) Venous Graft

A saphenous vein graft from the subclavian or the common carotid artery, may be used to by-pass the second portion of the V. A.

This technique does not require mobilization of the V. A. In case of an anterior radiculo-medullary branch, it can be spared more easily than with reimplantation.

Proximal implantation of the graft is preferentially done end to side onto the common carotid artery. The distal implantation is also done end to side onto the V. A., after unroofing of the transverse foramina on two or three levels. This has the advantage of providing a short but large by-pass with a straight and vertical graft course, which is not the case if the subclavian artery is the donor vessel.

d) Conclusion

Revascularization of the second portion of the V. A. has very few indications. Endarterectomy, and reimplantation are, in our opinion, improper techniques. Venous by-pass is the only technique to use at this level and the elective site of graft implantation onto the distal V. A. is at the C 1–C 2 level, even in the case of proximal lesions in the transverse canal.

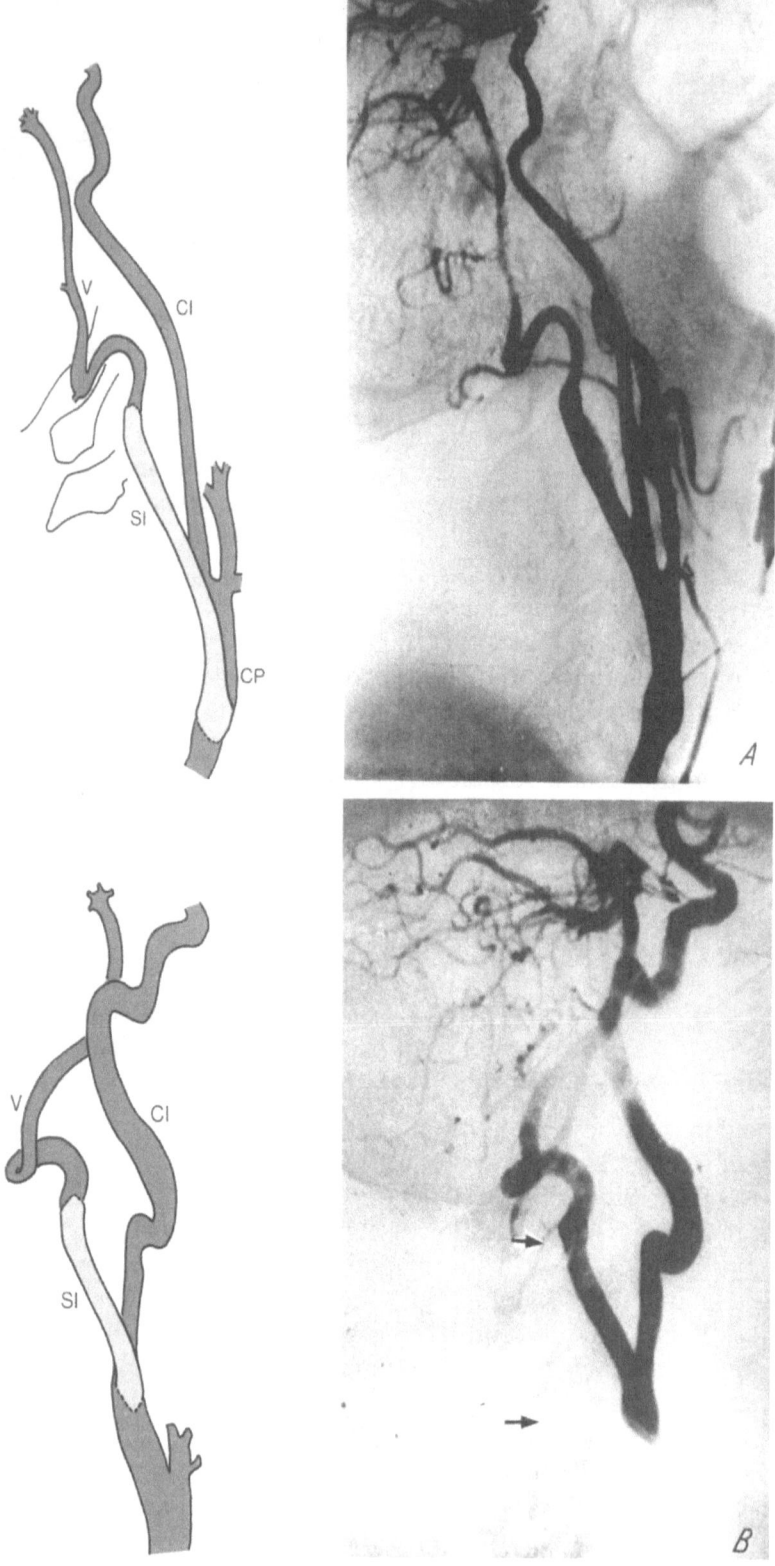

Fig. 68. Angiographic control of distal revascularization with a saphenous vein graft. **A)** Common carotid to V. A. at C 1–C 2. **B)** Internal carotid to V. A. at C 1–C 2. **C)** Subclavian to V. A. at C 1–C 2. **D)** Internal Carotid to V. A. at C 1 with exclusion

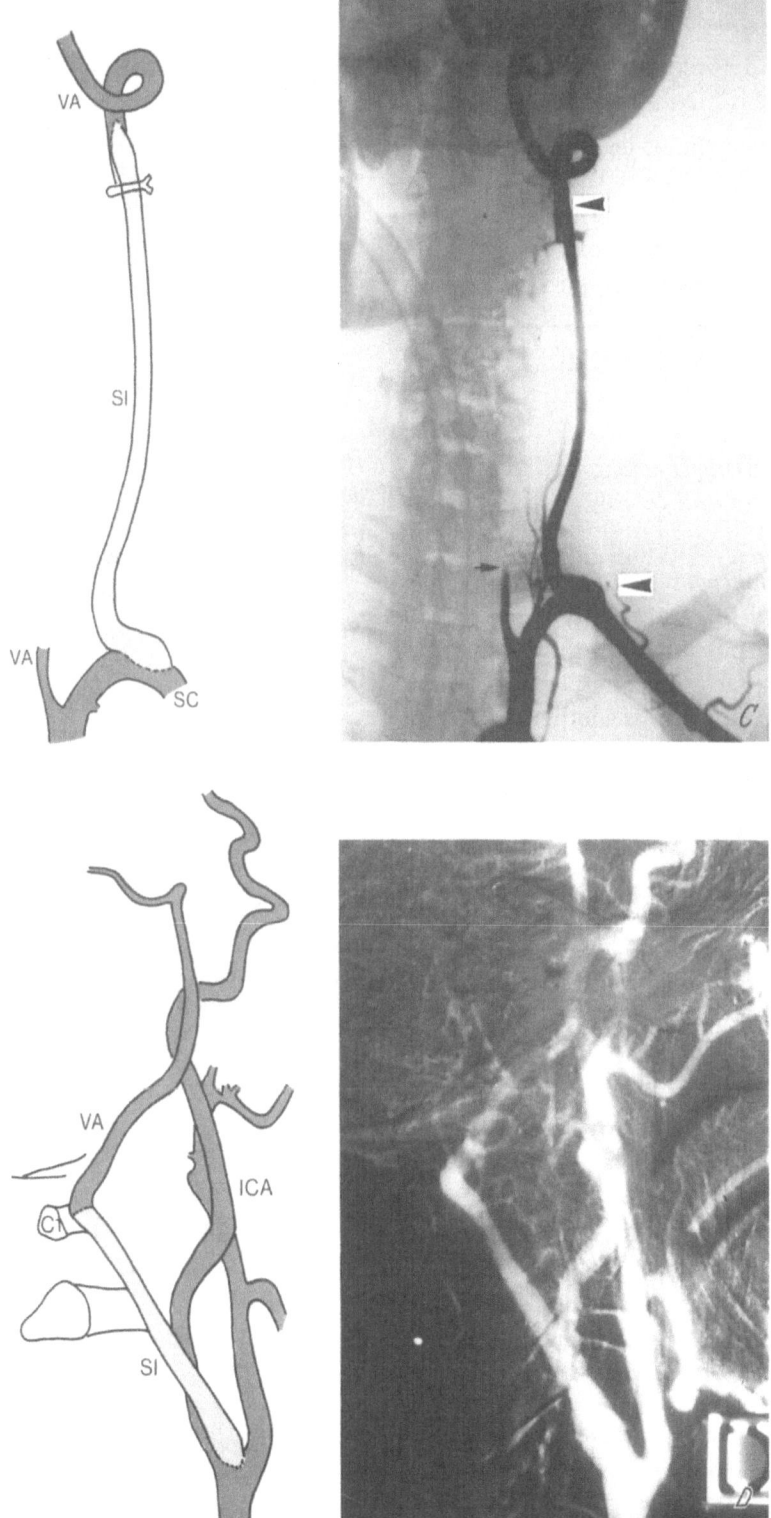

Fig. 68C and **D**

13.2.1.3 Reconstructive Technique for the Third Portion of the V.A.

Whatever the extent and severity of proximal lesions, the V.A. remains patent distally in almost every case, due to reinjection by a muscular network. Carotid-vertebral by-pass is the most frequently performed procedure, but alternative techniques may be useful in selected cases.

*a) Grafting Technique
(Figs. 68 and 69)*

a—1. Choice of graft material.
The saphenous vein is the preferred material for grafting. It is taken from the mid-portion of the thigh, where no, or few, valves are present.
The cephalic vein is another possibility, but, it is generally larger than the saphenous vein and may cause congruence problems.
Autologous arterial materials, such as an occluded internal carotid artery after endarterectomy, or the external carotid artery have rarely been utilized. In fact, this technique results in carotid transposition onto the V.A. (Corkill *et al.,* 1977, Kieffer *et al.,* 1984).
Prosthetic material has been used by Carney (1981), but without success.
The lack of a suitable vein graft is, in our opinion, a contra-indication to revascularization of the distal V.A., in the case of atherosclerotic lesions.

a—2. Distal implantation of the graft.
The C1–C2 interspace is the best site for distal revascularization, since it offers many advantages:
— the V.A. segment found here is always patent, even in cases of V.A. occlusion,

— the V.A. at this level is usually spared from atherosclerotic involvement,

— it is the widest interspace of the transverse canal, and at least a 2.5 cm segment of V.A. can be exposed without any bone resection. However, unroofing of the C1 transverse foramen can be performed without hesitation, whenever this segment appears too short.

From a technical point of view, distal anastomosis is more difficult than a proximal one. This is due to the small caliber and thin wall of the V.A. as well as the rather narrow surgical field. Some technical details which may appear minor, are in fact of considerable importance in order to perform this anastomosis with maximum comfort, and, therefore safety: protection of the accessory spinal nerve, enlargement of the field by dividing the S.C.M. muscle insertion on the mastoïd, extension of V.A. exposure, complete resection of the small deep muscles to facilitate needle passage, perfect control of the entire V.A. circumference to correctly apply the microclamps.

There is no reason in atherosclerotic pathology to implant the graft above C1. Exposure of the V.A. at this level is generally more troublesome and the available segment shorter.

The arteriotomy is extended on the V.A. so as to give perfect congruence with the vein graft tip which is slightly splayed. The reversed venous graft is anastomosed end to side onto the V.A. with two continuous sutures started at both angles of the anastomosis.
Microclamps are then removed and

back-flow into the venous graft is blocked by venous valves or a clamp.

End to end anastomosis has also been proposed by Kieffer *et al.* (1984) and Berguer (1985). This mode of anastomosis has some advantages:

— it necessitates a smaller exposure,

— it allows greater mobility of the distal end of the by-pass during head rotation.

But disadvantages appear even more important:

— poor congruence between the V. A. and the graft, with subsequent risk of intimal hyperplasia,

— exclusion of the proximal portion of the V. A. with subsequent thrombosis, and risk of spinal cord ischemia if a radiculo-medullary branch originates from the V. A.

a—3. Proximal implantation of the graft.

The site of proximal implantation is based on the dynamic consequences of head movements and existence of structural lesions of the carotid axis.

a—3.1) The dynamic consequences of head motion may explain graft failure despite a flawless anastomosis. Therefore, certain technical details must be respected:

— the graft by-pass must be as short as possible,

— the graft by-pass must be as vertical as possible, preventing tension during head rotation,

— the graft by-pass must be positioned as posterior in the neck as possible, so as to bring it the closest possible to the longitudinal axis of head rotation,

— the length of the graft must be carefully adjusted to avoid excessive tension during hyperextension,

— the graft course must run over the antero-lateral aspect of the internal jugular vein.

Opening of the C 1 or even C 2 transverse foramen may be useful in selected cases. We do not recommend our patients to wear any kind of collar postoperatively.

Taking all these elements into account, the most suitable site of proximal implantation appears in general to be on the common carotid artery, more or less close to its bifurcation.

a—3.2) Structural lesions of the carotid axis.

The common carotid artery is the preferred donor vessel. Graft implanted on it follows a smooth, regular course. It is the largest possible donor vessel in the vicinity of the distal V. A. Finally, it is rarely affected by extensive atherosclerotic lesions.

The use of the *internal carotid artery* necessitates clamping of a vessel directly supplying the brain. Moreover, except for the first centimeters, its caliber is much smaller than that of the common carotid artery. Atherosclerotic involvement is frequent and occurs essentially on the first centimeters. In our opinion, the internal carotid artery should not be used for treatment of atherosclerotic lesions; on the contrary, it may be preferred in other indications for revascularization if, according to the graft course aspect, it is the most appropriate implantation site.

The small diameter of the *external carotid artery* and its frequently severe and rapid involvement by atherosclerosis explain that this vessel should be avoided as much as possible. Furthermore, the graft implanted on it has a rather horizontal course, subjecting it to high tension during head rotation.

Exceptionally, the external carotid artery can be utilized to revascularize a small V. A. for better congruence reasons. It may also be indicated when clamping of the common carotid artery seems hazardous. However, in this last case, the subclavian artery is generally a better choice.

The subclavian artery has the major

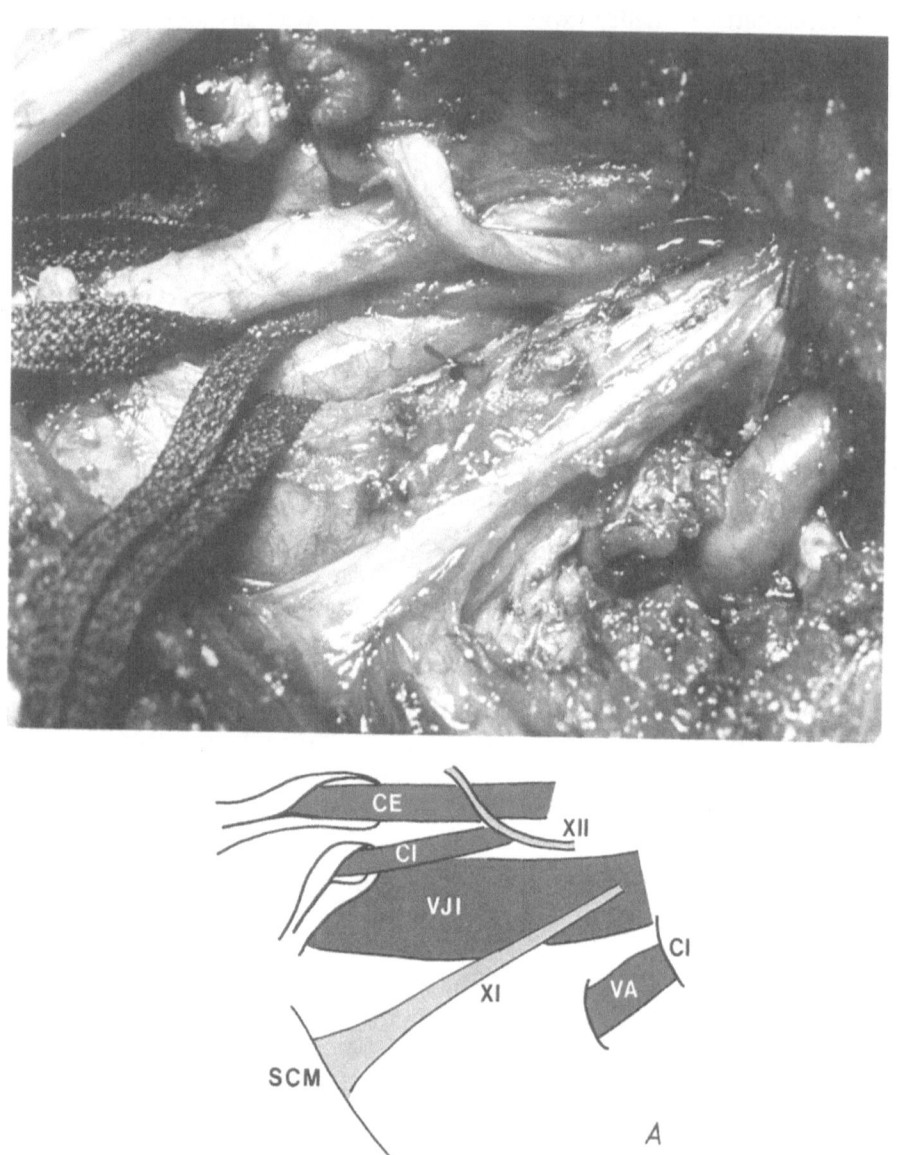

Fig. 69. Operative view of distal V. A. revascularization. **A)** Surgical field before anastomosis performance. **B)** Common carotid to V. A. by-pass at C 1–C 2. **C)** Internal carotid to V. A. by-pass at C 1–C 2

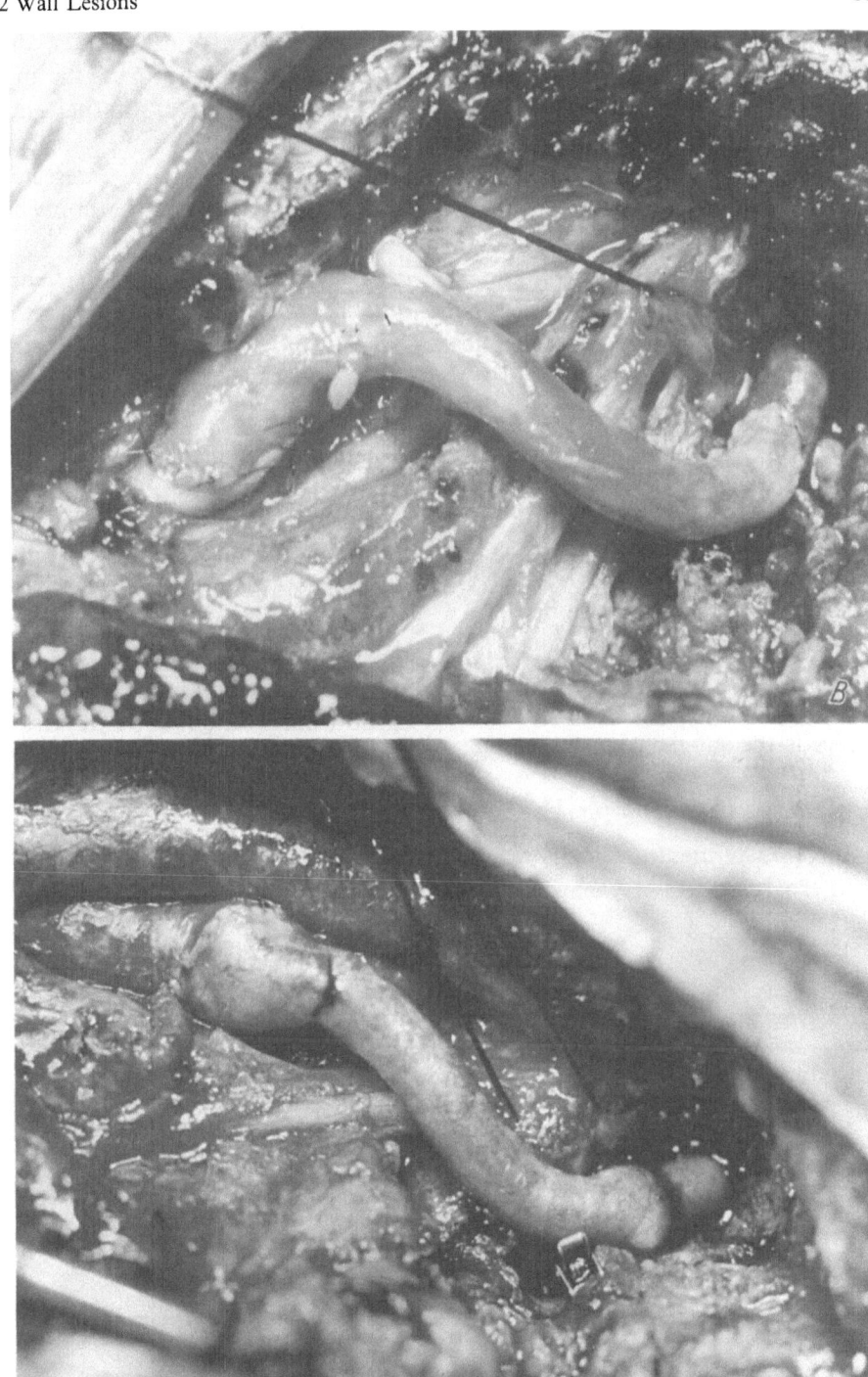

Fig. 69B and C

advantages of giving a vertical course to the graft, and of avoiding clamping of the carotid axis. However, it necessitates an extensive skin incision and a long dissection. Furthermore, it is frequently involved by the same atherosclerotic lesion as the V. A.

Therefore, the common carotid artery is to be preferred in every case, since this vessel affords the best technical possibilities and offers a source of high flow and high pressure into the by-pass. Other implantation sites are acceptable only if there is a major reason to refuse utilization of the common carotid artery:

— significant atherosclerotic involvement or, obviously, occlusion.

— ischemic hazard of clamping. If revascularization is indicated to treat atherosclerotic lesions, the second best choice is the subclavian artery.

b) Transposition onto the V. A.

As previously mentioned, the external or internal carotid artery may be used as a direct source of flow after distal section and mobilization. This might be proposed in case of internal carotid occlusion, but the same objections raised against use of these vessels for proximal graft implantation apply here.

c) Combined Treatment of Carotid and V. A. Lesions

Associated lesions of the internal carotid artery may influence the surgical technique.

Obviously, complete occlusion of the internal carotid artery reinforces the choice of the common carotid artery as the donor vessel, because of minimal risks of clamping in this case.

On the other hand, significant stenosis must be treated in the same surgical stage. According to the level of the carotid bifurcation and the risks of simultaneous clamping of both vessels, two different procedures can be selected.

c—1. Venous graft by-pass implantation on the proximal common carotid

Table 15. V. A. revascularization

Revascularization	hemodynamic ischemia prevention
	bilateral V. A. occlusion
	dominant V. A. occlusion
	bilateral V. A. stenosis
	dominant V. A. stenosis
Revascularization + exclusion	embolic ischemia prevention
	dissection
	aneurysm
	minor V. A. stenosis?
	underlying lesion treatment
	complex A. V. M
	"angiodysplasia"
	hypervascularized tumor
	V. A. embedding tumor

artery in a first step. The carotid-vertebral by-pass is then completed and left patent; following which the carotid artery is clamped above the graft implantation and a routine carotid endarterectomy is performed.

c—2. The second procedure includes primarily, carotid endarterectomy and then proximal implantation of the graft on the carotid arteriotomy.

d) Revascularization plus Exclusion (Table 15)

Since ulcerated atherosclerotic lesions of the V. A. are very rare, this indication for V. A. exclusion is exceptional. Conversely, this is widely used in treatment of other structural lesions in order to prevent embolus migration into the vertebro-basilar circulation. For the same reason, this procedure may be proposed to treat certain forms of tumor or arteriovenous malformations (**Fig. 70**).

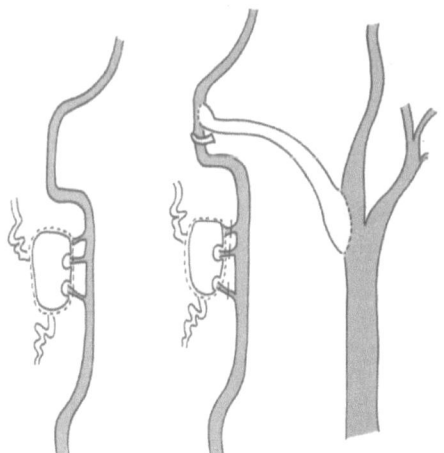

Fig. 70. Principle of treatment of hypervascular or surrounding V. A. lesions: V. A. revascularization distal to the lesion and exclusion of the underlying V. A. by a clip

e) Conclusion

Revascularization of the distal V. A. is therfore essentially realized by common carotid to V. A. venous by-pass. This is the most reliable technique affording high flow and high pressure into the vertebro-basilar system. Other techniques, particularly the use of other donor vessels, have very few indications when the common carotid artery cannot be utilized.

13.2.1.4 Indications of V. A. Revascularization in Atherosclerosis

Patients must be selected with caution, since the natural history of V. A. lesions is not very well documented. Three groups of patients should be considered for revascularization.

a) Significant Stenosis or Occlusion on the Dominant or on Both V. A.'s in Symptomatic Patients

Symptoms may be transient but repeated and disabling, or permanent but moderate, corresponding to sequelae of a vertebro-basilar stroke. In the former situation a marked decrease or disappearance of the transient ischemic symptoms can be expected with revascularization; in the latter, the aim is to prevent secondary deterioration, mainly from new ischemic events.

b) Multiple Carotid and Vertebral Artery Lesions

Simultaneous revascularization of homolateral carotid and vertebral arteries can be proposed in patients with significant lesions on both vessels whether they are symptomatic in one or both territories.

In those patients with multiple bilateral lesions, the brain supply must be considered as a whole; depending on the condition of the Circle of Willis, it may be more useful to revascularize a V. A. than a carotid artery having produced intracranial lesions, even if symptoms are in the carotid territory.

However, distal revascularization of an occluded V. A. in vertebro-basilar asymptomatic patients cannot generally be justified by the fact that since a homolateral carotid stenosis must be treated, the approach can easily be enlarged towards the V. A.

c) Patients at Risk During Carotid Artery Clamping

Preliminary V. A. revascularization may in some cases decrease the risk of carotid artery clamping. For instance, internal carotid and V. A. occlusion on one side associated with controlateral symptomatic internal carotid artery stenosis can be treated by V. A. revascularization before treatment of the controlateral carotid stenosis.

This indication may be peculiar to surgical teams who do not routinely use carotid shunt.

d) What V. A. Lesion Should Be Treated?

In case of bilateral V. A. lesions, only the dominant side should be treated.

If the V. A.'s are equivalent, the choice depends on the severity of the lesion and whether there is a homolateral carotid artery lesion.

e) What Procedure Should Be Chosen?

V. A. surgery suffers from a lack of studies with systematic post-operative control. Doppler scanning studies have proven insufficient to correctly verify proximal V. A. surgery. With digital intravenous angiography it is now easy to obtain a correct assessment of the surgical results. In contrast, distal revascularization must be controlled by arterial injection.

The preferred technique is reimplantation onto the common carotid artery for the first portion of the V. A. (Cormier and Laurian, 1976, Edwards and Mulheim, 1984), and venous graft by-pass between the common carotid artery and the V. A. at the C 1–C 2 level for the third portion (Laurian *et al.*, 1983).

Other techniques and revascularization of the second portion are very rarely indicated.

13.2.2 Revascularization for Non-atherosclerotic Lesions

13.2.2.1 Dissection

Since most V. A. dissections disappear or improve either spontaneously or under medical therapy, surgery must not be decided too early. Repeat angiography after at least 3 months, must previously be performed.

In fact, surgical treatment has very few indications, which are based on several criteria:

— clinical criteria: repetitive neurologic deficits evoking emboli, or progressive worsening,

— radiological data: occlusion of

several distal branches in the vertebro-basilar circulation on angiography and multiple areas of infarction on C.T. scan, equally suggesting emboli.

— Dissection in the form of aneurysm, which generally persists long after its discovery and carries a high risk of embolism,

— etiologic criteria: predisposing external or internal factors (see chapter Wall Lesion).

At present, surgical indications on V.A. dissections are very limited as are those on carotid artery dissections. Persisting aneurysm, dissection of any type with repeated embolic events, and persistent stenoses on multiple cervical vessels with cerebro-vascular insufficiency are the best surgical indications. The preventive treatment of a predisposing factor could be associated with treatment of the V.A. dissection, but better understanding of the role of these factors is needed.

The surgical procedure for dissection is usually exclusion or resection of the lesion, associated with the most appropriate type of V.A. revascularization. Since, a V.A. segment is excluded, a venous graft by-pass implanted beyond the exclusion site is the suitable procedure.

13.2.2.2 Fibromuscular Dysplasia (F.M.D.)

F.M.D. is a disease with various possible forms of evolution. Some cases may remained uncomplicated (Well and Smith, 1982), while others may evolve to dissection or arteriovenous fistula.

Since evolution is unpredictable, surgery must not be undertaken preventively. Consequently, only complications should be treated, in the same way as similar lesions of different origin.

13.3 Arteriovenous Malformations

Treatment of arteriovenous malformations is quite different according to the type of lesion: arteriovenous fistula or angiodysplasia.

Arteriovenous fistulas are now initially treated by endovascular techniques. Surgery is only discussed after failure of the radiological treatment.

Angiodysplasias must be considered as tumors with hypervascularity and invasive extension. Embolization helps reduce the blood supply but cannot achieve a complete cure. Surgery is thus the only curative, but it must not be proposed in every case.

13.3.1 Arteriovenous Fistulas

13.3.1.1 Indications

Some cases obviously need to be treated: arteriovenous fistula with vertebrobasilar insufficiency related to vertebral artery steal, or with cardiac

failure in the infant, or even cases accompanied by a poorly tolerated bruit. On the contrary, low flow fistulas with mild discomfort due to tinnitus do not justify high risk treatment.

In the elderly, embolization can be proposed if the procedure appears sufficiently safe, but surgery should generally not be performed, even if balloon techniques fail to achieve a correct cure. In young patients, treatment of low flow fistulas remains controversial. In no way is there a necessity to obliterate these fistulas while they are stable and the decision for treatment may be postponed until clinical, Doppler and angiographic controls have shown a worsening evolution.

When treatment is decided, surgery is always contemplated only after unsuccessful attempts of embolization.

Failures of endovascular techniques include incomplete occlusion of the fistula, persistent ectasy of the arterial wall at the site of the fistula, and balloon encroachment on the V. A. lumen, leading to narrowing or even occlusion. These failures of radiological techniques are more frequently observed with post-traumatic fistulas because of their particular anatomic features: these are fistulas with false aneurysm. Even if radiological techniques do not achieve correct treatment, they are mandatory before surgery to determine the exact site of the fistula. At a minimum, angiography with selective injection above or below an occluding balloon placed at different levels in the V. A. must be performed.

13.3.1.2 Surgical Technique (Table 16)

The V. A. is first approached above and below the fistula site. The main surgical problem is posed by the venous drainage through the perivertebral venous plexus, which can be impressively hypertrophied. Venous dilatation may also involve the cervical veins and epidural plexus since they communicate with the perivertebral veins. Cervical veins on the way to the V. A. can be ligated. The perivertebral veins must be controlled outside the periosteal sheath. Here, the rule of V. A. control with respect of the periosteal sheath should be even more rigidly adhered to than in other pathologic conditions. After this control has been achieved on both sides of the arterio-venous fistula site, the V. A. is clamped above and below by clips applied while the artery is still within its periosteal sheath. After V. A. clamping the draining veins largely collapse. Opening of the periosteal sheath can thus be done with easy venous control. The veins are coagulated progressively, upwards and downwards towards the

Table 16. Arteriovenous malformations

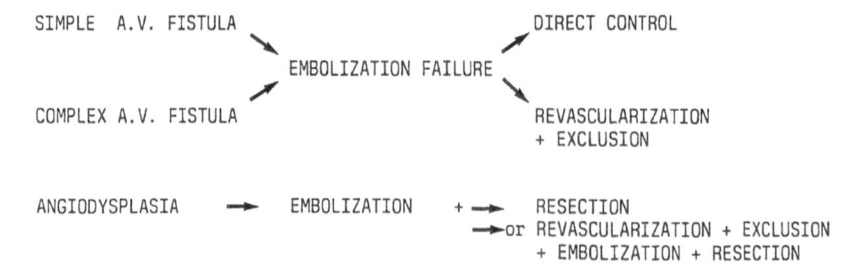

fistula site. Brief release of one clip helps confirm the site of communication, which usually consists of a small hole on the V. A. wall. An X suture point is generally sufficient to occlude it and to definitively close the fistula. Clips are then removed, allowing verification of correct closure. If necessary, complementary sutures are made.

13.3.1.3 Particular Forms

a) Arteriovenous Fistula Through a Radicular Branch

In some cases, the V. A. does not directly inject the fistula which is injected after a short segment of radicular or muscular branches.

Surgical approach to this form is identical to direct V. A. fistula, but control and closure are more easily achieved, by simple ligation of the collateral branches flush with the outer wall of the V. A. (**Fig. 71**).

b) False Aneurysm and Large Fistula

These forms are always of traumatic origin, as they imply a large defect in the arterial wall.

Correct repair cannot be achieved by direct approach unless the V. A. is definitively occluded in a deliberate

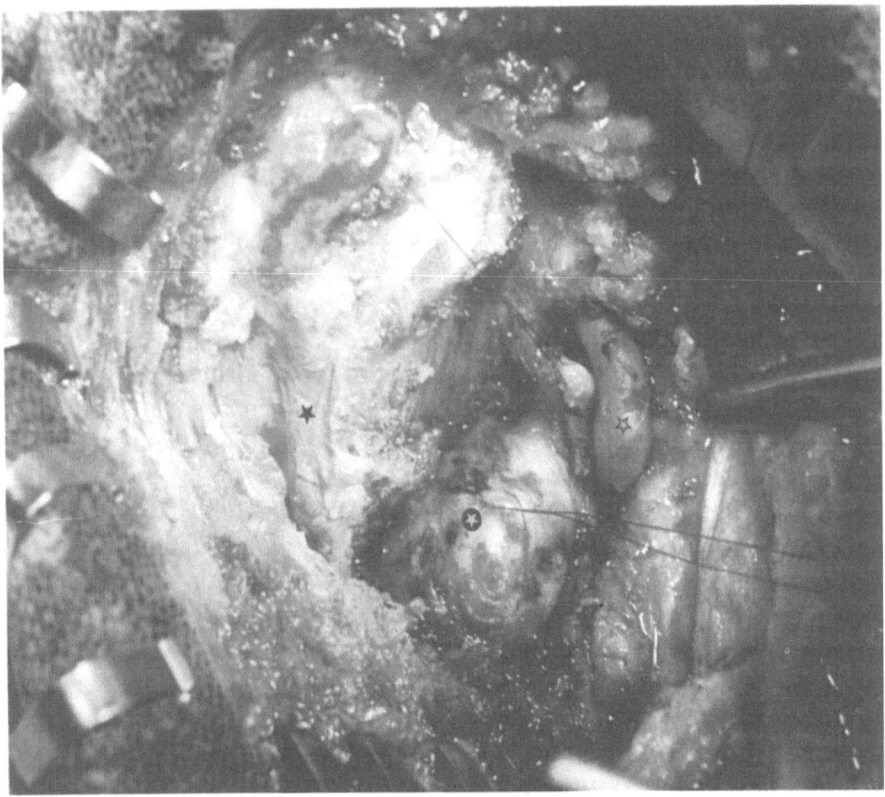

Fig. 71. Operative view of an arteriovenous malformation at C1–C2 presenting as a false aneurysm ● fed by 2 V. A. branches ☆ and one occipital artery branch ★

fashion. If this is acceptable there is no need for surgery, since balloon occlusion is far easier and safer to perform; moreover, it permits testing the tolerance of V. A. occlusion before definitive closure. Fistulas on hypoplastic V. A.'s in old patients are more likely to be treated in this way. In other cases, V. A. flow must be preserved by revascularization distal to the fistula; thereafter, the V. A. and the arteriovenous fistula can be occluded below the anastomosis.

c) Multiple Fistulas

Direct surgical approach in the case of multiple fistulas may be a long and difficult procedure, necessitating tedious progressive control of a long segment of the V. A. Distal revascularization associated with exclusion of the underlying V. A. is often a better choice. Since the V. A. still feeds the fistulas, no thrombosis occurs and selective embolization can be performed later.

13.3.2 Angiodysplasia

13.3.2.1 Indications

Angiodysplasia is a regional malformation involving various structures (muscles, vertebrae, ...). The request for resection of a cervical localization generally comes from cosmetic problems. More rarely, patients present with vertebro-basilar insufficiency or spinal cord symptoms. In the latter conditions, treatment seems reasonable. In contrast, if neurologic symptoms are lacking, the benefits or surgery are quite debatable. The cosmetic improvement is countered by the obliged resection of the muscles involved by the angiodysplasia. If complete removal of all the angiomatous tissue cannot be achieved, which is often unpredictable, evolution of remnants of the malformation may be dramatically precipitated with disastrous results. Correct assessment of the technical difficulties and of the muscular defects expected after resection must be made and discussed with the patient. It is sometimes wiser to refuse surgery than to give the hope of esthetic improvement and get the opposite.

13.3.2.2 Surgical Technique

If treatment is nevertheless decided, or required because of neurologic impairment, resection is performed after embolization of all supply from the external carotid and subclavian arteries. In extensive forms or those mainly supplied by the V. A., distal revascularization associated with V. A. occlusion and embolization may be discussed. This form of treatment without surgical resection has not yet been performed, but it is likely that it cannot obtain complete disappearance of all the arterio-venous shunts; if it did, surgical resection could be avoided (**Table 16**).

Surgical resection is conducted in the same way as for a tumor. The V. A. is controlled below and above the inferior and superior limits of the angiodysplasia. Then control of the V. A. is progressively carried out all along the involved segment. Collateral branches supplying the angiodysplasia are divided. At this point, vascularity is highly reduced and the angiodysplasia can be dissected out and removed "en-bloc".

However, the peripheral limits of the angiomatous mass are frequently not well defined. Sometimes not one but several juxtaposed angiomatous masses are found. Therefore, it may be difficult to be sure that excision is complete. Intra operative angiography is the only way to ascertain the quality of re-section. If intraoperative angiography is not available, a post-operative control must be systematically performed. Visualization of persisting arterio-venous shunts necessitates comple-mentary treatment by embolization or re-operation.

13.4 Tumor

13.4.1 Principles

The role of V. A. surgery in tumor removal can be deduced from the two ways in which a tumor can be related to the V. A.:

a) Proximity of the V. A.

The tumor may be flush with, displace, or compress the V. A., inducing variable degrees of stenosis; at maximum it may surround the vessel (embedded V. A.). Ideal results are achieved when the tumor is removed as completely as possible with V. A. flow restored or preserved. This goal can be reached safely if the V. A. is controlled in the initial steps of the procedure.

b) Vascular Supply from the V. A.

The tumor may receive part or all of its vascularization from V. A. branches. Any procedure dividing the vascular collaterals supplying the tumor before its removal requires control of the V. A. and its branches. Hypervascularized tumors are obviously more likely to benefit from this control.

13.4.2 Technique

Two techniques of V. A. surgery can be used in the treatment of tumoral lesions (**Table 17**).

13.4.2.1 Revascularization

Tumoral resection may necessitate, or be better achieved with, sacrifice of the

Table 17. Tumor

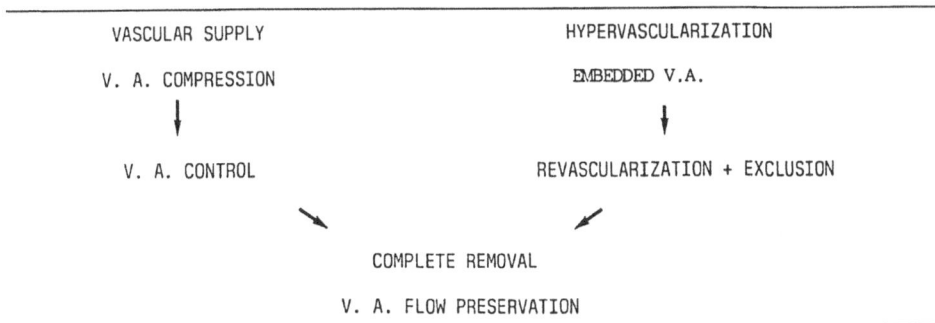

V.A. by any method of exclusion: clipping, ligation or balloon occlusion. This is mainly the case with an embedded V.A. or in hypervascularized tumors. In these tumors, exclusion may be performed to allow safe embolization of the underlying V.A.

If the V.A. is small, its occlusion should have no consequences as long as no anterior radiculo-medullary branch arises from it. If such a branch is identified, the V.A. flow must be preserved.

In the case of a large or dominant V.A. that must be occluded, revascularization of the V.A. is performed beyond the occlusion site. The technique is exactly the same as for the treatment of V.A. wall lesions (see chapter Wall Lesions). The elective site for distal revascularization is at the C 1–C 2 level. The feeding vessel for proximal implantation can be any part of the carotid axis, but, the internal carotid or the common carotid artery are to be preferred because of their larger diameter.

V.A. exclusion is associated with revascularization by clipping the V.A. just below the distal implantation of the by-pass graft, immediately allowing high flow through the by-pass and thus in the vertebro-basilar system.

Patency of the graft and its ability to supply the vertebro-basilar system are angiographically controlled. If the V.A. vascularizes the tumor, no retrograde thrombosis occurs after V.A. exclusion, thus V.A. embolization is possible. In the case of a poorly or non vascular tumor, thrombosis usually occurs in the following days or weeks. This possibility of delayed thrombosis must be taken into account if surgical

removal of the tumor is planned soon after V.A. exclusion or in the same surgical stage. In the case of persistent flow in the V.A., tumor resection must be preceded by control and ligation of the proximal V.A. below the tumor.

13.4.2.2 Direct V.A. Control

The most common technique is to directly control the V.A. and free it out from the tumor before removal of the latter.

The V.A. is approached below and above the tumor. Its control is realized after resection of the anterior branches of the transverse processes but care is taken not to open the periosteal sheath. At the tumoral level, the periosteal sheath is usually interrupted, with compression of the venous plexus, which is consequently under pressure. Therefore, injury to the periosteal sheath by too rapid mobilization of the tumor can lead to severe venous bleeding that may be difficult to arrest. The best method is thus to control the V.A. inside its periosteal sheath on both sides and at a distance from the tumor and then to progress towards it. Before starting to free the V.A. from the tumor, the periosteal sheath is opened and the venous plexus is collapsed using bipolar coagulation. At this time, the V.A. can be safely separated from the tumor and mobilized out if necessary. If an anterior radiculo-medullary branch is known to emerge near the tumor, V.A. mobilization should be as limited as possible, to avoid any stretching of this branch.

V.A. mobilization out of the tumor bed is facilatated by prior opening of the transverse canal above and below, thus avoiding any compression of the V. A. on the transverse processes. To summarize, tumor removal is preceded by V. A. control, which is done stepwise, beginning at a distance from both tumoral extremities and progressing toward the tumor.

An ultrasonic aspirator is a useful adjunct, particularly in poorly limited tumors closely related to the V. A.

a) Tumor of the First Portion of the V. A.

At this level, the V. A. is only one of the elements to control before tumoral resection; among the others, the subclavian artery, brachial plexus, phrenic nerve and thoracic duct are the most important. In extensive tumors, the lung apex must also be freed out and this may necessitate a complementary approach through thoracotomy.

The first portion of the V. A. is relatively mobile and often markedly displaced by tumor without significant compression. Notable exceptions are tumors of the upper part which may stretch the V. A. in bayonet fashion on the transverse process of C 6.

In the first portion of the V. A., there is no venous plexus, but usually two veins, which are ligated on each side of the tumor.

b) Tumor of Second Portion of the V. A. (Fig. 72)

In contrast, the V. A. is the main concern at this level. The nerve roots are also frequently involved, requiring their control as well.

Initial exposure of the V. A. and control of the venous plexus on both sides of the tumor is the basic principle. For a tumor extending up to the C2–C3 level, distal control of the V. A. is preferrentially performed first, between C 1 and C 2, before opening the C 2 transverse foramen.

An anterior radiculo-medullary branch is most frequently encountered in the lower part of this second portion.

c) Tumor of the Third Portion of the V. A.

Here, the accessory spinal nerve must be exposed and respected.

Above C 1, the usually well-developed venous plexus may present some difficulties.

The most troublesome problem is raised by tumors extending up to the foramen magnum, thus leaving no room for distal control of the V. A. If distal control is indispensable, it can be done intracranially after opening the posterior fossa. This implies penetration of the subarachnoidal space, which should not be accepted too easily since it increases the risk of post-operative complications. Furthermore, dissection of the V. A. at its dural penetration is somewhat difficult, mainly because of the continuity between the periosteal sheath and the dura mater.

This problem of distal control is well demonstrated by hour-glass tumors with both intracranial and cervical components.

A low origin of the P. I. C. A. must have been previously identified as well as other possible but less frequent anomalies in the V. A. course.

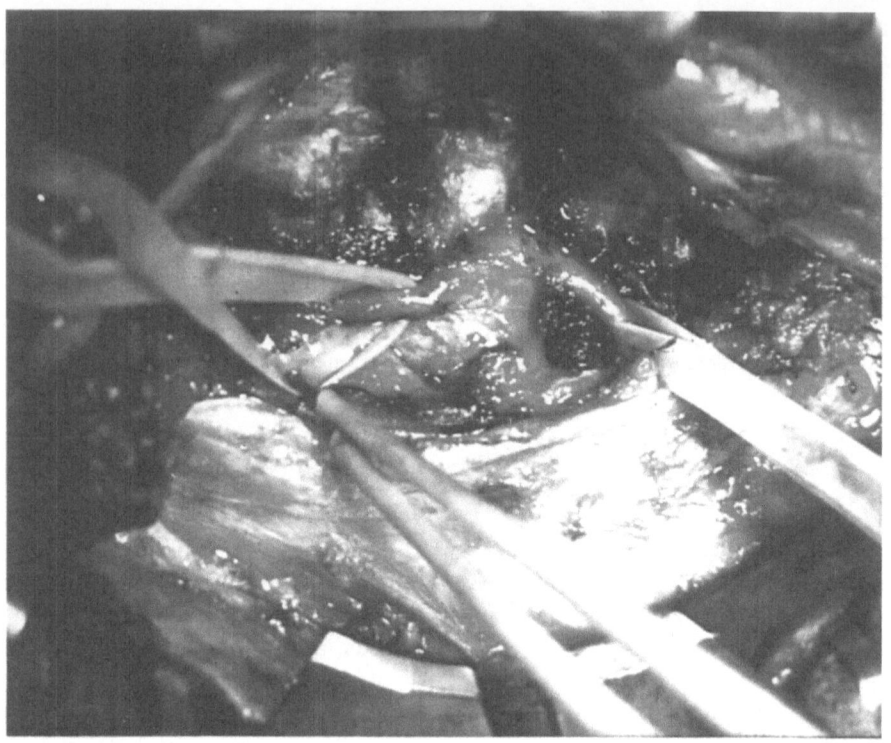

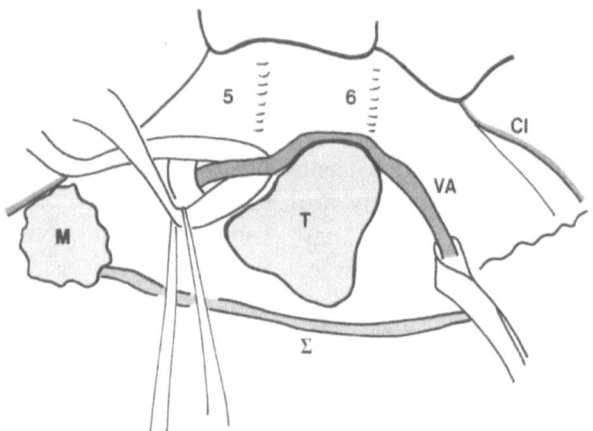

Fig. 72. Extradural hour-glass neurinoma before and after removal (C 5–C 6 level)

13.4.2.3 Particular Extensions

a) Hour-Glass Intraspinal Extension

Tumoral prolongation into the spinal canal through the intervertebral space is a common feature. There are different ways to deal with these tumors. However, based on the principle that it is preferable to suppress tumor vascularization before removal, and since the tumor is supplied by the V. A. and

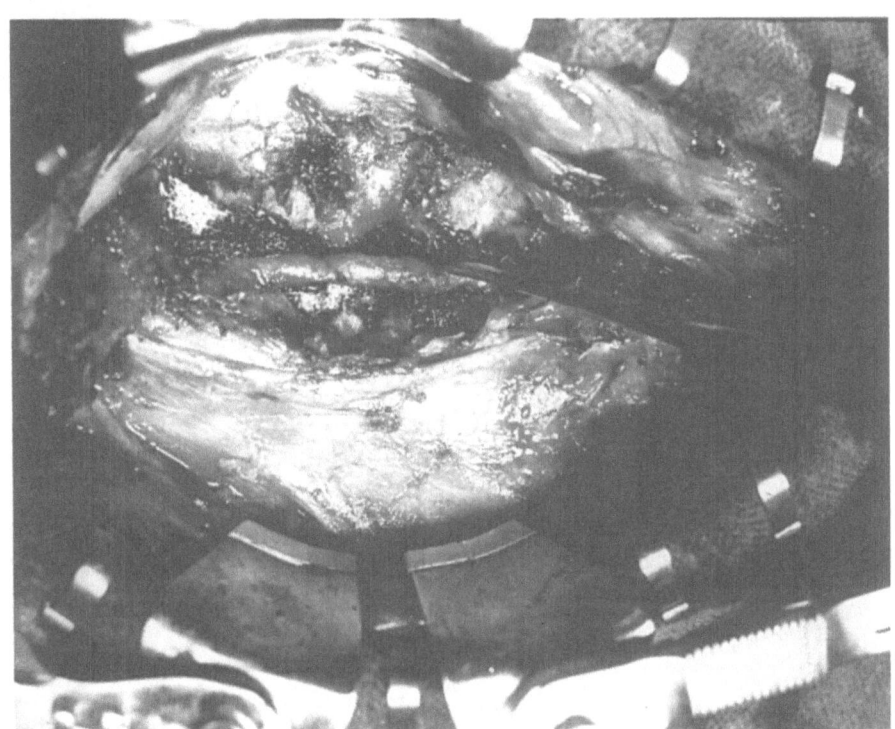

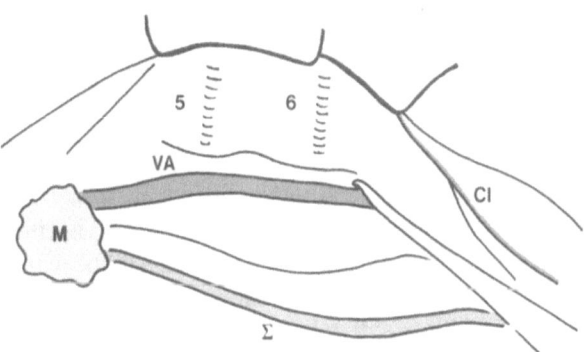

Fig. 72

other cervical arteries, it is consequently logical to attack the extra vertebral
component of these hour-glass tumors
intitially.

a—1. Resection through only the lateral
anterior approach (**Fig. 73**).

This is possible through the intervertebral foramen even in the case of
important intraspinal extension. The

limiting factors are adherences between
the tumor and the dural sac, intradural
extension, and certain locations of the
intraspinal prolongation as discussed
below:

— adherences between tumor and
dural sac. As the tumor removal progresses blindly toward the dural sac, it
may be hazardous to mobilize the

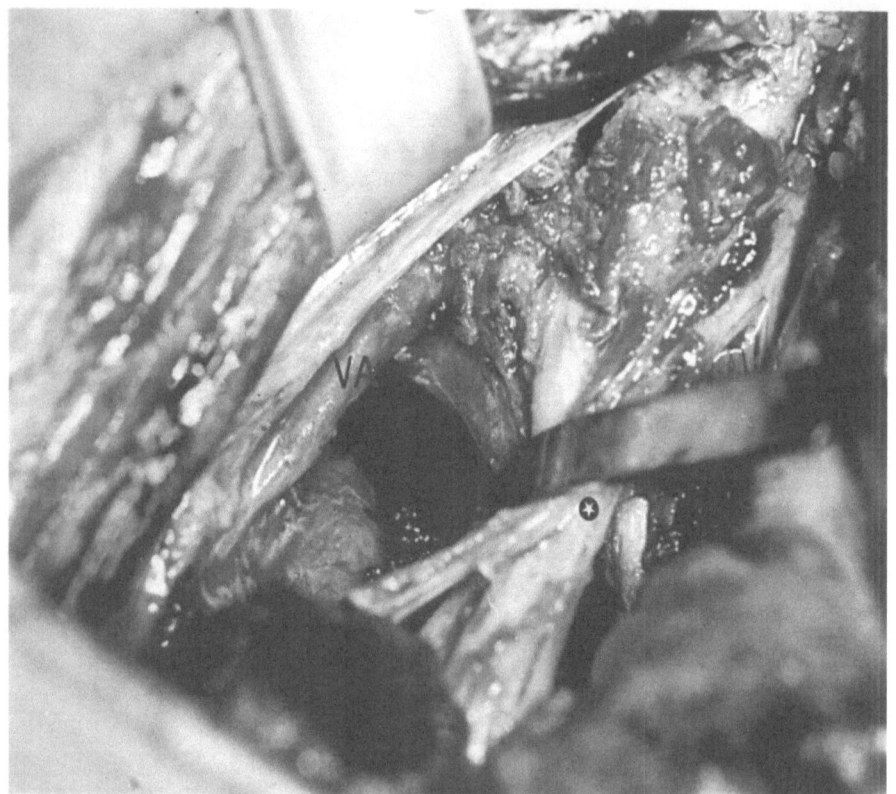

Fig. 73. Hour-glass extradural sarcoma at C5–C6 after removal through the naturally enlarged intervertebral foramen. Notice the brachial plexus retracted laterally ⊕

tumor, particularly if it is strongly adherent to the dura. The safest way is to follow the spinal nerve roots sheath until the dural sac is reached. At this time, either the dura can be adequately controlled and the removal is undertaken, or adherences are too firm and this part of the tumor is left in place and will be removed through a different approach,

— intradural tumoral extensions cannot safely be removed by the lateral anterior approach even with the use of the microscope, since the spinal cord is not correctly visualized behind the tumor,

— location of the intraspinal prolongation. Even if the dural sac is markedly displaced to the controlateral side by the tumor, there is no reason not to attempt its removal, but if the tumor spreads around the dural sac, particularly over its anterior and posterior surfaces beyond the midline, complete resection through the intervertebral foramen cannot reasonably be expected.

Removal through the intervertebral foramen may be facilitated by its enlargement, although the tumor itself may already have sufficiently eroded it. If necessary, enlargement is realized with a rongeur or drill on the anterior edge, removing part of the postero-lateral aspect of the vertebral bodies (Kamano *et al.*, 1980, Hakuba *et al.*, 1984, George and Laurian, 1985–1986). a—2. Resection through two combined surgical approaches.

Intraspinal prolongations can be removed by a complementary posterior approach through laminectomy. This obviously implies two different procedures with different positions, except at the level of the third portion of the V. A. At other levels, an initial lateral anterior approach is performed, with removal of the tumor as far as possible, through the intervertebral foramen. Thereafter, laminectomy is performed, with or without opening the dura depending on whether there is intradural extension. The two procedures may be performed in the same surgical stage so that if severe spinal cord compression exists, it can be released without delay. Here it should be stressed that removal of the intravertebral prolongation is greatly facilitated due to suppression of the vascular supply in the initial procedure.

a—3. Resection through only the posterior approach.

Above C 2, both the lateral anterior and posterior approach allow resection of the extraspinal tumor with V. A. control and removal of the intraspinal tumor through laminectomy. But in case of intradural extension, the posterior approach must be chosen, since only then, can correct control of the spinal cord be obtained. Therefore, the choice of approach implies a correct pre-operative assessment of tumor extension.

b) Hour-Glass Intracranial Extension

A lateral anterior approach affords, in most cases sufficient access for simultaneous exposure of both the cervical and the intracranial components of these tumors.

There are two main types of tumor with this feature: 1. Petrous bone tumors, of which the glomus jugulare tumor is the best example, extending through the jugulare foramen; and 2. intradural posterior fossa tumors, extending through the foramen magnum and/or the jugulare foramen.

In the first type, the lateral anterior approach extended over the mastoïd process and around the ear, in the lateral decubitus position, permits complete exposure of the lesion. If there is an intradural extension, it is advisable not to remove it at the same time, even though it might be technically possible. In this case, three surgical techniques are associated: cervical approach with V. A. control, infratemporal approach with facial nerve, sigmoid sinus and internal carotid artery control, and posterior fossa opening with brain stem and cerebellum exposure. Each has particular risks, which are cumulative if they are associated, particularly the risks of infectious complications and C. S. F. leak from air cell opening.

The second type of tumor can also be removed in the one surgical approach which may be the lateral anterior approach or the posterior approach. The first has the advantage of giving access to cervical prolongation, whatever its lower level, as well as to the posterior fossa without risk of air embolism. The second is limited inferiorly to the C 2 level and, if, a sitting position is chosen, air embolism is possible; but it gives better exposure of the intra-dural cervical part and the posterior fossa midline. Consequently, the lateral anterior route is preferred in the case of tumors located laterally and anteriorly in the posterior fossa and cervical area. Combined with sigmoid sinus division and an infratemporal approach, it gives fairly good access to the inferior clivus and the anterior part of the foramen magnum. On the contrary, for tumors developed posteriorly in the posterior fossa with cervical intradural exten-sions, the posterior route is a better choice.

c) Vertebral Body Involvement

By either the lateral anterior route or the anterior approach, the vertebral body can be resected in part or totality and any technique of bone grafting or arthrodesis may be performed there-after. The anterior approach gives a better view of the vertebral body beyond the midline, but the lateral anterior approach is safer, since work is done outside the jugulo-carotid track in a larger field.

d) Lung Apex Involvement

With the lateral anterior approach extended laterally, it is possible to follow any tumoral extension down to the first rib, which can be resected if necessary as in the treatment of the thoracic outlet syndrome. This re-quires control of the subclavian artery, the sympathetic elements, the thoracic duct and the lower nerve roots of the brachial plexus. Below the first rib, a complementary thoracic approach through thoracotomy is necessary. It is performed secondarily but in the same surgical stage.

13.5 External Compression

13.5.1 Principles

A clearly established relation between vertebro-basilar insufficiency and external compression of the V. A. justifies surgery to relieve it.

If a dynamic factor is present, the same head and neck movement as the one producing symptoms, must also induce the V. A. compression on angiography. Permanent external compression may explain symptoms of vertebro-basilar insufficiency if both V. A.'s are involv-ed or if it occurs on the dominant V. A.

Treatment of external compression of the V. A. varies according to its cause. In cases of cervical dislocation or spinal instability, reduction and fixation is generally sufficient.

In exceptional cases of compression at several levels, revascularization of the distal V. A. above the higher level of stenosis may be discussed. Exclusion of the V. A., flush with the inferior limit of the by-pass graft, is to be associated to afford higher flow through the anas-

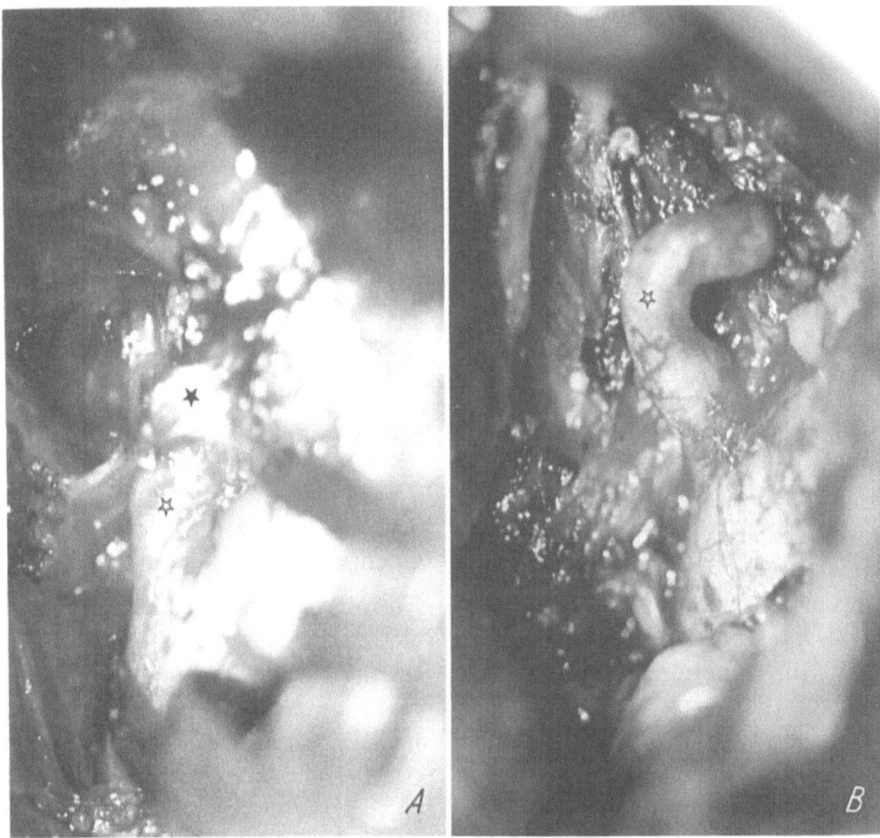

Fig. 74. V. A. external compression by the sympathetic nerve ★ crossing the anterior aspect of the juxta-ostial V. A. ☆ Operative view before (**A**) and after (**B**) compression release

tomosis and to prevent against the small but real possibility of embolism.

In other cases, the compressive agent itself must be resected by a direct approach (**Fig. 74**).

13.5.1.1 Spondylotic Compression

V. A. compression from an osteophytic spur may be released in two ways (**Table 18**).

a) One method of decompression is directed towards the osteophyte, without giving particular attention to the V. A. It is realized by an anterior approach with interbody graft fusion. This technique does not achieve complete liberation of the V. A., but for the authors supporting it (Bauer *et al.*, 1961), it is sufficient to suppress the stenosis. Furthermore the mobility of the two related vertebrae is limited by the fusion, alleviating postural interference. Lastly, intervertebral fusion prevents recurrence of the osteophyte.

b) The second method is, in contrast, directed towards the V. A., with the main objective of freeing it. In our opinion, the lateral anterior approach gives the best access to achieve this goal. The transverse foramen is opened

Table 18. Spondylotic compression

Interbody graft fusion	V. A. direct control
Bone graft	osteophyte resection foramen opening tissue scar resection
Vertebral mobility limitation Recurrence prevention	direct V. A. decompression sympath. N. irritation alleviation

above and below the level of compression which may be considered sufficient in the case of postural compression.

However, correct technique also requires resection of the osteophytes, with small rongeurs or an air drill. This implies previous control of the V. A. kept within its periosteal sheath so as to protect the vessel during the manoeuvers of osteophyte removal. This control may be rather difficult because of frequent and tight adherences between the periosteum and the osteophyte.

For most authors, complete freeing of the V. A. requires opening of the periosteal sheath in order to resect the connective tissue scar surrounding the V. A., which is thought to play a role in the genesis of symptoms by sympathetic irritation (see chapter External Compression). The microscope may be useful at this time to cope with the venous plexus and to avoid injury of the arterial wall.

13.5.1.2 Other Causes of V. A. Compression

Fibrous bands and ligamento-muscular elements are divided and detached from the periosteal sheath, to which they are more or less adherent. Usually the nearest transverse foramen above the compression which may be the lowest in the case of compression of the first portion of the V. A. must be opened. The anterior branch of the transverse process below the compression generally acts in such a way that it imposes a bayonet course on the V. A. Therefore, simple resection of the fibrous band or of the longus colli tendon would suppress only one of the two stenosing agents. Correct decompression frequently requires resection or opening of one or two transverse foramina.

13.5.2 Conclusion

Management of any external compression of the V. A. can be compared with that of sciatica. Just as in surgery for sciatica, every element participating in compression must 1. be recognized before surgery to correctly establish the indication and then 2. be identified during surgery to relieve its compressive effect by the most adequate method. For instance, unroofing of the transverse foramina on both sides of the compression site is frequently a useful adjunct to removal of the primary compressive agent.

13.6 Intraoperative Embolization

Approach and control of the V. A. may be used for direct puncture for catheterization when this is not possible by the conventional method.

There are two reasons for failure of V. A. catheterism through femoral or brachial puncture. One is occlusion of the artery, either spontaneous or following surgical ligation; the other is tortuosity or plicature of the vessel. This latter reason is now exceptional due to recent progress in interventional neuroradiology using tiny balloon-tipped catheters.

Another indication for direct surgical exposure for V. A. catheterization is to permit the use of a large catheter.

Sundt *et al.* (1980) and Smith *et al.* (1983) exposed the V. A. at the base of the cranium to insert a balloon catheter for angioplastic dilatation of the intracranial V. A. and the basilar trunk. We used a similar technique to perform embolizations with solid particles. These solid particles require a larger catheter than I. B. C. embolization, and because of its size, this catheter is less easily manipulated. Shortening of the catheter by using a point of entry as close as possible to the lesion may allow an embolization which otherwise would be impossible.

For maximum shortening of the catheter, the V. A. is best exposed and punctured above C1. In this way, the V. A. loops at C2 and C1 are avoided, and the catheter may be led straight to the basilar trunk.

If a proximal thrombosis or kinking is the reason for direct puncture, the level of C1–C2 is preferred for easier exposure: however above this level, one loop remains in the transverse foramen of C1 and one above the arch of the atlas.

Finally, if a cervical spinal cord lesion is to be embolized, the level of puncture is chosen after discussion with the neuroradiologist. It is usually better not to expose the V. A. just at the level of the lesion but rather at some distance from it.

Whatever the level, the V. A. must be completely controlled with opening of its periosteal sheath and coagulation of the venous plexus.

Puncture through the periosteal sheath would cause difficulties in closing the puncture hole after the procedure, and carry the risk of a post-operative arteriovenous fistula.

Prior to puncture, 7/0 polypropylene monofilament suture is passed around the chosen catheterization site, so that it can be closed easily at the end of the procedure. A U or X stitch can be prepared; but it is more useful to realize a purse string suture, which allows tightening the arterial wall arounds the catheter during the procedure. This avoids any blood oozing in a field which cannot easily be controlled during the embolization. The field is usually packed with wet sponges and the catheter fixed by a 2/0 suture on the medial aspect of the S. C. M. muscle. Since this catheter is used to introduce the embolizing catheter, all subsequent manipulations are done out of the field by the neuroradiologist.

14. PERSONAL EXPERIENCE

Since we directed our interest to V. A. surgery, seven years ago, we have performed 151 operations on the cervical V. A.

Table 19 lists types of lesions for which this surgery was indicated. V. A. wall lesions and tumors were the two principal indications. The other possible indications (A. V. M., external compression, trauma) were both less commonly observed and far less frequently considered for surgery.

Table 19. Personal series

	Proposed for surgery	Accepted for surgery
Wall lesion	(90)	(75)
atherosclerosis	71	71
dissection, dysplasia	19	4
Tumor	(59)	(54)
tumor	58	53
infection	1	1
External compression	(17)	(6)
osteophyte	11	2
trauma	4	2
others	2	2
Arteriovenous malformation	(33)	(9)
spontaneous	16	3
traumatic	13	2
angiodysplasia	4	4
Trauma	(22)	(1)
external compression	4	2
arteriovenous fistula	13	2
dissection	4	0
laceration	1	1
Interventional radiology	(6)	(6)
embolization	5	5
catheter removal	1	1
Total	227	151

Table 20. Type of surgery

	Wall lesion	tumor	A. V. M.	Others
Revascularization	71	2	1	0
Direct control	4	53	8	12

Table 21. Level of surgery

	Wall lesion	Tumor	A. V. M.	Others	Total
1st Portion	47	11	0	2	60
2nd Portion	1	15	6	5	27
3rd Portion	27	28	3	6	64

Table 20 shows the type of surgery applied to each group of lesions. Revascularization was principally but not exclusively, proposed for treatment of V. A. wall lesions. Direct surgical control of the V. A. was realized in the other cases.

The levels at which the V. A. was approached are listed in **Table 21**. A marked predominance is noted for the first and third portions. For the first portion of the V. A., this is due to the high frequency of atherosclerotic stenosis at the V. A. ostium, since proximal V. A. reimplantation is the usual treatment. The incidence of surgery on the third portion is due to distal V. A. revascularizations and tumors which have a marked predominance at this level.

In the entire series, mortality was limited to one case: a patient who died two days after surgery from a Sylvian infarct. The patient had been operated for a hemangiopericytoma at the level of the second portion of the V. A., without any technical or anesthetic complication. No clear explanation was found for this accident. There was no cardiac anomaly or carotid atherosclerotic lesion which could have been the source of a cerebral embolism.

Morbidity was also very low, if we exclude the frequent occurrence of two incidents: a transient Horner's syndrome whatever the level at which surgery is performed, and an almost obligatory hypoesthesia or anesthesia in the second cervical nerve territory after surgical approach to the third portion. One post-operative hematoma required re-operation three days after a distal V. A. revascularization. It was thought to be secondary to excessive neck movements with subsequent distension of the suture at the distal graft implantation site.

Painful tension of the S. C. M. muscle

for two months was observed in one case, probably due to irritation of the accessory spinal nerve.

Lymph accumulation after approach to the proximal V. A. was noted in 4 cases; this disappeared progressively and spontaneously in two weeks to two months. In two other cases, lymph oozing through the suture line required maintenance of post-operative drainage until drying of the skin suture (up to five days).

14.1 Wall Lesions

Atherosclerotic lesions are the most frequent structural lesions encountered on the V. A., and the most frequently treated by surgery. In our surgical series, all but four wall lesions were atherosclerotic stenosis or occlusion (**Table 22**). In addition, there were four cases of atherosclerotic occlusion in which V. A. revascularization at C 1–C 2 level was attempted but was not possible, due to insufficient caliber of the V. A.

Table 22. Wall lesion

Atherosclerosis*	(67)
stenosis	34
occlusion	33
Others	(4)
aneurysm	3
dissection	1
* Approached but not revascularized	(4)
Total	75

14.1.1 Clinical Background

In the last three years, 371 patients with various symptoms of cerebral ischemia were referred directly to the department of Neurosurgery of Lariboisière Hospital in Paris.

Among these, 120 cases were attributable to the vertebro-basilar territory. 24 cases were not investigated because the patient's neurologic and/or general condition was too poor.

96 were completely explored with Doppler, ultrasound, angiographic and cardiac investigations:

— 26 had negative results: either no or insignificant anomalies on angiography, with normal cardiac investigations,

— in 59 cases, angiography demonstrated a significant lesion, i. e. occlusion, greater than 75% stenosis, or evidence of a dissecting hematoma or fibromuscular dysplasia,

— cardiac lesions considered likely to be the source of cerebral emboli were discovered in 11 cases (**Table 23**).

These cases were referred after ischemic events of various types (transient: T. I. A., or permanent and more or less regressive: stroke) and locations (brainstem, cerebellum, occipital lobe and spinal cord). **Table 24** indicates the relative frequency of each, with the corresponding results of the cardiovascular investigations.

Table 23. V. B. ischemia. Investigations

				Stenosis	N = 23
		Angiography	N = 59	Occlusion	N = 29
Positive	N = 70			Dis. dys.	N = 7
		Cardiac inv.	N = 11		
Negative	N = 26				

Dis. dys.: Dissection and fibromuscular dysplasia. Cardiac inv.: Cardiac investigations.

Table 24. V. B. ischemia. Clinical datas

	Angiography				Cardiac investigations
	ST	OCC	DISS	—	
T. I. A. N = 35	8	12	4	10	1
Stroke N = 61					
brain stem	8	12	3	8	3
cerebellum	4	4	—	3	2
occipital	2	1	—	5	5
spinal cord	1	—	—	—	—
	23	29	7	26	11

ST: stenosis; OCC: occlusion; DISS: dissection of dysplasia; —: no or non significant anomaly.

Investigations performed to search the possible cause of a vertebro-basilar ischemic event were thus positive in 72% of the cases, which is comparable to the 75% positive investigations for carotid ischemia in the same series.

Embolism of cardiac origin is slightly more frequently suggested in carotid ischemia than in vertebro-basilar ischemia, 24 and 15% respectively. Finally, among the cases with positive angiography, stenosis is more common than occlusion in carotid ischemia, in contrast to what is seen in vertebro-basilar ischemia. In carotid ischemia, stenosis accounts for 60% of the cases with positive angiographic investigations, while in vertebro-basilar ischemia, it represents only 39%. Moreover, this predominance of occlusion in vertebro-basilar ischemia is observed not only with stroke but also in cases with T. I. A.

Therefore, since reliable surgical techniques for V. A. revascularization exist, complete investigations for any type of vertebro-basilar ischemia are at least as important as for carotid ischemia.

The higher frequency of occlusion discovered after vertebro-basilar ischemia tends to confirm that emboli from ulcerated stenosis are less likely to occur from the vertebral than from the carotid arteries. Conversely, a hemodynamic mechanism can be more frequently incriminated in the vertebral circulation. As expected (see chapter Pathophysiology), embolism of cardiac origin was essentially observed in occipital stroke (5 of 8 cases of occipital strokes and 5 of 11 cases of ischemia of cardiac origin). Eight cases in this series, were considered for surgery and treated by V. A. revascularization. The remaining cases were treated conservatively for various reasons: unilateral lesion, lesion on the minor V. A., associated extracranial and intracranial lesions, spontaneous healing of dissection, poor general condition of the patient. Some with associated carotid and vertebral artery lesions were treated surgically on the carotid lesions.

The 63 other cases treated surgically on the V. A. were either directly referred from another center for surgical treatment after demonstration of a significant lesion on angiography or are cases treated in our hospital prior to 1983.

14.1.2 Surgical Series

14.1.2.1 Non-atherosclerotic Lesions

Only four of 20 cases of non atherosclerotic lesions were treated surgically:
— Nine dissecting hematomas, more or less regressive under medical therapy.
— Three aneurysms of various origin.

— Nine cases with angiographic aspect characteristic of fibromuscular dysplasia (including one with a dissecting hematoma) (**Figs. 75, 76** and **77**).

a) Dissection

Among the nine cases with dissecting hematoma, one presented with occlu-

Table 25. V. A. dissection

No.	Sex	Age	Etiology	Lesion and localization	Surgery
1	f	46	Sp	ST C1–C2 bilat	–
2	m	49	T	ST + An C6–C7	–
3	f	30	Sp	ST C2–C6 + AVM cerebel.	–
4	f	40	Sp	ST C4–C5 bilat + ICA	+R
5	m	43	T	O C4–C7	–
6	m	35	T	ST C1–C2 bilat	–
7	f	52	T	ST C3–C7	–
8	f	40	Sp	ST C3–C4	–
9	m	34	FMD	O C4–C7	–
10	m	59	T	An C3	+R
11	m	42	Sp	An C1	+R

Etiology: T: traumatic, Sp: spontaneous, FMD: fibromuscular dysplasia. Lesion: ST: stenosis, O: occlusion, An: aneurysm. Surgery: R: revascularization.

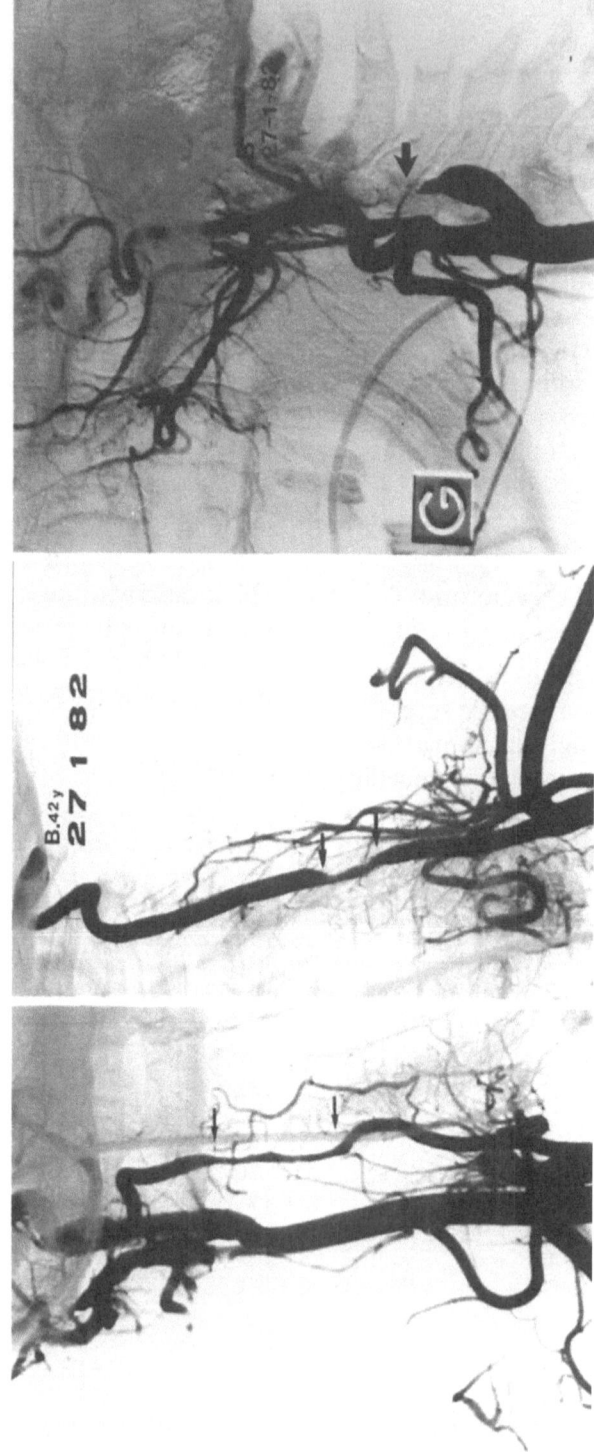

Fig. 75. Spontaneous dissection of both V. A.'s and the left internal carotid artery. V. A. stenosis in the transverse portion and internal carotid artery occlusion. Common carotid to V. A. at C1–C2 venous graft with V. A. exclusion on the left side

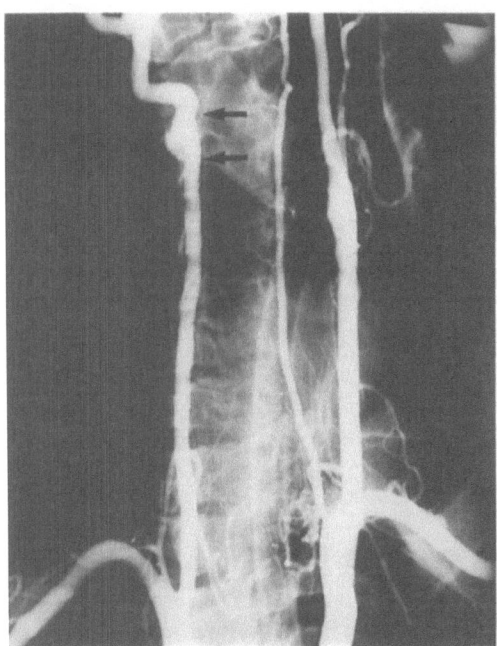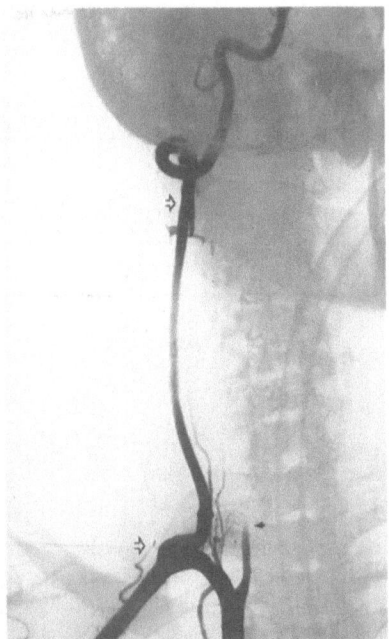

Fig. 76. Dissecting aneurysm at C 3 of traumatic origin. Left: before treatment. Right: revascularization from the subclavian artery plus exclusion. Note the partial thrombosis of the V. A. (black arrow) under the clip

sion, in all probability related to fibromuscular dysplasia, since the V. A. controlaterally and ipsilaterally below the occlusion showed characteristic angiographic features. Minor cervical trauma was found in the recent history of four patients; in the other four, no explanation could be given.

Only one patient went to surgery; she presented with bilateral V. A. stenosis and an internal carotid artery occlusion with no regression during three months observation. In the eight other cases, lesions were either stenotic and regressive (six cases) including two bilateral stenoses, or occlusive and persistent (two cases) but on the nondominant V. A. Therefore, surgery was not proposed in those cases.

b) Aneurysm

Two were probably secondary to dissecting hematoma, one spontaneous and one traumatic.

The third was observed in the context of Recklinghausen's disease.

Table 26

		1st Portion	2nd Portion	3rd Portion
Dissection				
stenosis	6	1	3	2
occlusion	2	1	1	—
Aneurysm	3	1	1	1
Dysplasia	9	—	3	6

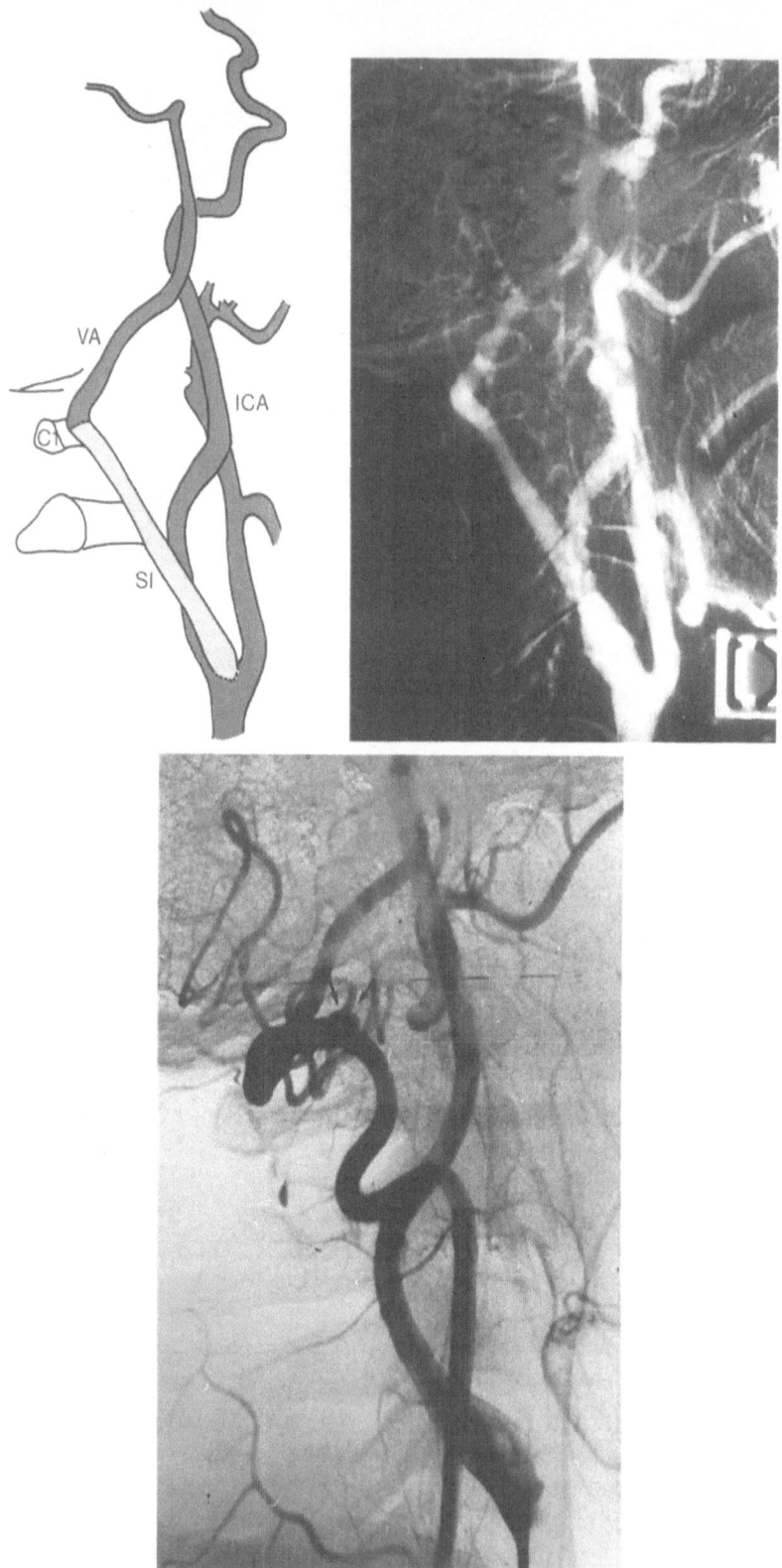

Fig. 77. Spontaneous aneurysm at C1. Lower: before treatment. Upper: revascularization by internal carotid to V. A. at C1 by-pass plus exclusion

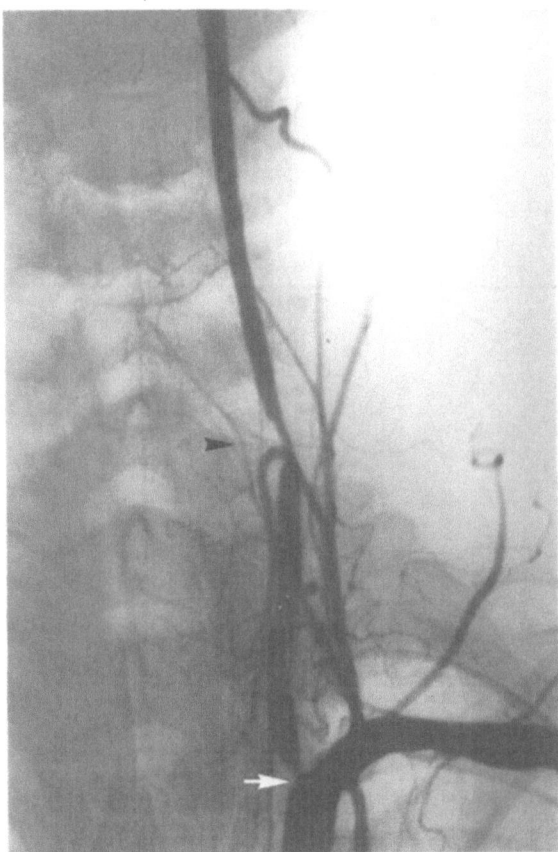

Fig. 78. Ostial stenosis on the left dominant V.A., associated to external compression by a fibromuscular band at C6. Treatment by distal revascularization from the common carotid artery

Two of these 3 cases, one at the C3 level, the other above C1, were operated on with revascularization and exclusion of the distal V.A. since embolism from the aneurysm appeared to be the mechanism of their ischemic manifestations. The third, located on the first portion, was treated by re-implantation of the proximal V.A. onto the common carotid artery.

c) Fibromuscular Dysplasia

In the last nine cases, the angiographic appearance was typical of fibromus- cular dysplasia. Identical angiographic features was noted on the internal carotid artery in three cases, and one or several associated intracranial aneurysms were identified in two cases. In only two cases were the character-istic anomalies, extensive on the cer-vical V.A.; in the others, they were limited to a short segment near C2. Unilateral occlusion, probably second-ary to a dissecting hematoma, was ob-served in a case with bilateral lesions. No patient of this group was proposed for surgery on the cervical lesion.

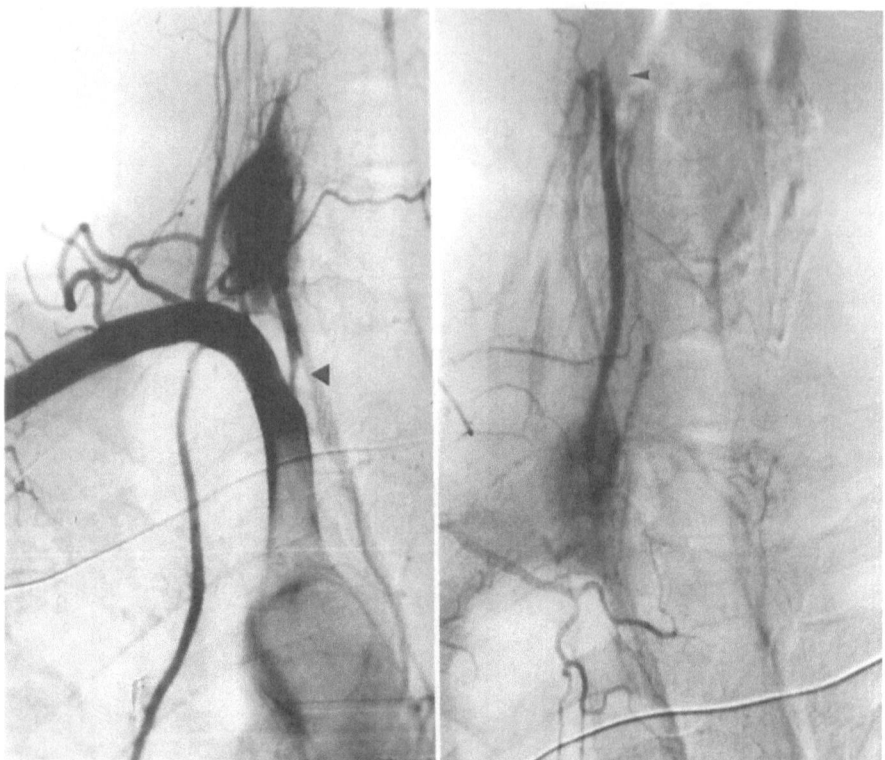

Fig. 79. Pre-occlusive stenosis at the ostium. Slow filling of the V. A. up to C 3. Thrombectomy and reimplantation on the common carotid artery

14.1.2.2 Atherosclerotic Lesions

V. A. revascularization was performed as frequently for occlusive as for stenotic atherosclerotic lesions, in 33 and 34 cases respectively.

As indicated in **Table 27**, proximal reimplantation was mainly proposed for stenosis: 31 of 46 cases. The remaining 15 cases presented with occlusion on one side and stenosis on the other (13 cases) or with recent occlusion (2 cases). In the first 13 cases, revascularization was performed on the side with stenosis. In the two cases with occlusion, surgery was performed in the acute phase and included thrombectomy and

reimplantation on the common carotid artery (**Fig. 79**).

Conversely, distal revascularization was mainly performed in cases of occlusion: 18 of 21 cases. Only three cases in which stenosis extended up to the second portion of the V. A. were treated in this way. In fact, two were pre-occlusive stenosis (**Fig. 78**).

Whatever the level, V. A. revascularization was only performed in cases with bilateral anomalies, as indicated in **Tables 27** and **28**. On the side contralateral to the revascularization, the V. A. was either occluded, or stenosed or atretic (**Fig. 80**).

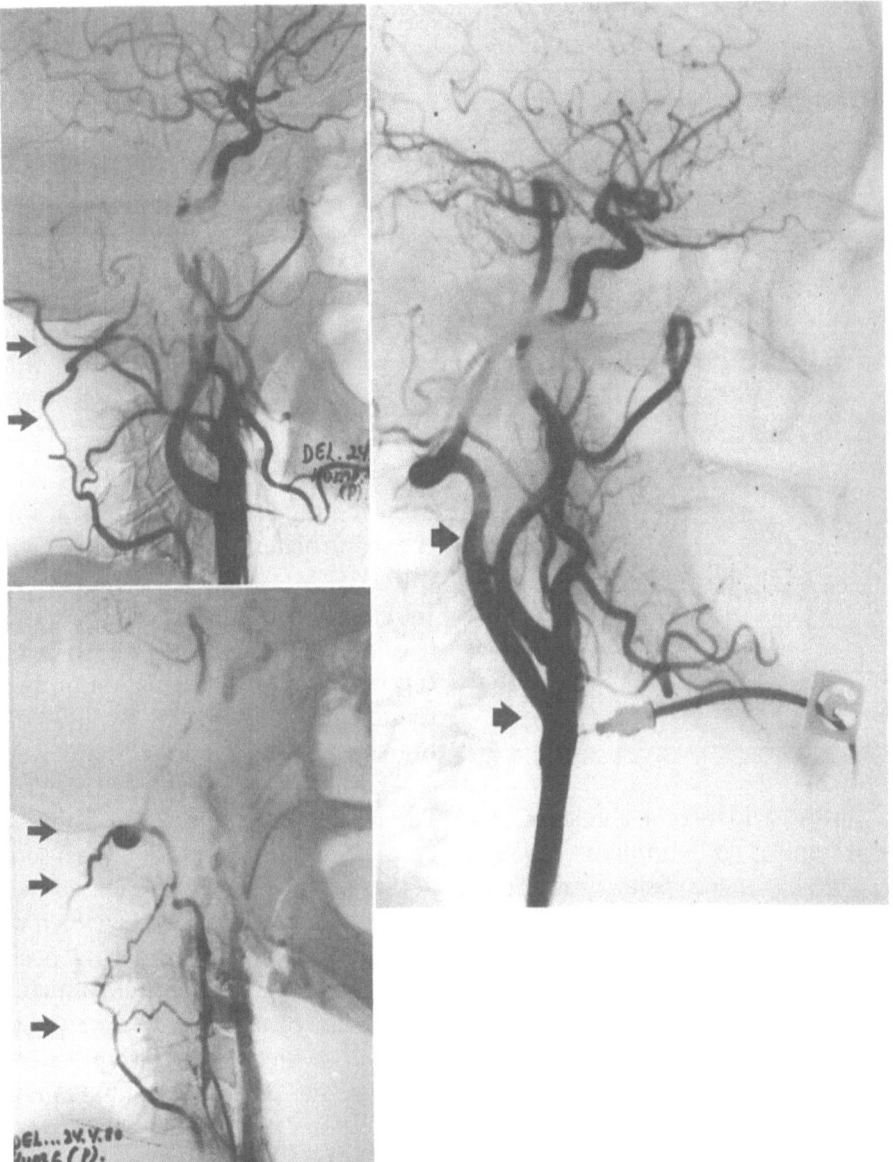

Fig. 80. Bilateral V. A. occlusion. Complete stroke. Brain stem infarct. Common carotid artery to V. A. at C 1–C 2 saphenous vein graft on the right side

No unilateral lesion was considered for surgery if the controlateral V. A. was of good caliber and disease free. Moreover, of 67 cases, 34 (51%) were associated with a lesion of one or both carotid arteries.

Furthermore, surgery was only performed if symptoms could be attributed to insufficient V. A. flow rather than embolism, even in cases of stenosis. Consequently, no case with unilateral stenosis was accepted for surgery. In

Table 27. Atherosclerotic lesions

Level of V. A. surgery	1st Portion	3rd Portion
O bilat	—	7
ST bilat	25	—
O + ST	13	7
O + atret	2	4
ST + atret	6	3
ST or O ICA	21	13

O: occlusion; ST: stenosis; bilat: bilateral; atret: atretic V. A.; ST or O ICA: associated internal carotid artery stenosis or occlusion.

Table 28. V. A. surgery. Atherosclerosis

Occlusion	bilateral	7	N = 33
	+ stenosis	20	
	+ atretic V. A.	6	
Stenosis	bilateral	25	N = 34
	+ atretic V. A.	9	

our series, evidence of a relation between stenosis and symptoms, through an embolic mechanism, was never clearly demonstrated, except in two cases (George and Laurian, 1983). In those cases, occlusion developed secondarily, without any new symptoms, although a partially regressive brainstem infarct had revealed the stenosis. In another case, referred after a mild Wallenberg's syndrome, the V. A. was occluded at the C 1 level with a concave upper limit to the injected contrast, suggesting embolus; angiography was repeated at 1, 2, and 6 months. At 1 month, the V. A. was no longer occluded and had completely recovered its normal caliber. No proximal V. A. lesion was noted and cardiac investigations were normal. None of these three cases required surgical treatment, since the controlateral V. A. was of good caliber.

In cases of occlusion, the technical feasibility of distal revascularization can be assessed by evaluation of distal reinjection of the V. A. by muscular branches arising from the occipital and ascending or deep cervical arteries. Patency of the distal V. A. is common in cases of proximal occlusion. In a series of 68 occlusions, 16 presented with filling of the proximal V. A., which was interpreted as indicating a distal occlusion (**Fig. 81**). In the remaining 52 cases, the proximal V. A. was never injected which was interpreted as evidence of ostial occlusion. Among these cases, a distal reinjection was seen in 40; in fact this number was probably underestimated, since carotid angiography was not performed in all cases and thus the occipital artery was not always injected.

Distal V. A. reinjection through muscular branches is generally of moderate quality, with a weak and delayed filling of the basilar trunk. This fact is taken into account when estimating the pos-

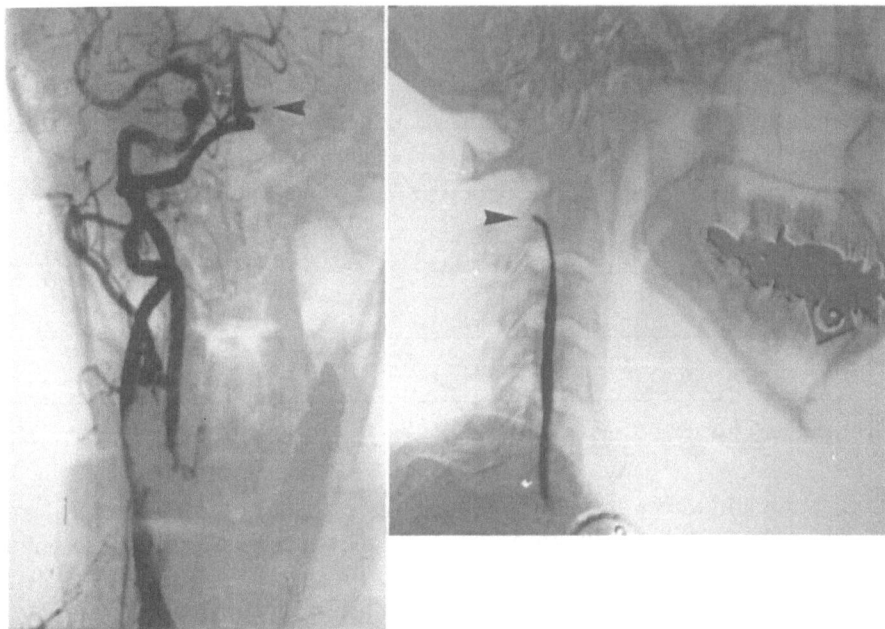

Fig. 81. Distal thrombosis of the left V. A. Contrast stagnation in the proximal part. Controlateral V. A. of good size with retrograde filling of the last centimeter of the thrombosed V. A. (arrow)

sible benefits of surgical V. A. revascularization. However, it also explains that the exact diameter of the V. A. cannot be correctly evaluated; the caliber of the controlateral V. A. is often a good way to estimate that of the occluded V. A., but if the controlateral V. A. is not filled, (in case of bilateral occlusion) this data is obviously not available. In four such cases where surgical revascularization was nevertheless attempted, the V. A. appeared too small (less than two millimeters) to allow high flow under high pressure, and the by-pass was not performed.

14.1.3 Surgical Techniques

Two main techniques were employed to revascularize the V. A.: reimplantation for the first portion, and grafting techniques, utilized at all levels but essentially on the third portion (**Tables 29** and **30**).

14.1.3.1 Reimplantation

The V. A. was most frequently reimplanted on the posterior wall of the common carotid artery (37 cases). If this vessel is thrombosed, the subclavian artery may be used instead, in which case, reimplantation without graft interposition requires a longer segment of V. A. Two cases were treated by direct V. A. reimplantation on the subclavian artery.

In our series, there was no case of reimplantation of the second portion of the V. A. onto the carotid artery, nor of

Table 29. Techniques of V. A. revascularization. Wall lesions

	1st Portion		2nd–3rd Portion
	Reimplant.	Graft	Graft
C.C.A.	37	5	19
I.C.A.	—	—	1
E.C.A.	—	—	3
S.C.A.	2	2	1
Total	39	7	24

Endarteriectomy + patch = 1.

mobilization and direct anastomosis of the external carotid artery onto the third portion of the V. A.

14.1.3.2 Endarteriectomy

Endarteriectomy plus patch is an almost abandoned technique. We used it in one case of ostial stenosis. The lesion was quite limited in length, and carotid artery clamping would have been hazardous because of severe middle cerebral artery stenosis.

14.1.3.3 Grafting Techniques

A segment of saphenous vein, taken from the thigh where no valves are present, is the most suitable grafting material. It was used in all but one patient, who had had a previous surgical stripping. In this case, the cephalic vein should be employed.

In all cases, the graft was implanted by side to end anastomosis proximally, and by end to side distally.

a) Proximal Implantation

For the first and second portion of the V. A., the choice of the donor vessel is limited to the common carotid artery and the subclavian artery. The common carotid artery is usually preferred because of its better wall quality for suturing and its easier exposure. Revascularization of the proximal V. A. using grafting techniques onto the common carotid artery and the sub-clavian artery was performed in 5 and 2 cases respectively.

For the third portion, there are four possible vessels: the external carotid, the internal carotid, the common carotid and the subclavian arteries.

The external carotid artery is a small vessel on which atheromatous stenosis develops frequently and rapidly. Therefore, it was used in only three cases. In the first case, the V. A. was small (2 mm in diameter) and the external carotid artery was the most congruent vessel (**Fig. 82**). In the second case, the external carotid artery seemed to be of good caliber and free of any atherosclerotic lesion. However, six months later, atheromatous stenosis developed on the external carotid artery trunk proximal to the anastomosis and the graft had to be prolonged and

Table 30 A. Proximal revascularization. Wall lesions

No.	Sex	Age	Lesion	Surgery
1	f	56	A ST BI	R CCA
2	m	52	A ST BI	R CCA
3	m	58	A ST BI	R CCA
4	f	61	A O+ST	R CCA
5	f	30	A O+AT	G CCA
6	m	70	A O+ST	R CCA
7	f	48	A O+AT	R CCA
8	m	65	A ST BI	R CCA
9	m	72	A ST+AT	R CCA
10	f	72	A ST BI	G CCA
11	m	43	A O+ST	R CCA
12	m	75	A ST BI	R CCA
13	f	45	A ST BI	R CCA
14	m	69	A ST BI	R SCA
15	m	59	A ST+AT	R CCA
16	m	55	A O+ST	G CCA
17	m	61	A O+ST	R CCA
18	f	59	A ST BI	R CCA
19	f	28	An	R CCA
20	m	61	A ST BI	R CCA
21	m	60	A ST BI	R CCA
22	m	72	A O+ST	R CCA
23	f	48	A ST BI	R CCA
24	m	52	A ST BI	R CCA
25	m	76	A ST BI	R CCA
26	m	58	A ST BI	G CCA
27	m	63	A O+ST	R CCA
28	m	50	A ST BI	G CCA
29	m	68	A ST BI	R CCA
30	f	65	A ST BI	R CCA
31	m	62	A ST BI	R CCA
32	f	66	A ST BI	R CCA
33	m	62	A ST BI	R CCA
34	m	68	A ST BI	R CCA
35	m	47	A ST+AT	R CCA
36	m	53	A O+ST	R CCA
37	m	70	A ST BI	R CCA
38	m	69	A ST+AT	R CCA
39	m	68	A ST BI	R CCA
40	m	42	A ST BI	R CCA
41	m	53	A ST+AT	R CCA
42	m	61	A O+ST	G CCA
43	f	61	A O+ST	G SCA
44	m	49	A O+ST	R SCA
45	m	46	A ST+AT	patch
46	f	48	A O+ST	R CCA
47	m	59	A O+ST	G CCA

A: atherosclerosis, An: aneurysm, O: occlusion, ST: stenosis, AT: atresia, BI: bilateral, R: reimplantation, G: venous graft, patch: endarterectomy + patch, CCA: common carotid artery, SCA: subclavian artery.

Table 30B. Distal revascularization. Wall lesions

No.	Sex	Age	Lesion	Surgery
1	m	51	A O BI	CCA VA
2	m	53	A O BI	ECA VA
3	m	71	A O BI	CCA VA
4	m	46	A O+ST	ECA VA
5	m	48	A ST+AT	CCA VA
6	m	58	A O+AT	CCA VA
7	m	62	A O BI	CCA VA
8	m	56	A O+ST	CCA VA
9	m	58	A O BI	CCA VA
10	m	57	A O BI	CCA VA
11	m	56	A O+ST	CCA VA
12	m	51	A O+ST	CCA VA
13	f	61	A O+ST	CCA VA
14	f	59	A O+ST	CCA VA
15	m	47	A O BI	CCA VA
16	m	31	A O+AT	CCA VA
17	m	58	A O+AT	CCA VA
18	m	71	A O+ST	CCA VA
19	m	50	A ST+AT	CCA VA
20	m	67	A O+AT	ECA VA
21	m	66	A ST+AT	CCA VA
22	m	59	An C3	SCA VA
23	m	27	AVM C3–C5	ICA VA
24	m	42	An C1	ICA VA C1
25	f	40	DISS BI	CCA VA
26	m	5	tumor C4	ICA VA C1+CCA VA

A: atherosclerosis, An: aneurysm, AVM: arteriovenous malformation, DISS: dissection. CCA VA: common carotid to V. A. venous graft by-pass, ECA VA: external carotid to V. A. venous graft by-pass, ICA VA: internal carotid to V. A. venous graft by-pass, SCA VA: subclavian to V. A. venous graft by-pass, ICA VA C1: internal carotid to V. A. at C1 level venous graft by-pass.

implanted on the common carotid artery, with an ultimately good clinical and anatomic result. In the third case, the external carotid artery was chosen because multiple atherosclerotic lesions of the cervical vascular axes suggested that clamping of the carotid artery would be hazardous. The first angiographic control at eight days, showed good results but a six months control has not yet been done on this recent case.

The internal carotid artery was never selected in revascularization for atherosclerotic lesions. It was, however, used in other indications in three cases. One was an aneurysm located adjacent to the transverse foramen of C 1. This was treated by revascularization of the V. A. above the posterior arch of the

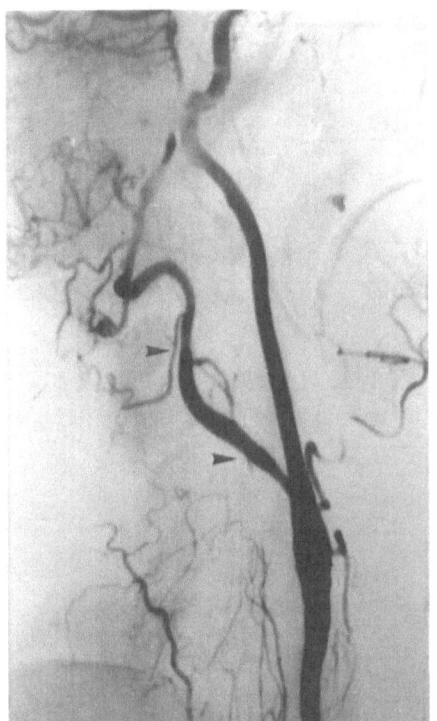

Fig. 82. Bilateral V. A. occlusion. Vertebrobasilar insufficiency. External carotid to V. A. at C 1–C 2 saphenous vein graft on the right side

atlas and exclusion of the V. A. with a clip placed below the graft implantation (**Fig. 77**).

The two other cases involved proximal implantation on the internal carotid artery and were done for tumor in one case and A. V. F. in the other (see chapter 14.2 Distal Revascularization).

One distal revascularization was realized by graft implantation on the subclavian artery. In this case, there was an aneurysm at the C 3 level and no posterior communicating artery on angiography. To avoid clamping of the carotid axis, the subclavian artery was selected with good result at three years (**Fig. 76**).

The common carotid artery is the most suitable vessel for proximal implantation. It was by far the most frequently utilized vessel (20 cases). Angiographic control showed good immediate and six-month results in all cases, i. e. a large caliber graft with smooth contours and good filling of the basilar trunk and its branches (**Fig. 80**).

b) Distal Implantation

On the proximal V. A., the distal graft implantation site was chosen beyond the distal limit of the atherosclerotic lesions in such a way that the graft would exhibit a smooth course.

In one case, distal implantation was done on the second portion of the V. A. The V. A. was occluded at the ostium, and reinjection by muscular branches had kept the V. A. patent down to the C 6 level. However, on angiographic control after grafting at the C 5 level, the V. A. wall appeared irregular on the three vertebral segments above the anastomosis, indicating the implantation site should have been more distal (**Fig. 83**).

On the third portion of the V. A., distal implantation was usually performed between C 1 and C 2 (22 cases). One case of aneurysm was implanted above C 1 (**Fig. 77**).

14.1.3.4 Associated Vascular Surgery

When internal carotid artery and V. A. lesions occurred on the same side, both vessels were treated, either in the same or in separate surgical procedures.

33 internal carotid artery and one innominate carotid artery atherosclerotic

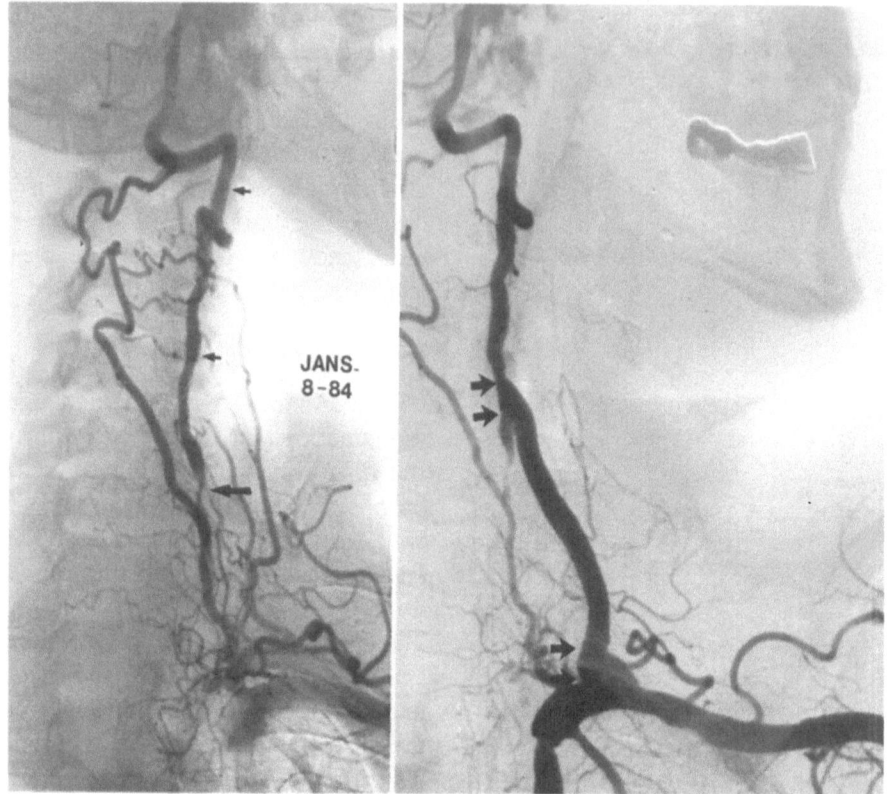

JANS.
8-84

Fig. 83. Bilateral occlusion. Vertebro-basilar insufficiency. Subclavian artery to V. A. at C 4–C 5, saphenous vein graft. Good feature of the graft but the V. A. remains irregular between C 5 and C 2

lesions were associated with the V. A. lesions. In eight cases, there was an internal carotid artery occlusion, and revascularization was performed utilizing the common carotid artery. In the other 26 cases, stenosis of the internal carotid artery or the innominate artery was treated in one stage with the V. A. revascularization (18 cases) or in a separate procedure (8 cases).

14.1.4. Clinical Data

All cases in the surgical series, were symptomatic, but not all had symptoms attributable to the vertebro-basilar territory.

V. A. revascularization, especially when distal, was performed in some cases before surgical treatment of a controlateral carotid or V. A. lesion.

This protocole was proposed when it seemed hazardous to clamp the controlateral vessel because of the multiplicity of cervical vessel lesions.

Revascularization of the V. A. was also considered after ischemic manifestations in the carotid territory if there was no possibility of treatment on the

Table 31. Wall lesions

V. B. ischemia	Distal lesion	Proximal lesion	Dissection dysplasia
T.I.A.	10	24	3
Stroke	7	6	1
I.C.A. or doubtful	4	16	

carotid arteries. The resulting large caliber by-pass is, in our opinion, preferable hemodynamically to a micro extra-intracranial anastomosis. However, this revascularization of the V. A. was not always possible, since in two such cases, the V. A. was seen to be of insufficient caliber (less than 2 mm). The anastomosis in these cases would not have been larger than the already existing muscular branches reinjecting the V. A., and the venous by-pass was therefore not performed.

In cases with vertebro-basilar symptoms, these symptoms were either transient (52%) or permanent and more or less regressive (19%). **Table 31** indicates in what proportions these symptoms were observed prior to each type of revascularization.

14.1.5 Anatomic Results

Revascularization was verified by angiography at eight days and six months after surgery and then each year by ultrasound and Doppler effect. Angiography was repeated only if the annual control showed an abnormality. The overall patency rate, in our series, was 100% on short term controls and 98% on long term follow-up.

On the first portion of the V.A., no technical failure occurred. On the third portion, one case of common carotid to V. A. venous graft appeared occluded three years post-operatively, whereas previous controls had not discovered any abnormality. This graft thrombosis ocurred uneventfully and was discovered on the third annual non-invasive control and confirmed angiographically. No explanation for this late occlusion was found; we can only speculate on the possibility of mechanical compression during excessive rotation of the head and neck.

In one case of external carotid to V. A. venous by-pass, marked stenosis developed secondarily on the external carotid artery proximal to the anastomosis. Its discovery on the six-month post-operative angiographic control led to prolongation of the venous graft onto the common carotid artery with good results.

Finally, we must mention again the rather poor result seen on angiographic control of the unique revascularization on the second portion of the V.A. Reoperation to perform a more distal revascularization was not considered necessary, since the controlateral V.A. was operated on for ostial stenosis.

14.1.6 Clinical Results

There was no operative mortality in our series. One patient died three years post-operatively from a traffic accident. There was no late case of fatality of cardiac origin.

Morbidity was limited to that classically observed in V. A. surgery: transient Horner's syndrome, hypoesthesia in the second cervical nerve territory, and regressive lymphatic oozing.

In one case with distal V. A. revascularization for bilateral V. A. occlusion, painful tension of the S. C. M. muscle was observed post-operatively, but disappeared progressively over the following two months. Irritation of the accessory spinal nerve during surgery is the likely explanation.

When surgery was indicated for T. I. A., marked improvement (no new T. I. A.) was noted in 93% of the cases. In one case, the frequency and importance of vertebro-basilar symptoms seems not to have been modified by surgery.

Revascularization performed after stroke, was not followed by new ischemic symptoms in any case. In the entire series, no ischemic stroke was observed post-operatively, with a follow-up of 6 months to eight years.

In non vertebro-basilar symptomatic cases, treatment efficiency was demonstrated by perfect tolerance of surgery on the controlateral vessels and increase in cerebral blood flow of up to 25%.

14.2 Distal Revascularization

This chapter briefly reviews all the cases of distal revascularization, which include not only structural lesions (atherosclerosis, aneurysm and dissection) but also one case of tumor and one case of multiple arteriovenous fistulae.

In the tumor case, the patient was a 5

Table 32. Revascularization

	1st Portion	3rd Portion
Atherosclerosis	45	21
Dissection dysplasia	1	3
A.V.F.	—	1
Tumor	—	2
	46	27

year boy with a benign tumor (osteoblastoma) involving the third and fourth vertebrae. For reasons of the patient's age and disease, and in order to allow bilateral embolization, both V. A.'s were revascularized. On one side, an internal carotid to V. A. venous by-pass was performed with implantation at the C 1 level of the V. A., and on the other side, a common carotid to V. A. venous graft was implanted at the C 1–C 2 level. The tumor was then completely removed with a combined bilateral lateral anterior approach. The entire procedure was perfectly tolerated and results remain excellent at three years.

The case with multiple vertebro-vertebral arteriovenous fistulae pre-

Table 33. Distal revascularization

	CCA	ICA	ECA	SCA
Atherosclerosis	18	—	3	—
Aneurysm	—	1*	—	1
Dissection	1	—	—	—
A. V. F.	—	1	—	—
Tumor	1	1*	—	—

* V. A. revascularization at C1 level.

sented with severe and long standing vertebro-basilar insufficiency. Direct embolization could not be realized. The V. A. was revascularized with a venous graft implanted on the internal carotid artery and then excluded by a clip at C 2 just below the anastomosis. The V. A. was then safely embolized and the three fistula sites were occluded. In two weeks, most of the symptoms of vertebro-basilar insufficiency disappeared. This patient has now remained asymptomatic for four years.

The complete series of distal revascularizations included 27 cases (**Table 32**). Of them, seven were associated with exclusion of the underlying V. A. in order to prevent embolism in the vertebro-basilar system: three cases of aneurysm or dissection, one case of atherosclerotic stenosis and three cases (one tumor with bilateral revascularization and one A. V. F.) prior to radiological embolization.

Proximal implantation of the venous graft was on the external carotid artery in three cases, on the internal carotid artery in three cases, on the subclavian artery in one, and on the common carotid artery in 20. Distal implantation was on the V. A. at the C 1–C 2 level in 25 cases, and above C 1 in two.

14.3 Arteriovenous Malformations

14.3.1 Etiology

A. V. M.'s involving the V. A. were observed in 33 cases.

According to etiology, the cases of A. V. M. can be divided into three main groups; traumatic A. V. F., spontaneous A. V. F., and angiodysplasia.

14.3.1.1 Traumatic A. V. F.: 13 Cases

Injury was iatrogenic in eight cases: unintentional puncture of the V. A. (6 cases) or local surgery (2 cases). Five patients sustained an accidental injury: direct (bullet in 3 cases) or indirect (severe craniocerebral trauma in the other 2 cases) (**Fig. 84**).

These fistulas were preferentially localized at C 5–C 6.

Symptoms were discovered immediately after trauma in fistulas of iatrogenic origin, but only after several days or weeks in the others.

On angiography, complete steal from the homolateral V. A. was present in all cases. Venous drainage was into the perivertebral venous plexus and cervical veins in 12 cases. The thirteenth case was a vertebro-jugular fistula with a false aneurysm at the communication site.

Table 34. Arteriovenous malformations

No.	Sex	Age	Etiology	Localization	Surgery
1	f	23	Sp	C1 C2	0
2	f	14	Sp	C1 C2	0
3	m	5	Sp	C1 C2	0
4	f	16	Sp	C1 C2	0
5	m	25	Sp	C1 C2	0
6	f	39	Sp	C1 C2	0
7	f	48	Sp	C1 C2	0
8	f	30	Sp	C1 C2	0
9	f	70	Sp	C1 C2	0
10	m	50	Sp	C1 C2	0
11	m	10	Sp	C6 C7	0
12	m	8	Sp	C6 C7	0
13	m	27	Sp	C6 C7	0
14	f	33	Sp(?)	C1 C2	+
15	m	27	Sp	C3 C5	+R
16	m	38	Sp	C3	+
17	m	44	T punct	C6	+
18	m	35	T surg	C2	0
19	m	72	T surg	C7	0
20	f	66	T punct	C6	0
21	f	29	T punct	C5	0
22	m	53	T punct	C5 C6	0
23	m	55	T punct	C5 C6	0
24	m	70	T punct	C7	0
25	m	26	T bullet	C3	0
26	m	29	T bullet	C1	0
27	f	33	T traffic	C5 C6	0
28	f	35	T traffic	C4	0
29	m	29	T bullet	C1	+
30	f	16	A	C2 C6	+
31	m	16	A	C4 C5	+
32	f	24	A	C1 C2	+
33	m	26	A	C2 C4	+

Sp: spontaneous, Sp(?): doubtful traumatic origin, T: traumatic, punct: puncture, surg: surgery, A: angiodysplasia, R: revascularization + exclusion + embolization.

14.3.1.2 Spontaneous A. V. F.: 16 Cases

Spontaneous occurrence was assumed in the absence of prior injury. Age ranged from 3 to 70 years with a mean age of 20; both sexes were equally represented, with 8 females and 8 males.

These fistulas were mostly located at C 1–C 2 (11 cases) and supplied directly by the V. A. in all but one case (case No 14—**Table 34**). This last case was

Table 35. Arteriovenous malformations

	1st Portion	2nd Portion	3rd Portion
Spontaneous	3	2 (2)	11 (1)
Traumatic	2	8 (1)	3 (1)
Angiodysplasia	—	3 (3)	1 (1)
Total	5	13 (6)	15 (3)

( ): Cases treated surgically.

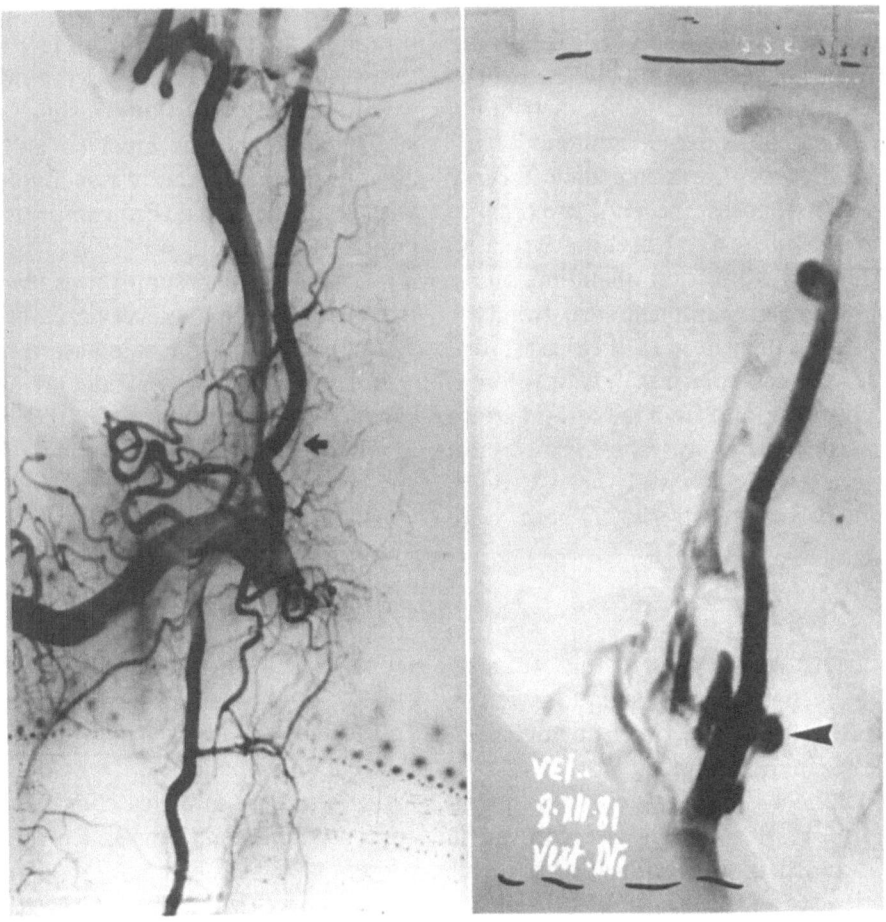

Fig. 84. Arteriovenous fistula at C 6 level following puncture. Surgical treatment after embolization failure (left)

revealed by a cervical bruit below the mastoid tip, four years after severe trauma with hyperextension of the neck. The A. V. F. presented an aneurysmal pouch supplied by two V. A. branches at C 1 and C 3, as well as by the occipital artery, and it drained into the epidural venous plexus. After failure of embolization, it was cured surgically. The traumatic origin of this A. V. F. cannot be ascribed with certainty, although the likely mechanism is dissection from the V. A. branch at C 1–C 2, with secondary development of an aneurysm and, finally, A. V. F. Five cases were located at C 5–C 6–C 7 and fed by a collateral, probably radicular, artery. Cases were evenly distributed between both sides (9 right and 7 left). The V. A. was the main pedicle in every case. In 11 cases, the V. A. proximal to the fistula was pseudo-dysplasic, exhibiting significant dilatation.

More or less complete steal from the V. A. was present in 13 of 16 cases; steal from the controlateral V. A. was found in four cases and from the carotid artery in one. In six cases, other cervical arteries were involved (deep cervical and occipital arteries). There were multiple fistulas in one case, with three main sites of communication between C 3 and C 6 (**Fig. 85**).

Venous drainage was into the vertebral and cervical veins in 10 cases and into the vertebral veins and spinal venous plexus in five. In one case, venous drainage was mainly through a radiculo-medullary vein.

14.3.1.3 Angiodysplasia: 4 Cases

These pseudo-tumoral angiomas were observed in the paravertebral area and involved the soft tissues, mainly the muscles. One case extended to the deep occipital muscles, one to the jaw and two cases extended towards the outer ear. In one case, the skin overlying the site of angioma was involved and in another a vertebral body was involved with resulting spinal cord compression (**Fig. 86**).

The main vascular supply was always from the V. A.; but in every case, other sources of vascular feeding were present from external carotid and subclavian artery branches. In the case involving a vertebral body, the angiodysplasia was also fed by the controlateral V. A.

14.3.2 Symptomatology

Whatever the type of fistula, tinnitus was the most frequent symptom. It was present in all the cases of angiodysplasia, in 12 traumatic cases and in 6 spontaneous cases. A continuous murmur with systolic reinforcement was heard in the cervical area in all patients.

Spontaneous fistulas were also revealed by neurologic manifestations: vertebro-basilar insufficiency in two cases and medullary ischemia in one.

In the cases of angiodysplasia, reasons referring the patient were essentially esthetic, except in the case with spinal cord compression. This last case also presented with a Klippel Trenaunnay syndrome with multiple localizations on the arms and legs.

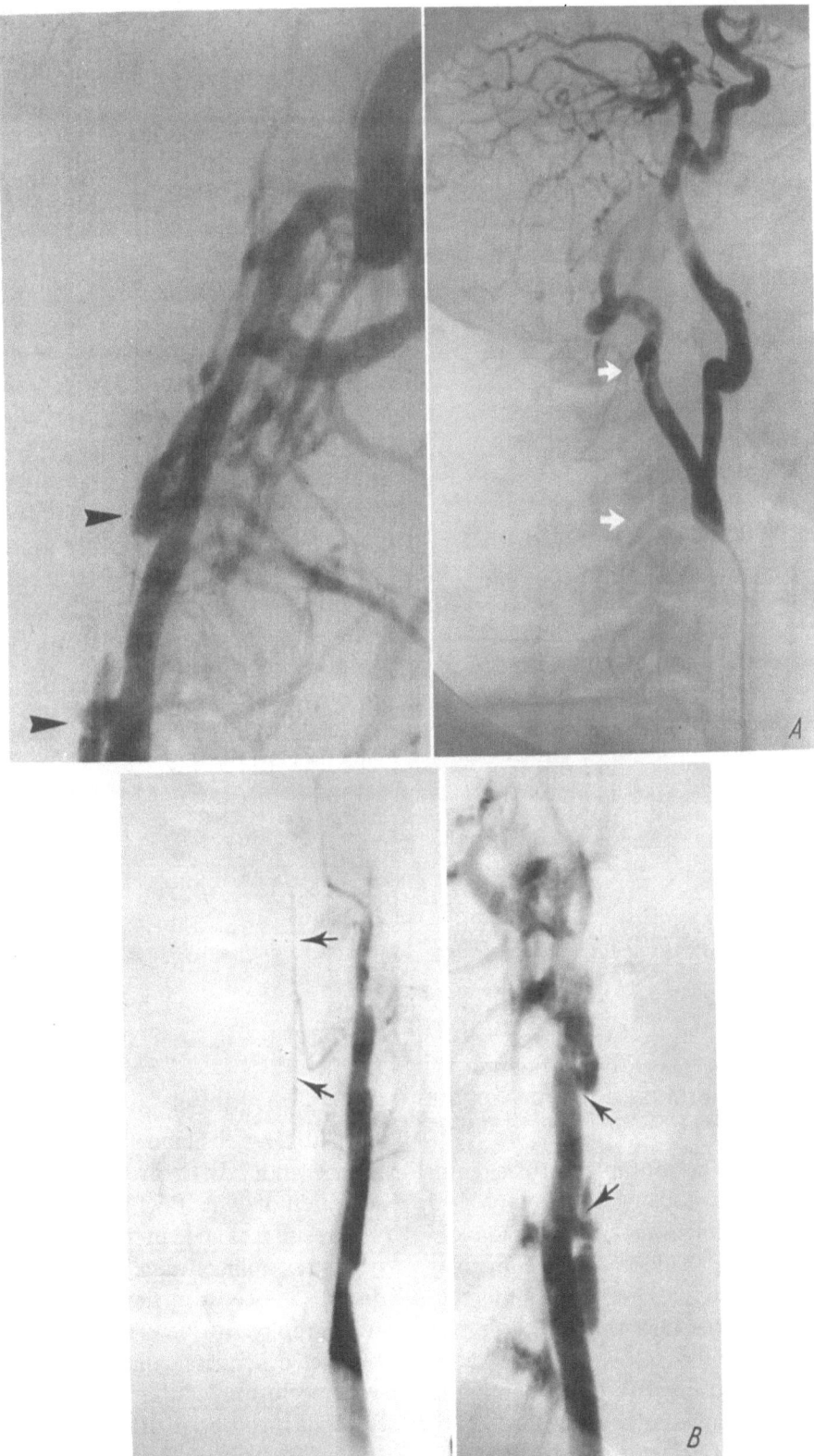

Fig. 85. Multiple spontaneous ărteriovenous fistula. Vertebro-basilar insufficiency. **A)** V. A. revascularization at C 1–C 2 by a saphenous vein graft implanted on the internal carotid artery with exclusion of the underlying V. A. **B)** After embolization, the V. A. remains patent with an anterior radiculo-medullary branch arising at C 3–C 4

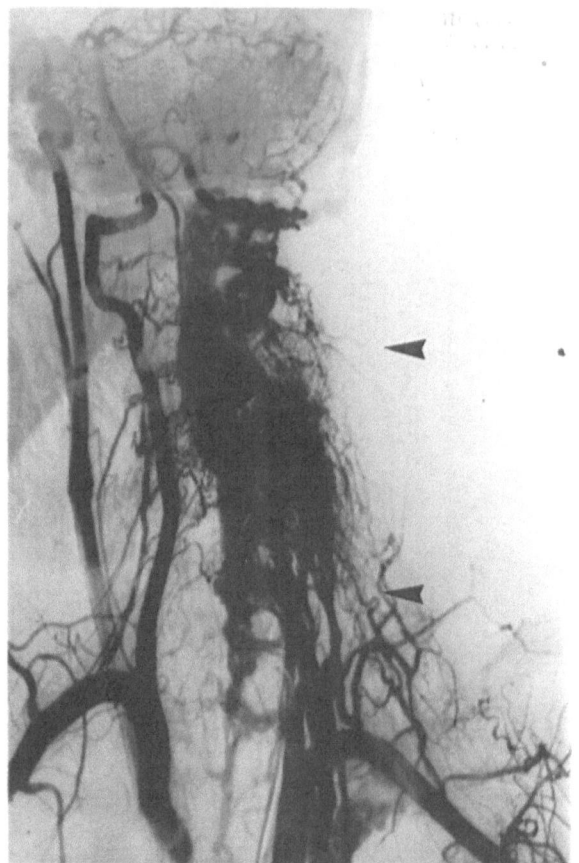

Fig. 86. Angiodysplasia involving the vertebral body of C 4 and supplied by both V. A.'s and many branches from the subclavian artery. Failure of the surgical resection (see text)

14.3.3 Treatment

14.3.3.1 Traumatic and Spontaneous A. V. F.

In simple or multiple fistulas, initial treatment was always attempted by technique of interventional radiology, principally balloon occlusion. Nevertheless, in five cases no treatment was proposed because the A. V. F.'s were well tolerated. One of these closed spontaneously. In the remaining 24 cases, endovascular occlusion of the fistula was performed, with an excellent result in 12 cases: complete occlusion of the fistula by a balloon in 10 cases, a coil in one and I. B. C. in one, with preservation of V. A. flow in all.

The result was good in three cases, with persistance of a residual aneurysm after disappearance of the balloon on angiography.

In three other cases, the result was fair with occlusion of the fistula but associated thrombosis of the V. A.

In the last six cases, endovascular techniques failed. One case was not further treated. The other five were proposed for surgery. Surgical treatment was realized by direct approach in four cases, with occlusion of the fistula by suture of the site of arteriovenous communication and preservation of the V. A. flow; one of these cases (case No. 14, **Table 34**) was treated by ligation of the three branches arising from the V. A. and the occipital artery, and resection of the aneurysm, located between the laminae of C 1 and C 2. The patient was a young woman who had suffered from backpain for four years. Symptoms improved after the first partial embolization, recurred 10 months later, and completely disappeared after surgery. It is thought that these symptoms were related to hypertension in the epidural venous plexus which was the main drainage of the fistula (**Fig. 21**).

One case with multiple fistulas was treated by revascularization using a saphenous vein graft between the internal carotid artery and the V. A. at the C 1–C 2 level. The V. A. was clipped just below the anastomosis, allowing embolization of the three sites of communication, 10 days following surgery. Complete disappearance of the arteriovenous shunts was obtained, with, rather surprisingly, no further thrombosis of the V. A. An anterior radiculomedullary branch arose from the involved V. A. Despite angiographic study with V. A. balloon occlusion at various levels, this branch could not have been identified prior to surgery, but was discovered after embolization. This branch is a possible explanation of the persistent V. A. patency. It should be mentioned that this patient suffered from long standing severe vertebrobasilar insufficiency, which completely resolved in the weeks following treatment (**Fig. 85**).

14.3.3.2 Angiodysplasia

All four cases of angiodysplasia were treated surgically after embolization of the vascular supply from the external carotid and subclavian arteries. A V. A. balloon occlusion test was performed in each case.

In three of these cases, the tissue involved by the angioma was removed "en masse", including in one case, three separate angiomatous masses, involving the V. A. Angiographic control showed excellent results in one case, with complete normalization. In the other two, no persistent arteriovenous shunts could be seen, but hypervascularization remained in the deep cervical area. In the case with excellent result, the angiodysplasia was resected with the surrounding tissue, including the skin and the outer ear which necessitated subsequent plastic repair. In the two other cases, the superficial tissues were left in place for esthetic reasons, since the cutaneous angioma extended to the lower cervical region.

The fourth case had a long and complex history. The patient was a 16-year-old boy with Klippel Trenaunnay syndrome and an angioma involving the fourth vertebral body and left paravertebral muscles. Both the V. A. and the left subclavian artery fed this angiodysplasia. A direct approach was proposed after embolization. The left V. A. was clipped above the level of the angioma and the underlying V. A. was completely controlled with division of all branches supplying the angioma. Resection of the angioma was then attempted, but severe hemorrhage from the right side necessitated suspension of the procedure. Bleeding was stopped with great difficulty, and a postoperative hematoma required re-operation on the second day. Ten days later, angiography showed the angioma was fed by new and more numerous branches from the subclavian artery and the controlateral V. A. Re-embolization was performed, but control six hours later was highly discouraging, since a still more important vascular network had developed and injected the angioma as if embolization had not been performed (**Fig. 86**). Despite the presence of consumptive coagulopathy, direct puncture of the angioma with direct I. B. C. emboliza-

tion was performed but there was no significant clinical or angiographic effect. No other treatment was proposed. The patient survived almost two years with progressively worsening tetraplegia and development of new cervical and brachial angiomas.

This patient illustrates the risks of unleasing an irreversible evolution in these particular forms of angiomatous disease.

As this patient was treated early in our experience, we did not propose what might have been the curative treatment: bilateral occlusion of the V. A.'s with revascularization on one side, followed by complete embolization of all the vascular pedicles, including those from the two V. A.'s. However, it is not certain that this would have been sufficient, considering the extraordinary evolutivity of this lesion.

14.4 Tumor

58 tumors involving the V. A. have been observed in the last five years. 53 were operated on with control of the V. A.

In five cases, surgery was either refused by the patient (one case of fibrous dysplasia) or not proposed for medical reasons: one case of Hodgkin's disease, one of Paget's disease, one thyroid carcinoma metastasis and one sarcoma; chemotherapy and/or roentgentherapy were administered in these four cases. One case of infection, (actinomycosis) presenting with features similar to those of tumor, should be added to this series. It appears at the bottom of **Table 36** and is briefly reported at the end of this chapter.

Table 36 lists all the patients, with indication of the main clinical data: sex, age, tumor location in relation to the V. A., anatomic form, histologic type, and treatment.

Ages ranged from 5 to 77 years and males predominated with a sex ratio (M/F) of 1.5.

Localization predominated on the third portion of the V. A. (30 cases) which included more cases than both the first and second portions together (12 and 16 cases respectively).

Table 37 details the relation between tumor location and the histologic type.

Table 36. Personal series

No.	Sex	Age	V. A. Portion	Hour-glass	Surgery	Histology
1	m	65	2	0	+B G	hemangiopericytoma
2	f	51	2	0	+	neurinoma
3	m	23	1	0	+	hemangiopericytoma
4	f	18	2	+	+	sarcoma
5	m	16	1	+	+La B G	neurinoma
6	f	18	3	0	+	sarcoma
7	m	13	2	0	+	sarcoma
8	f	18	3	0	0	hodgkin
9	f	44	3	+ IC EC	+P F	paraganglioma
10	m	16	2	0	+B G	osteoblastoma
11	m	46	3	+ IC EC	+P F	thyroid meta.
12	m	53	1	0	+	carcinoma
13	m	35	3	+ IC EC	+P F	paraganglioma
14	m	55	3	+ IC EC	+P F	meningioma
15	m	56	3	+ IC EC	+P F	paraganglioma
16	m	47	2	+	+La	paraganglioma
17	m	33	3	0	+	hemangiopericytoma
18	f	73	3	+ IC EC	+P F	meningioma
19	m	20	1	0	+	hemangioma
20	f	53	3	+ IC EC	+P F	meningioma
21	m	12	1	0	+	hemangioma
22	m	40	3	+	+La	neurinoma
23	f	23	3	+	+	neurinoma
24	f	45	3	+ IC EC	+P F	paraganglioma
25	m	24	3	+ IC EC	+P F	paraganglioma
26	m	27	3	+ IC EC	+P F	meningioma
27	m	14	3	+ IC EC	+P F	meningioma
28	m	5	2	0	+B G REVA	osteoblastoma
29	m	30	3	0	+	osteoid osteoma
30	f	17	2–3	+	+La	chordoma
31	m	23	3	+ IC EC	+P F	neurinoma
32	f	42	3	+ IC EC	+P F	paraganglioma
33	m	55	1	0	+	carcinoma
34	m	58	1	0	+	carcinoma
35	f	30	2	+	+La	neurinoma
36	m	39	3	+ IC EC	+P F	paraganglioma
37	f	22	3	+	+	neurinoma
38	m	30	1	0	+	neurinoma
39	m	25	3	+	+La	neurinoma
40	m	63	2	0	+	neurinoma
41	m	26	3	+ IC EC	+P F	paraganglioma
42	f	18	2	+	+	hemangioma
43	f	20	2	+	+B G	neurinoma
44	f	58	2	0	+	neurinoma
45	m	35	1	+	0	sarcoma
46	f	42	1	+	0	thyroid meta.

Table 36 (continued)

No.	Sex	Age	V. A. Portion	Hour-glass	Surgery	Histology
47	m	72	3	0	0	paget
48	f	19	3	0	0	fibrous dysplasia
49	f	39	1	0	+	neurinoma
50	f	56	3	+ IC EC	+P F	paraganglioma
51	f	30	2	+	+La	sarcoma
52	f	56	3	+ IC EC	+P F	meningioma
53	m	6	2–3	+	+La B G	rhabdomyosarcoma
54	m	30	3	0	+	neurinoma
55	m	77	2	+	+	neurinoma
56	m	72	2–3	+	+La	chondroma
57	f	35	1	+	+	sarcoma
58	m	31	3	0	+	osteogenic chondroma
59	f	16	3	0	+	actinomycosis

IC EC: intra extra-cranial, B G: bone graft, La: laminectomy, P F: posterior fossa craniectomy, REVA: revascularization, meta.: metastasis.

Table 37. Tumor. Type

	C1–C2	C6–C2	OST–C6
Neurinoma	6	6	3
Paraganglioma	9	1	—
Meningioma hemangiopericytoma	7	1	1
Carcinoma sarcoma	1	4	4
Osseous tumor	4	4	2
Others	3	—	2
	30	16	12

14.4.1 Anatomic Form (Table 38)

Tumor extension frequently exhibited an hour-glass form: 18 cases were hour-glass cervical tumors with extension through the intervertebral foramen. Neurinomas predominated (8 cases); but 5 hour-glass forms of sarcoma and one each of chordoma, chondroma,

Table 38. Tumor. Localization

Hour-glass	Cervical	18
	Intracranial	17
Paravertebral		16
Osseous		7

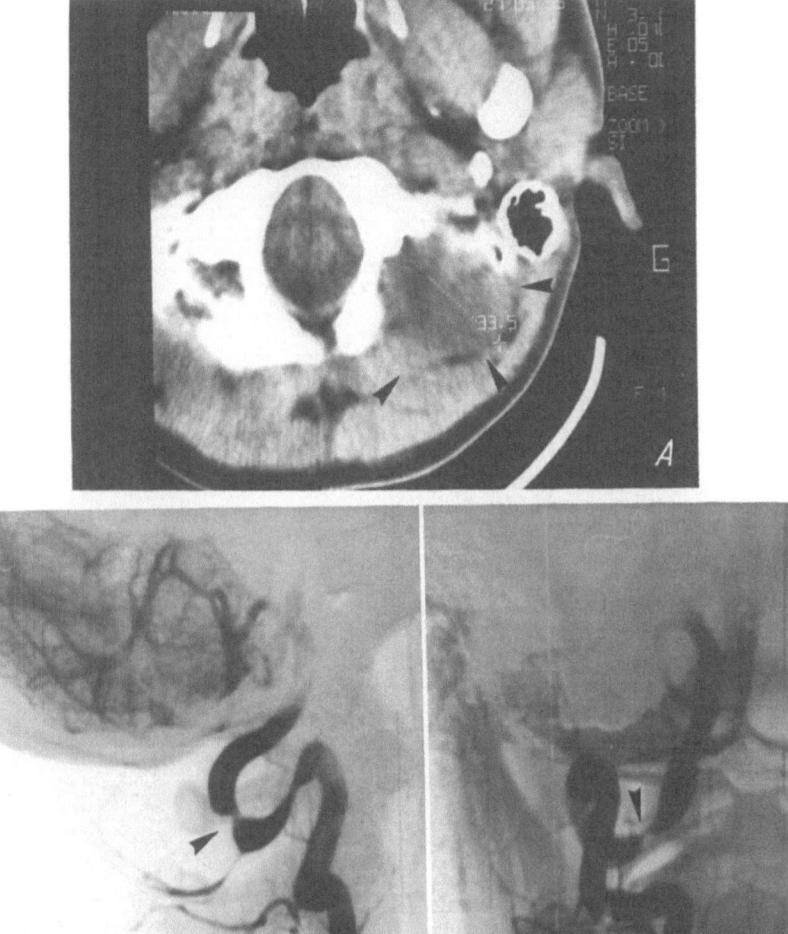

Fig. 87. A) C. T. scan: hour-glass neurinoma above C 1. B) Angiography: marked inferior displacement and severe stenosis of the V. A. above the arch of atlas

hemangioma, metastasis and paraganglioma were also observed (**Figs. 87, 88**, and **90**).

17 cases were hour-glass intracranial and cervical tumors, with extension through the jugulare foramen, mainly observed in case of paraganglioma (9 cases), and/or the foramen magnum most often seen in the case of meningioma (6 cases); one case of posterior

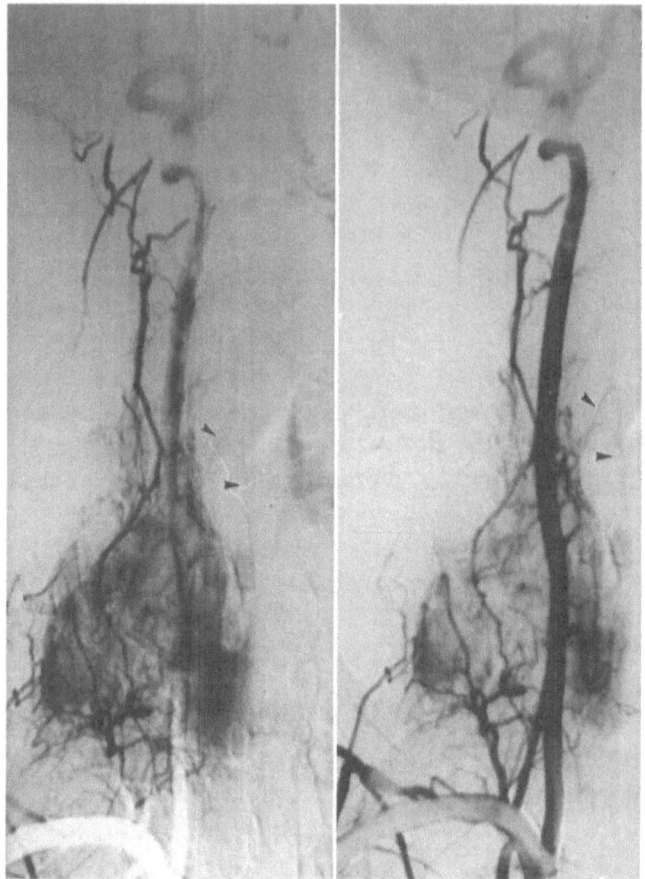

Fig. 88. Hypervascular hour-glass neurinoma at C5–C6. Mild V. A. shift. Anterior radiculo-medullary branch at C5

fossa neurinoma extruded through the jugulare foramen, and one case of thyroid carcinoma metastasis invaded the petrous bone and the upper cervical area (Fig. 89).

Seven tumors were strictly osseous; the tumor may originate from the vertebral body and extend laterally towards the transverse process, such as in two cases of osteoblastoma; or it may develop primarily from the transverse process which occurred, for example, in one case of osteogenic chondroma. It

should be noted that a histologically osseous tumor may not be classified as osseous according to its anatomic form. For instance, a case of chondroma presented with an hour-glass form and therefore was not classified as osseous. On the contrary, a lesion involving bony structures, such as may be seen in Hodgkin's disease, is classified as an osseous tumor (Figs. 90, 91 and 92).

16 cases were extravertebral tumors developed in the paravertebral soft tissues. Examples of this are neuri-

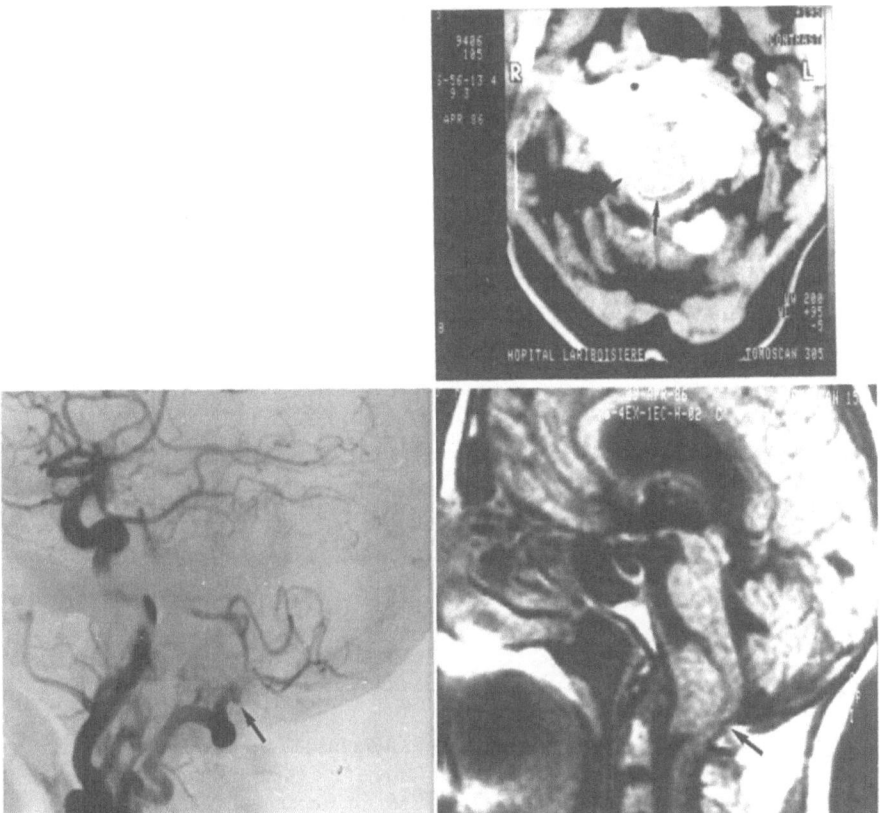

Fig. 89. Foramen magnum meningioma with internal and superior displacement of the V. A. above C 1

nomas (6 cases), hemangiopericytomas (3 cases) and sarcomas (2 cases).

Five tumors related to the first portion of the V. A., involved the lung apex: three carcinomas, one neurinoma and one chondroma.

14.4.2 Histologic Type

The histologic types are given in **Tables 37** and **38**.

The most frequent tumor was the neurinoma, which exhibited various anatomic forms. Of 15 cases of neurinoma, 8 were of hour-glass cervical form, one was of hour-glass intracranial and cervical form, and 6 were strictly extravertebral.

Other histologic types were less frequent. However, paragangliomas and meningiomas had a higher incidence than the other tumors, 10 and 6 cases respectively. These were essentially observed in relation to the third portion of the V. A.

The great variety of histologic types in our series must be emphasized. Most

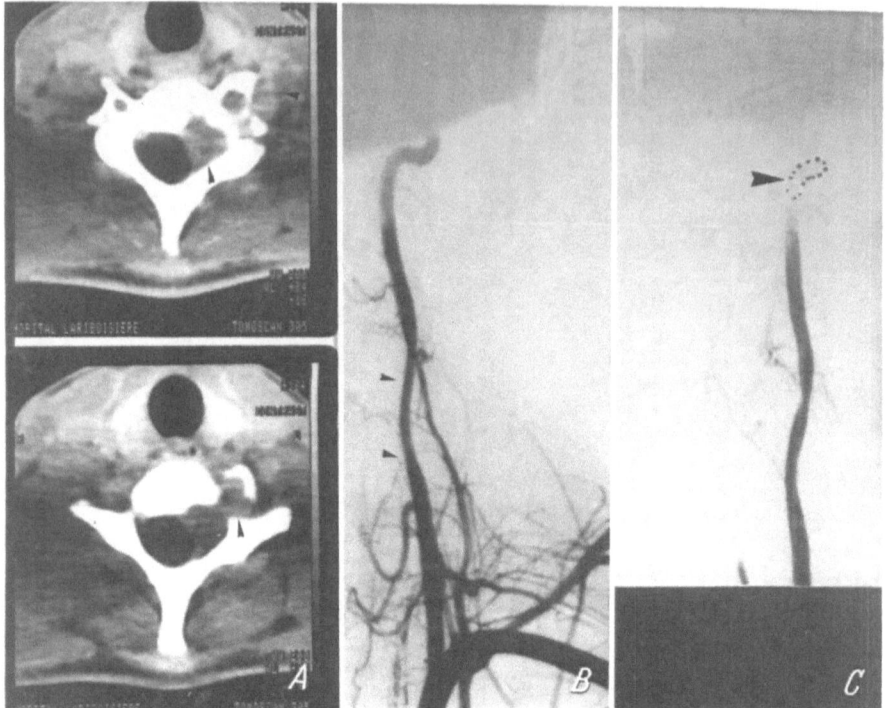

Fig. 90. A) C. T. scan: hour-glass hemangioma on the dominant V. A. side. Notice the difference in size between the 2 transverse foramina. Removal through the enlarged intervertebral foramen. B) Angiography: moderate shift and stenosis at C5–C6. C) Angiography under balloon occlusion: anterior radiculo-medullary branch arising at C6

were benign, and the V. A. surgical techniques helped achieve complete cure; some, in contrast, were malignant, and V. A. surgery allowed an attempt of extensive removal before complementary treatment by radiotherapy and/or chemotherapy.

14.4.3 Angiographic Data

As emphasized in the chapter Tumor, the relation between any tumoral process and the V. A. must be evaluated in several respects. The results of this analysis are given in **Table 39**.

Any tumor in our series has at least one positive answer to the four following questions:

— Does the tumor displace the V. A.?

— Does the tumor compress or even occlude the V. A.?

— Is there an important vascular supply from the V. A.?

— Does an anterior radiculomedullary branch arise from the V. A. close to the tumor?

47 tumors developed so close to the V. A. that they displaced or compressed

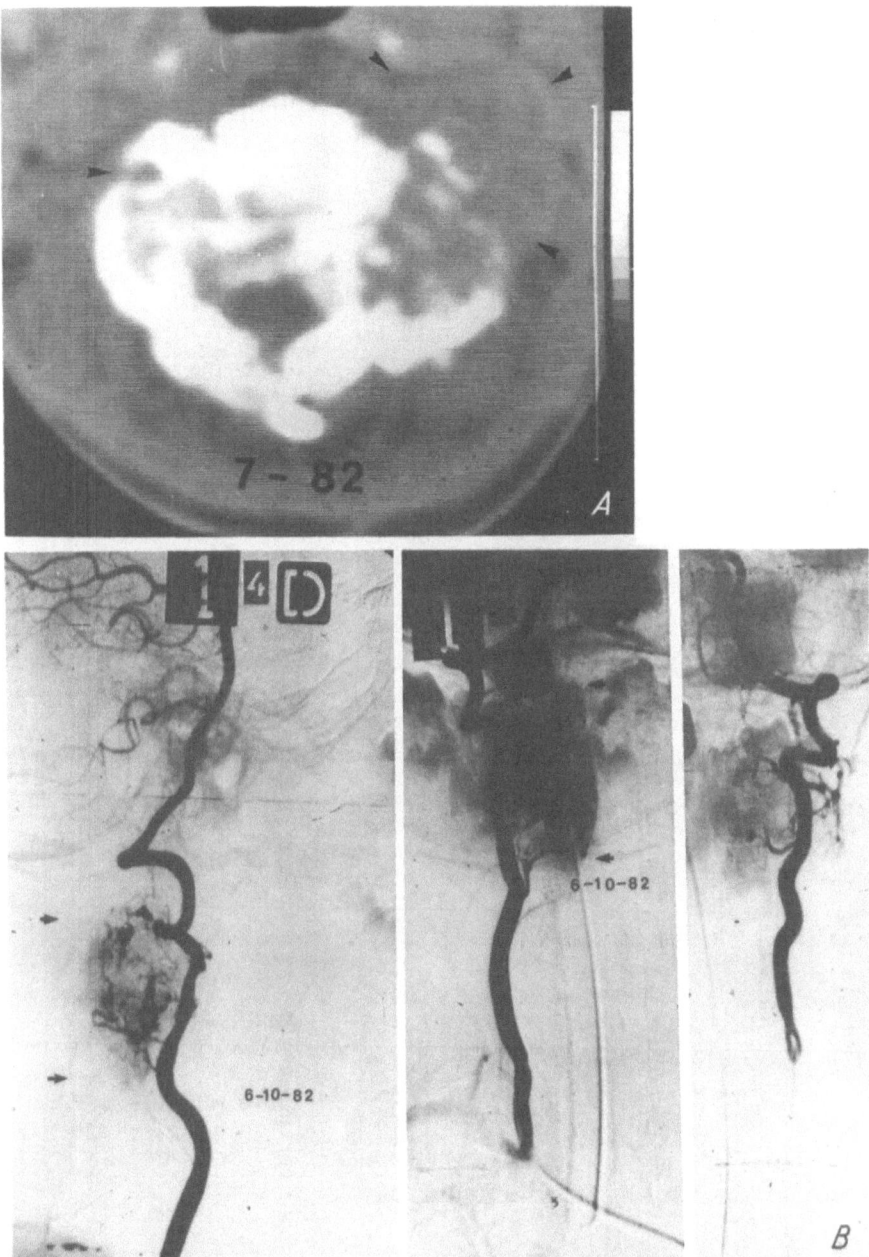

Fig. 91. A) C. T. scan: osteoblastoma involving almost completely the C 3 and C 4 vertebrae and specially both transverse foramina. **B)** Angiography: hypervascularization from both V. A.'s. **C)** Angiography: treatment by bilateral distal V. A. revascularization plus bilateral exclusion. Embolization of both V. A.'s. Finally complete surgical removal in a one-staged bilateral surgical approach. **D)** Operative view: V. A. revascularization on one side by a common carotid to V. A. at C 1 saphenous vein graft

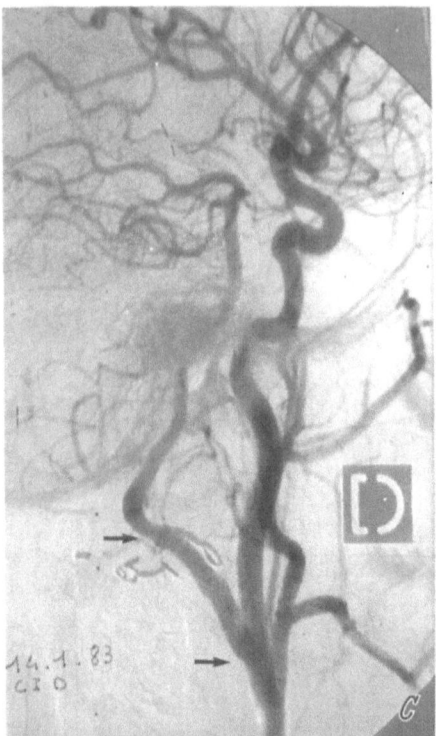

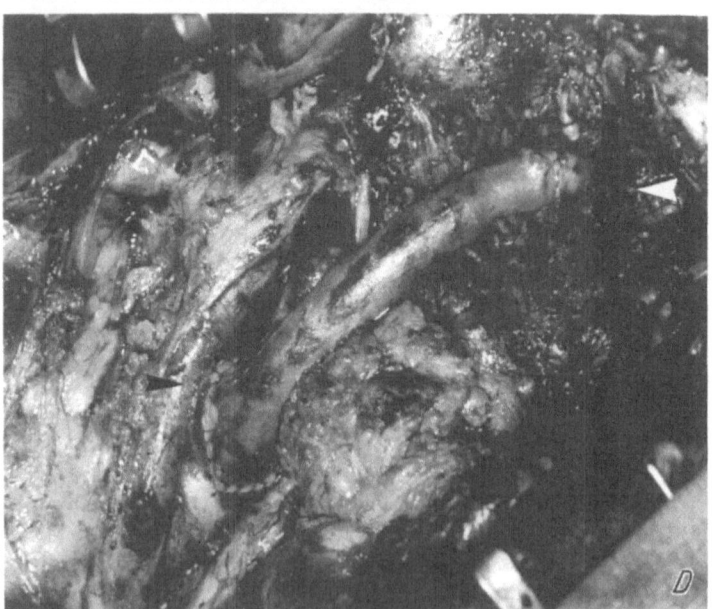

Fig. 91 C and D

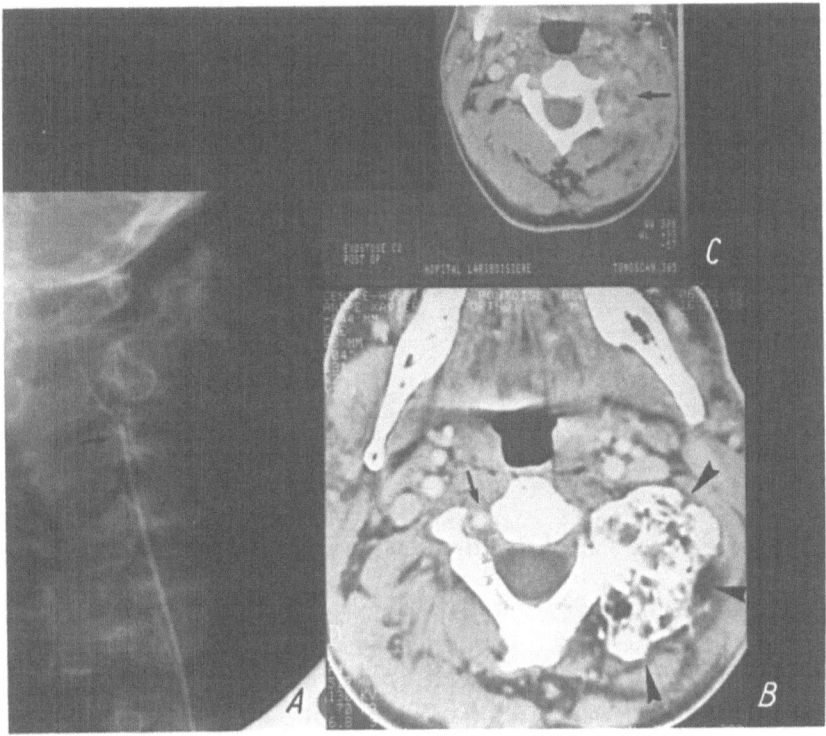

Fig. 92. A) C. T. scan: osteogenic chondroma of the C 2 left transverse process. **B)** Angiography: complete occlusion of a hypoplastic V. A. at the tumoral level. **C)** Post-operative C. T. scan

Table 39. Tumor. Angiography

	C1–C2	C6–C2	OST–C6	Total
Shift	10	15	10	35
Stenosis	6	5	1	12
Hypervascularization	16	10	9	35
Rad. med. artery	0	6	0	6

it; among them, 24 were hypervascularized, mainly from the V. A. 11 cases were adjacent to the V. A. but did not modify its course, although they received major vascularization from the V. A. (**Figs. 87** and **88**).

Of 12 cases with V. A. compression, four presented with complete occlusion: one Hodgkin's disease, one Paget's disease, one fibrous dysplasia, and one osteogenic chondroma. It is probably not merely coincidental that all these tumoral occlusions occurred at the C 2 level (**Fig. 92**).

Finally, in more than 10% of the cases, an important feeding branch to the spinal cord emerged in the vicinity of the tumor.

Table 40. Tumor. Surgery

	C1–C2	C6–C2	OST–C6
V. A. Approach			
lateral anterior	23	16	10
posterior	4	—	—
Complementary technique			
laminectomy	2	5	1
post. fossa craniectomy	17	—	—
revascularization	—	1	—
bone graft	—	5	1
thoracotomy	—	—	4

14.4.4 Surgery (Table 40)

In every case, the V. A. was controlled in the initital steps of the surgical procedure. For this control, the lateral anterior approach was used in 49 cases. In the remaining four cases, all at the C 1–C 2 level, the posterior approach was preferred (3 meningiomas with posterior fossa opening to remove the intracranial intradural extension, and one osteoid osteoma of the lateral mass of C 1).

Pre-operative embolization was performed in 23 cases, i. e. in two-thirds of the cases on which angiography showed hypervascularization.

In 39 cases, a complementary technique for V. A. control was utilized.

Laminectomy was associated in 11 cases. In eight cases, it was performed in the same surgical stage but through a separate posterior approach. In three cases, at the third portion level, the posterior approach was used to control the V. A. and thus laminectomy was performed through the same approach. Craniectomy of the posterior fossa was associated in 17 cases: Three by the same posterior approach as the V. A. control, 10 by the lateral anterior approach, and four by a separate route (a posterior approach for the craniectomy and a lateral anterior route for the V. A. control).

Intervertebral bone graft was used in six cases by the same approach as the V. A. and was completed in two cases by arthrodesis.

Revascularization was performed in one case of osteoblastoma in a 5-year-old boy. The two V. A.'s were revascularized above the tumor and then excluded by a clip just below the anastomosis, allowing embolization of the two V. A.'s and subsequent complete removal of the tumor. An anterior and posterior bone graft fusion completed the procedure.

Thoracotomy was used in four cases (3 carcinomas and one neurinoma) to completely remove an apical lung extension.

14.4.5 Results

Removal appeared macroscopically complete in all cases without any particular morbidity. Morbidity was limited to the usual, transient, symptoms observed in any V. A. surgery and in the case of neurofibroma, to a sensory-motor deficit in the territory of the involved nerve.

One patient died two days post-operatively from an unexplained Sylvian infarct. This 70-year-old patient was operated for a hemangiopericytoma of the second portion of the V. A. with no complication during surgery.

There was no incidence of V. A. injury and V. A. flow was preserved or restored in all cases.

14.4.6 Infectious Process

One case of actinomycosis was observed in a 16-year-old female, with a four years history of an inflammatory mass in the right side of the upper neck. Direct puncture and antibiotics had failed to cure this lesion. It was located mainly at the C 1–C 2 level, with involvement of the right atloido-occipital joint. It stretched the V. A. without stenosis and was not injected on angiography.

This mass was removed by the lateral anterior approach. The V. A. between C 1 and C 2 and above C 1, as well as the atloido-occipital joint, were freed of all fungal abscesses. Complete cure was achieved by complementary treatment with antibiotics.

14.5 External Compression

14.5.1 Compression of the V. A.

The cases of external compression of the V. A. were of different etiologies as shown in **Tables 41** and **42**.

The most frequent cause was tumor. Of a total of 47 cases, the V. A. was displaced in 35, stenosed in 8 and occluded in 4.

The second most frequent etiology was trauma. In the four cases in this group, there was V. A. displacement in one, stenosis in two, and bilateral occlusion in one. The displacement was due to a bullet, one stenosis was due to scar tissue following a cervical hematoma, the other stenosis was due to a luxation at C 5–C 6, and the occlusion was secondary to a complete vertebral luxation at the C 4–C 5 level (**Fig. 93**).

The third etiology observed in our series was osteophytic compression, seen in two cases. Nine additional cases with V. A. loops overlying osteophytes, with little or no encroachment on the V. A. lumen were not considered for surgery. In the two surgical cases, one had bilateral stenosis with, on one side,

Table 41. External compression

No.	Sex	Age	Etiology	Localization	Surgery
1	f	25	scar	C6–C7	+
2	m	19	bullet	C6–C7	+
3	m	68	osteophyte	C4–C5	+
4	m	65	osteophyte	C4–C5	+
5	m	25	fibrous band	C5	+
6	m	68	sympath. nerve	C7	+
7	m	67	luxation	C4–C5	−
8	m	26	luxation	C5–C6	−

External compression series except tumor and non operated osteophyte.

Table 42. External compression

	Symptomatic	Surgery
Tumor	47	—	43
Trauma	4	1	2
Osteophytes	11	2	2
Fibrous bands	1	1	1
Symphathetic N.	1	1	1

angiography. There was no symptomatic case in the tumoral group, and only one in the traumatic group. Two cases in the osteophytic compression group, an almost complete occlusion at the C3–C4 level during head rotation. The other had unilateral compression at C4–C5, but on the dominant V.A.

Finally, there were two particular cases: 1. a case of bilateral fibromuscular compression at the entry of the V.A. into the transverse canal at the C4 level; 2. a V.A. plicature at C7 with pre-occlusive aspect on angiography due to compression by the sympathetic nerve (**Fig. 94**).

In the entire series of external compression cases, only five were symptomatic. All five presented with intermittent symptoms during head and neck movements, correlating with severe compression of the V.A. on

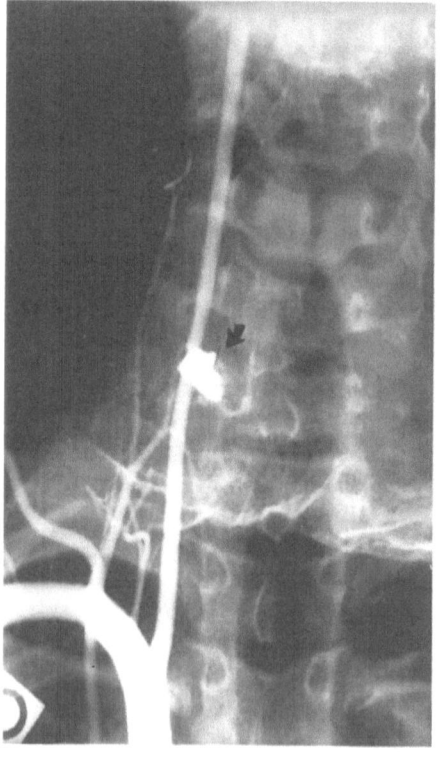

Fig. 93. V.A. compression by a bullet at C7 level

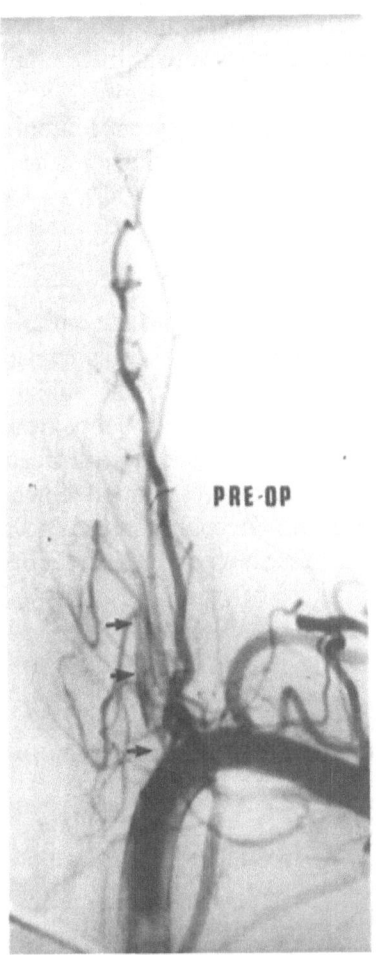

PRE-OP

Fig. 94. Pre-occlusive compression of the ostial V. A. by the sympathetic nerve

one case with compression by fibrous bands and one with compression by the sympathetic nerve were symptomatic (**Table 42**).

49 cases were treated surgically, including 43 tumors, the five symptomatic patients and the case with V. A. displacement by a bullet.

Relevant technical details in these last 6 cases are as follows:

— Traumatic cases: one case was due to compression by scar tissue following a cervical hematoma produced by sustained hyperextension of the neck during coma after suicide attempt. The V. A., as well as the cervical nerve roots of the brachial plexus were progressively exposed and freed from the ostium to C 6.

The second case was a bullet with the tip inside the lateral aspect of the body of C 7 and the base pressing on the V. A. The V. A. was exposed on both sides of the bullet and gently retracted before bullet extraction; this required making a groove around the bullet tip with an air drill while protecting the V. A. (**Fig. 93**).

— Osteophytes: in one case, the V. A. was exposed between two transverse foramina and the osteophytes were removed with the adjacent intervertebral disc. An interbody fusion with an iliac bone graft was then realized.

In the second case, the transverse foramina above and below the osteophytes were opened and the arthritic spurs removed. The disc was left intact in this case.

In both cases, the periosteal sheath was opened and all the scar tissue surrounding the V. A. was released.

— Fibrous bands: the V. A. was exposed from C 6 to C 4. The bayonet shape of the V. A. course was evident as it ran over the transverse process of C 5 and then passed under the hypertrophied fibrous anterior scalenus muscle insertion before entering the C 4 transverse foramen. The fibrous band was divided and then in addition to unroofing the transverse foramen of C 4, the transverse process of C 5 was resected.

— Sympathetic nerve: the first portion

of the V. A. was exposed from the subclavian artery to C6. This revealed a marked plicature of the V. A., which was severely compressed and displaced posteriorly by the sympathetic nerve as it crossed the vessel anteriorly to join the stellate ganglion (**Fig. 74**). The sympathetic nerve was divided and all associated fibrous elements were removed, restoring normal contours and a smoothly curved course to the V. A.

14.5.2 Compression by the V. A.

V. A. loops are particularly frequent on the first portion. In the transverse portion, a V. A. loop may erode the lateral aspect of a vertebral body or pedicle, simulating intervertebral foramen enlargement by tumor. We observed one case with particularly important loops on both sides all along the transverse portion of the two V. A.'s. This patient presented with a history of many years of neck pain and pyramidal signs in both lower extremities but without any motor impairment. It was considered that the irritation to the spinal cord exerted by the V. A. loops was not sufficient to indicate surgical treatment at the time of presentation. Such surgical treatment could consist of revascularization above the last loop with exclusion of the underlying V. A. (**Fig. 95**).

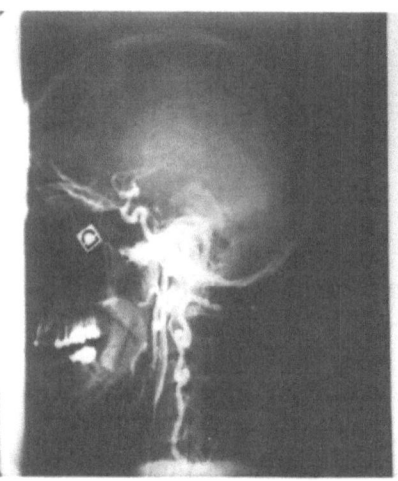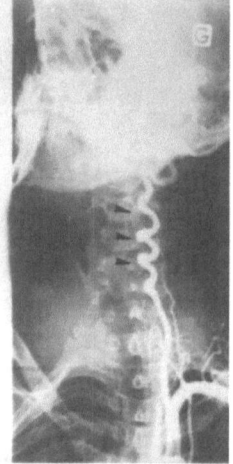

Fig. 95. Bone erosion by bilateral loops with enlargement of the intervertebral foramina simulating an hour-glass tumor

14.6 Trauma

V. A. injury was demonstrated in 22 patients, but only five cases were treated surgically. As mentioned in the chapter Trauma, injury to the V. A. may be consecutive to penetrating or non penetrating trauma, producing various lesions at different levels (**Tables 43** and **44**).

Table 43. Trauma. V. A. lesions

	Laceration	A.V.F.	Ext. comp.	Dissect.
Penetrating injury				
surgery	1	2	—	—
jugular puncture	—	5	—	—
carotid puncture	—	1	—	—
gunshot	—	3	1	—
Non penetrating injury				
hyperextension	—	2	1	4
fracture-luxation	—	—	2	—

Table 44. Trauma. Topography

Localization	1st Portion	2nd Portion	3rd Portion
A.V.F.	2	8 (2)	3 (1)
Ext. comp.	—	4 (2)	—
Dissection	—	2	2
Laceration	—	—	1 (1)
Total	2	14 (4)	6 (2)

( ): Cases treated surgically.

14.6.1 A. V. F.

A. V. F. was the most frequent complication in our series, with 13 cases. All but two were secondary to penetrating injury. Eight of these penetrating injuries were of iatrogenic origin: six followed attempts of jugular or carotid puncture, and two occurred during surgical approach for mastoidectomy and sympathectomy. Three cases followed gunshot wounds. In the two A. V. F.'s after non penetrating injury, a mechanism of cervical hyperextension could be demonstrated, but without vertebral fracture or luxation.

Onset of symptoms was immediate after injury in every fistula of iatrogenic origin, but was delayed several days or weeks in the other cases. In the A. V. F. series (chapter 14.3), case No. 14, not included here, is probably of traumatic origin. However, this A. V. F. appeared four years after cervical trauma with hyperextension, and this long delay makes the etiology less clear.

Two cases were treated surgically. One was a vertebro-jugular fistula with false aneurysm at C2 following a stab wound. The second was a vertebro-vertebral fistula at C 6 following attempts to puncture the internal jugular vein. Surgery was proposed after radi- ological balloon occlusion had failed to correctly treat the fistula.

14.6.2 External Compression

External compression was due to fracture luxation in two cases, bullet in one and prolonged hyperextension with cervical hematoma in one. This last mechanism was seen in a young woman who attempted suicide by drugs and remained in coma for 36 hours with hyperextension of the head and neck. She presented with palsy of the 6th and 7th cervical nerves and vertebro-basilar insufficiency during head rotation. Since symptoms persisted, surgical exploration was performed one month following trauma to remove the scar surrounding the nerve roots and the V. A.

The case with bullet compression was also treated surgically. The tip of the bullet was in the lateral wall of the body of C 7 while the base compressed the V. A.

The two cases of fracture luxation did not require a V. A. approach. One was a luxation at C 5–C 6 imposing a bayonet course to the V. A. at this level, causing no significant stenosis. The second was a 68-year-old man who fell down stairs and presented with severe brain injury and tetraplegia from complete luxation of the spine between C 4 and C 5. Bilateral occlusion was demonstrated initially and persisted even after reduction of the luxation. This patient died on the 14th day following trauma.

14.6.3 Dissection

Of a total of nine dissecting hematomas of the V. A., four cases were related to minor trauma with hyperextension. In two, the lesion was located at C 1–C 2, and in the other two it was at C 6. The following case is demonstrative: a 46-year-old man fell while skiing, landing on his head. He experienced left sided headaches for 24 hours and left sided IX to XII cranial nerve palsy appeared on the second day. When the patient was referred, 8 days later, the neurological symptoms had partially regressed. Complete angiographic investigations showed a dissecting aneurysm at the C 6 level. After six weeks of anticoagulant therapy, a second angiography was performed. The ectasia on the arterial wall had almost disappeared and was more smoothly contoured. Heparin was discontinued and replaced by anti-platelet agents. The six-month angiographic control demonstrated the complete healing of the dissection. Other cases of dissection were observed after motor vehicle accidents (2 cases) and table tennis (1 case). None required V. A. surgery, since the wall lesion disappeared or markedly regressed in all cases.

14.6.4 Laceration

Finally, it was necessary to repair a wall laceration produced on the V. A. above the arch of the atlas during posterior fossa opening for a cerebello-pontine angle tumor. The V. A. was controlled and clamped before repair with a small venous patch. Angiographic control two years after surgery showed normal, regular, V. A. contours.

14.7 V. A. Surgery and Interventional Radiology

In six cases (**Table 45**), V. A. surgery was used to facilitate or replace endovascular techniques.

Table 45. V. A. neuroradiology

No.	Sex	Age	Lesion	Localization	Treatment
1	f	34	AVM	spinal cord	embol. C1 C2
2	f	24	AVM	spinal cord	embol. C1
3	m	24	AVM	spinal cord	embol. C1 C2
4	m	22	AVM	thalamus	embol. C1
5	f	39	An	V. A.	occlusion
6	m	26	AVM	Galen's vein	catheter removal

AVM: arterio-venous malformation, An: aneurysm, embol.: embolization.

14.7.1 Indications

In four of these cases, it permitted treatment of arteriovenous malformations, three on the spinal cord and one in the thalamus (**Figs. 96** and **97**).

In a fifth case, surgery was proposed for occlusion of the V. A. with a clip, as distally as possible in order to decrease blood pressure in an intracranial V. A. aneurysm which could not be approached either surgically or radiologically.

In the sixth and last case, the aim was to reduce the length of a balloon catheter which had been ligated and fixed subcutaneously in the axilla after endovascular treatment of a malformation of the great vein of Galen; secondarily, this catheter had migrated within the subclavian and the vertebral artery where it was blocked with multiple loops.

In the five cases of intraoperative embolization, conventional methods failed because of proximal thrombosis in two cases and tortuosity of a small V. A. in three.

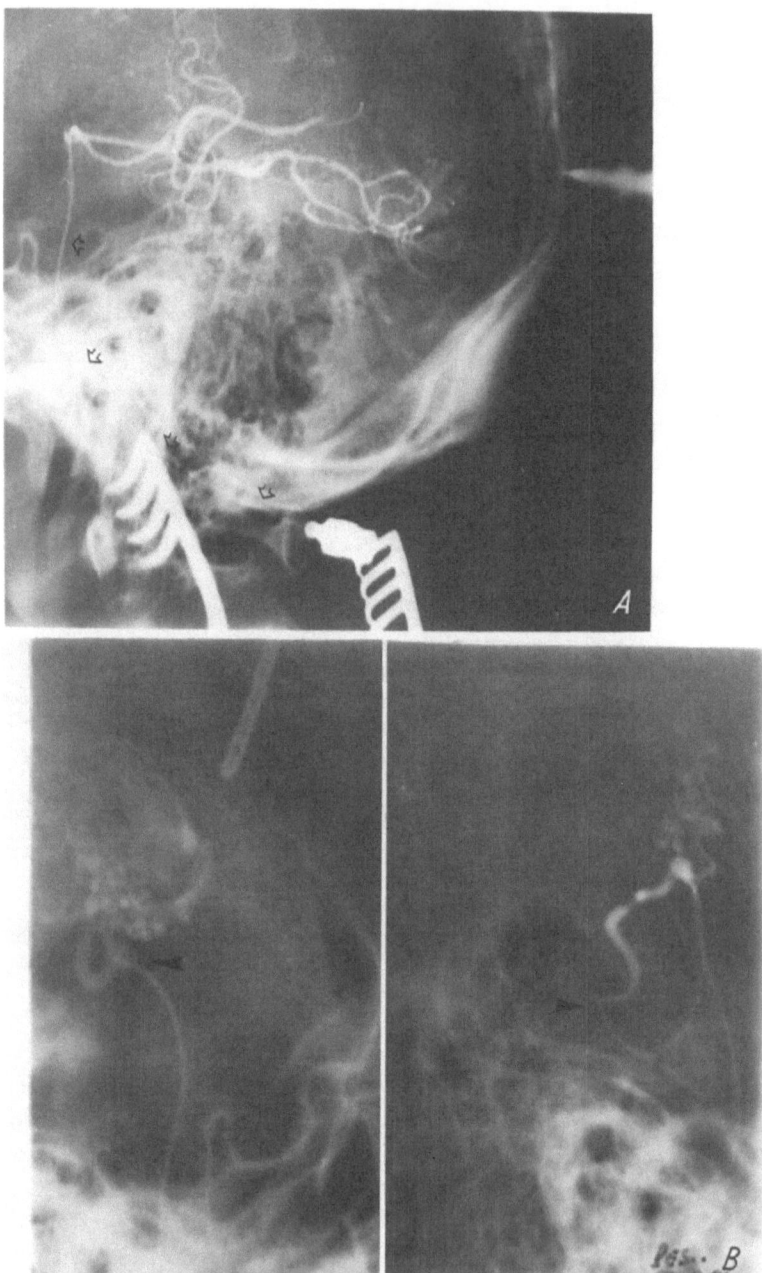

Fig. 96. A) Intraoperative embolization of a thalamic arteriovenous malformation through the V. A. exposed above C1. **B)** Selective injection and embolization of perforating arteries

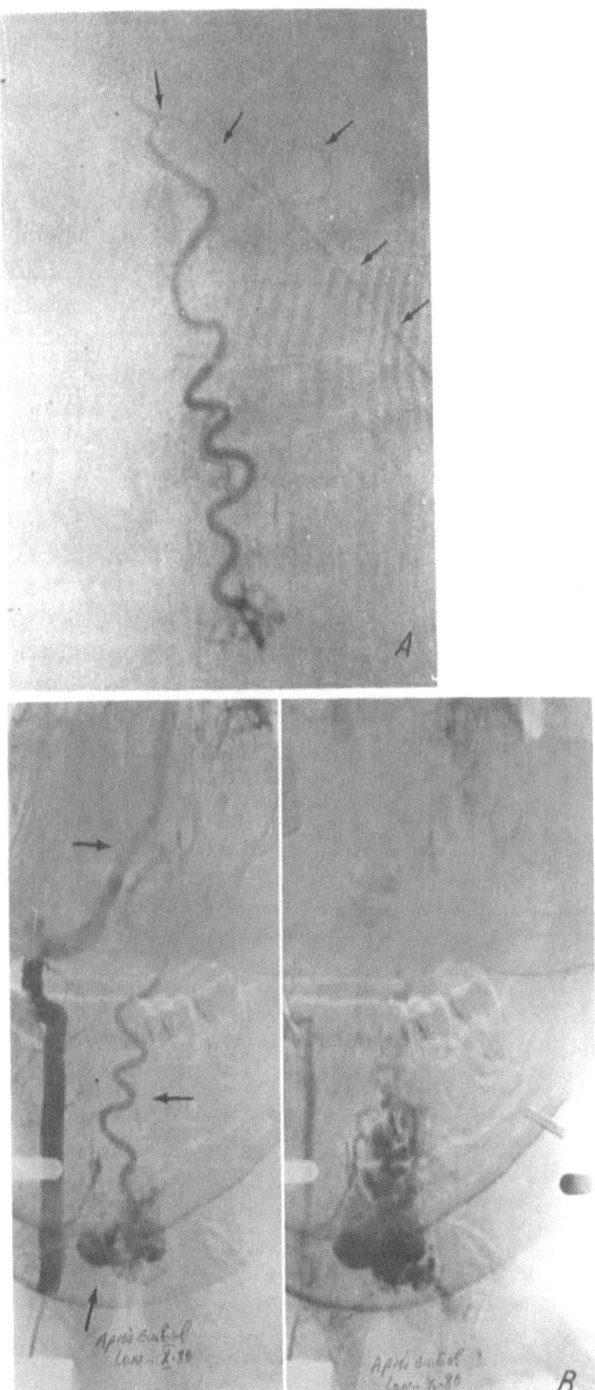

Fig. 97. Intraoperative embolization (**A**) of a spinal cord arteriovenous malformation (**B**) through the V. A. exposed between C 1 and C 2

14.7.2 Technique

V. A. exposure was performed above C1 in two cases of arteriovenous malformation (the thalamic and one spinal cord malformation) and in the aneurysm case, between C1 and C2 in the other spinal cord malformation, and at C5–C6 to extract the looped catheter.

In the first four embolization cases, the reduction of the catheter length and avoidance of V. A. loops, simplified and greatly facilitated the embolization procedure for the neuroradiologist. In no other way, could embolization have been done safely. It must be stressed that because endovascular techniques have improved dramatically since these V. A. exposure for embolization were performed, most such exposures would no longer be necessary. V. A. loops are now far more rarely a problem, and even thrombosis can be overtaken by direct distal puncture and catheterization.

14.7.3 Results

V. A. flow was always preserved. Puncture holes were closed by an X stitch suture in the first four cases.

In case No. 6, the V. A. was exposed at C5–C6, where the catheter tail was situated. The artery was then clamped with Heifetz clips, and a small arteriotomy (1 cm in length) was performed. Twenty centimeters of the catheter were pulled from the artery and then cut, leaving two centimeters to suture to the prevertebral fascia. The arteriotomy was closed around the catheter by a purse string suture.

Angiographic controls did not show any abnormalities on the arterial wall, neither at the site of puncture in the four embolization cases, nor at the arteriotomy site in case No. 6.

15. CONCLUSION

Cervical vascular surgery has in general been limited to the carotid arteries and vertebral artery surgery has been considered as an unusual challenge or adventure.

At the present time, the surgical approach, exposure and control of the V. A. on any portion of its cervical course is a reliable technique whatever the level. The ostial portion must therefore no longer be considered the only site for V. A. surgery.

Precise techniques now permit V. A. exposure in a field sufficiently large to allow any surgical procedure, just as on any other vessel.

Treatment of wall lesions, and above all, those due to atherosclerosis, is the main application of V. A. surgery. The particular anatomic features of the vertebral arteries explain that techniques of revascularization are specific for this vessel.

However, structural lesions are only part of the pathologic conditions that may involve the V. A. In comparison to the internal carotid artery, the V. A. is less frequently involved by atherosclerosis, but various other processes, are most frequent. The anatomic situation of the V. A. leads to a wide variety of pathology. The V. A. runs in a bony canal adjacent to the vertebrae. Therefore, any process extruding from the vertebrae, such as tumors or osteophytes, or displacing the vertebrae, such as luxation or fracture, may interfere with the V. A.

The V. A. is crossed by the nerve roots just as they emerge from the intervertebral foramen. Any process involving the nerve roots, particularly hour-glass tumors, must also involve the V. A.

The V. A. is surrounded by a venous plexus, which makes it similar to the internal carotid artery within the cavernous sinus. Abnormal communications between the artery and surrounding veins are therefore not surprisingly observed on both vessels.

In addition, the V. A. participates in the vascular supply of many cervical tumoral and vascular lesions.

In contrast the internal carotid artery lies in a free anatomic space, is accompanied only by the vagus nerve, and has no perivascular plexus at the cervical level. Moreover, it gives no collateral branch until its entry into the petrous bone.

Tumor, external compression and arteriovenous malformations are consequently frequent indications for V. A. surgery, while these indications are rare on the internal carotid artery.

The need for reliable and safe surgical techniques for the V. A. is therefore at least as great as for the internal carotid artery. The lateral anterior approach is the preferred surgical approach to the

V. A. Other routes proposed in the past are less appropriate, although they may be considered in particular cases alone or associated with the lateral anterior approach.

We have now performed more than 150 surgical approaches to the V. A. for various indications, with excellent results, no mortality and very limited morbidity. In our opinion, assuming mastery of the anatomy of the deep cervical area and precise surgical techniques, V. A. surgery should be considered a routine procedure.

However, the choice of the most appropriate procedure remains difficult and controversial. The frequent anatomic variations and anomalies, as well as the variability of each V. A.'s importance in the vertebro-basilar supply (including the spinal cord) explain the difficulties. The controversial aspects of V. A. surgery belong to the general problem of surgery for cerebral ischemia. If from a technical point of view, internal carotid artery and V. A. surgery are considered equally feasible, a more rational approach to the treatment of cerebral ischemia will result. Such an approach begins with complete investigations of both the carotid and vertebral systems after any cerebral ischemic event, whatever its localization. There is no justification for continuing to consider the cerebral vasculature as consisting of two separate entities: the carotid artery supplying the forebrain and the V. A. supplying the hindbrain. Practical reasons based on the lack of surgical possibilities were partly responsible for this way of thinking. Cerebral vascularization must be considered as a whole, originating from the branches of the circle of Willis, itself supplied by both the carotid and vertebral systems.

In fields other than cerebral ischemia, V. A. surgical techniques have also made important contribution, examples of which are achievement of more complete tumoral removal and better possibilities for treatment of arteriovenous malformations.

The V. A. should no longer be feared or forgotten in the discussion of surgical procedures in the neck. The quills of the hedgehog, to which the V. A. has been compared (Walt, 1984), can now be neutralized.

REFERENCES

1. Aaslid R, Markwalder TM, Nornes H (1982) Non invasive transcranial Doppler ultrasound recording of flow velocity in basal cerebral arteries. J Neurosurg 57: 769–774

2. Aaslid R (17–19 april 1986) Brain hemodynamics: importance of the Circle of Willis. Meeting of Society for Neurovascular Surgery, Chicago

3. Ackerman RH, Correia JA, Alpert NM (1981) Positron imaging in ischemic stroke disease using compounds labeled with oxygen 15: initial results of clinicophysiological correlations. Arch Neurol 38: 537–551

4. Ackerman RH, Alpert NM, Correia JA (1984) Positron imaging in ischemic stroke disease. Ann Neurol 15 [suppl]: 126–137

5. Adachi B (1928) Das Arteriensystem der Japaner, Bd I. Kenkyusha Tokyo

6. Adeloye A, Anomah NU, Latunde OE (1970) Traumatic aneurysm of the first portion of the right vertebral artery. Br J Surg 57: 312–314

7. Alajouanine TH, Castaigne P, Cambier J, Lianantonakis E (1958) Le rôle des positions anormales et prolongées de la tête et du cou dans le déterminisme de certains accidents vasculaires du tronc cérébral. B Soc Med Hop Paris, 74: 21–26

8. Alajouanine T, Lhermitte F, Gautier JC (1960) Transient cerebral ischemia in atherosclerosis. Neurology 10: 906–914

9. Alexander W (1882) The treatment of epilepsy by ligature of the vertebral arteries. Brain 5: 170–187

10. Alexander JJ, Glagov S, Zarnis CK (1986) Repair of a vertebral artery dissection. Case report. J Neurosurg 64: 662–665

11. Al Meffy O, Marano G, Rayarraman S, Nugent GR, Rodman N (1979) TIA due to increased platelet aggregation and adhesiveness ultra structural and functional correlation. J Neurosurg 50: 449–453

12. Alpers BJ, Berry RB, Puddison RM (1959) Anatomical studies of the circle of Willis in normal brain. Arch Neurol Psych 81: 409–418

13. Alpers BJ, Berry RB (1963) Circle of Willis in cerebral vascular disorders. Arch Neurol 8: 298–411

14. Alpert JN, Gerson LP, Hall RJ, Hollman GL (1982) Reversible angiopathy. Stroke 13: 100–105

15. Alves AM, Black C (1972) Post-traumatic extracranial aneurysms of the vertebral artery. Int Surg 57: 422

16. Anderson RE, Shealy CN (1970) Cervical pedicle erosion and rootlet compression caused by a tortuous vertebral artery. Radiology 96: 537–538

17. Anderson RA, Sondheimer FK (1976) Rare carotid-vertebro-basilar anastomoses with notes on the differentiation between proatlantal and hypoglossal arteries. Neuroradiology 11: 113–118

18. Aronson NI (1961) Traumatic arteriovenous fistula of the vertebral vessels. Neurology 11: 817–823

19. Avellanosa AM, Glasauer FE, Young OH (1977) Traumatic vertebral arteriovenous fistula associated with cervical spine fracture. J Trauma 17: 885–888

20. Avman N, Ozkal E, Erdogan A (1975) Vertebral angiography and microsurgery in the management of dumb-bell cervical neurinomas. Surg Neurol 4: 327–329

21. Bach ST (1970) Cervical chordoma. Report of a case and brief review of the literature. Acta Oto Laryng 69: 450–456

22. Bachman DM, Kim RM (1980) Transluminal dilatation for subclavian steal syndrome. AJR 135: 995–996

23. Bahar S, Chiras J, Carpean JF, Meder JF, Bories (1984) Spontaneous vertebro-vertebral arteriovenous fistula associated with fibromuscular dysplasia. Report of two cases. Neuroradiology 26: 45–49

24. Barbieri A (1867) Dell'Arteria Vertebrale. Milan

25. Baron JC, Bousser MG, Guillard A, Comar D, Castaigne P (1981) Reversal of focal "Misery Perfusion Syndrome" by extra intracranial by-pass in hemodynamic cerebral ischemia. Stroke 12: 454–459

26. Baron JC, Steinling M, Tanaka T (1981) Quantitative measurement of CBF, oxygen extraction fraction (OEF) and CMRO 2 with the ^{15}O continuous inhalation technique and position emission tomography (PET): experimental evidences and normal values in man. J Cereb Blood Flow Metab 1: 5–6

27. Barré M (1926) Sur un syndrome sympathique cervical postérieur et sa cause fréquente: l'arthrite cervicale. Rev Neurol 33: 1246–1248

28. Bartal AD, Levy MJ(1972) Excision of a congenital suboccipital vertebral arteriovenous fistula. Case report. J Neurosurg 37, 452–456

29. Barton JW, Margolis MT (1975) Rotational obstruction of the vertebral artery at the atlantoaxial joint. Neuroradiology 9: 117–120

30. Bauer RB, Sheeha S, Meyer JS (1961) Arteriographic study of cerebral vascular disease. II: cerebral symptoms due to a kingking tortuosity and compression of carotid and vertebral arteries in the neck. Arch Neurol 4: 119–131

31. Bayley P, Cushing H, Eisenhardt L (1928) Angioblastic meningiomas. Arch Pathol 6: 953–990

32. Belan A, Vesels M, Vanek I, Weiss K, Peregrin JH (1982) Percutaneous transluminal angioplasty of fibromuscular dysplasia of the internal carotid artery. Cardiovasc Intervent Radiol 5: 79–81

33. Bellot J, Guerardi R, Poirier J, Lacour P, Debrun G, Barbizet J (1985) Fibromuscular dysplasia of cervico cephalic arteries with multiple dissections and a carotido-cavernous fistula. A pathological study. Stroke 16: 255–261

34. Benhamou AC, George B, Merland JJ, Bories J, Natali J (1979) Traitement par abord chirurgical direct d'un faux anévrysme traumatique artério-veineux vertébro-jugulaire interne au niveau du tubercule de l'atlas. J Chir Paris 116: 659–662

35. Beraneck L (1984) Erosion d'un trou de conjugaison cervical par une boucle de l'artère vertébrale. Rev Rhum 51: 439

36. Bergstrom K, Lodin H (1966) Arteriovenous fistula as a complication of cerebral angiography. Report in three cases. Br J Radiol 39: 263–266

37. Berguer R, Andaya LV, Bauer RB (1976) Vertebral artery by-pass. Arch Surg 111: 976–979

38. Berguer A, Feldman AJ, Wilner HI, Lazo A (1982) Arteriovenous vertebral fistulae. Cure by combination of operation and detachable intravascular balloon. Ann Surg 96: 65–68

39. Berguer R, Feldman AJ (1983) Surgical reconstruction of the vertebral artery. Surgery 93: 670–675

40. Berguer R (1985) Distal vertebral artery by-pass: technique, the "occipital connection" and potential uses. J Vasc Surg 2: 621–626

41. Berquist E (1971) Bilateral arteriovenous fistulae. A complication of vertebral angiography by direct percutaneous puncture. Br J Radiol 44: 519–523

42. Berthelot JL, Couffinhal JC, Coquillaud JP, Andreassian B (1982) Fistule artério-veineuse vertébrale. Technique chirurgicale par voie postérieure para-médiane. Neurochirurgie 28: 315–318

43. Bjork VO (1966) Iatrogenic vertebral arterio-venous fistula. Thorax 21: 367–368

44. Bladin PF (1974) Dissecting aneurysm of carotid and vertebral arteries: a clinical and angiographic study of early diagnosis, natural history and pathophysiology of cerebral lesion. Vasc Surg 8: 203–223

45. Bladin PF, Merory J (1975) Mechanisms in cerebral lesions in trauma to high cervical portion of the vertebral artery rotation injury. Proc Anst Assoc Neurol 12: 35–41

46. Blank RH, Connar RG (1974) Arterial complications associated with thoracic outlet compression syndrome. Ann Thorac Surg 17: 315–323

47. Boldrey R, Maas L, Miller ER (1956) The role of atlantoid compression in the etiology of internal carotid thrombosis. J Neurosurg 13: 127–139

48. Bohmfalk GL, Story JL, Browne WE, Marlin AE (1979) Subclavian steal syndrome. Part 1: proximal vertebral to common carotid artery transposition in three patients and historical review. J Neurosurg 51: 628–640

49. Bohmfalk GL, Story JL, Browne WE, Marlin AE (1979) Subclavian steal syndrome. Part 2: intraoperative vertebral artery blood flow measurement. J Neurosurg 51: 641–643

50. Bonduelle M, Ruscalleda J, Zalzal P (1973) Dysplasie fibromusculaire avec fistule artério-veineuse de l'artère vertébrale extra-crânienne. Rev Neurol 128: 204–206

51. Bonte FJ, Stokely EM (1981) Single photon tomographic study of regional cerebral blood flow after stroke: concise communication. J Nucl Med 22: 1049

52. Boreadis AG, Gershon-Cohen J (1956) Luschka joints of the cervical spine. Radiology 66: 181–187

53. Bosniak MA, Morton A (1964) Cervical arterial pathways associated with brachiocephalic occlusive disease. AJR 1: 1232–1236

54. Bostrom K, Liliequist B (1977) Primary dissecting aneurysm of the extracranial part of the internal carotid and vertebral arteries. Neurology 17: 179–186

55. Boudin G, Barbizet J (1958) Les accidents nerveux des manipulations du rachis cervical. Rev du Prat 8: 2235–2243

56. Boudin G, Guillard A, Romion A (1974) Dysplasies fibro-musculaires des artères carotides et vertebrales. Ann Med Int 125: 863–875

57. Boudot L (1864) Des résections des apophyses transverses des vertèbres. Thèse Médecine. Strasbourg, n° 812

58. Boyle AC (1971) The rheumatoid neck. Proc R Soc Med 64: 1161–1165

59. Bradac GB, Kaerbach A, Bolck-Weischedel, Finck GA (1981) Spontaneous dissecting aneurysm of cervical cerebral arteries. Neuro-Radiology 21: 149–154

60. Brodribb AJ (1970) Vertebral aneurysm in a case of Ehlers-Danlos syndrom. Br J Surg 57: 148–151

61. Brown AS, Donaldson AA (1971) Clinical vertebral artery cerebral blood flow measurement. Em Neurol 6: 274–276

62. Brunon J, Goutelle A (1974) Traitement chirurgical de l'insuffisance vertébro-basilaire par compression extrinsèque de l'artère vertébrale extra-crânienne. Neurochirurgie 2: 127–145

63. Brunon J, Gaillarde AM, Schott B (1974) Insuffisance vertébro-basilaire par pseudarthrose des pédicules de l'axis. Lyon Med 232: 655–659

64. Buonanno FS, Rykett IL, Brady TJ (1983) Proton N. M. R. imaging in experimental ischemic infarction. Stroke 14: 178–182

65. Buscaglia LC, Crowhurst HD (1979) Vertebral artery trauma. Ann J Surg 138: 269–272

66. Callow AD (1985) Evaluation of operative risk by computer tomographic scan and echo. B. In: Courbier R (ed) Basis for a classification of cerebral arterial diseases. Excerpta Mecial Current Clinical Practice. Series 22, pp 29–39, Amsterdam

67. Camp PE (1984) Carotid to distal vertebral artery by-pass for vertebro-basilar ischemia. J Neurosurg 60: 187–189

68. Caplan LR, Sergay S (1976) Positional cerebral ischemia. J Neurol Neurosurg Psychiat 39: 385–391

69. Caplan LR (1980) "Top of the basilar" syndrome. Neurology 30: 72–79

70. Caplan LR (1981) Vertebrobasilar disease. Time for a new strategy. Stroke 12: 111–114

71. Carney AL, Emmanuele R, Anderson EM (1976) Surgery of the vertebral artery. Medicam AV Productions, Chicago

72. Carney AL, Anderson EM (1978) Carotid distal vertebral artery by-pass for carotid artery occlusion. Clin E E G 9: 105–109

73. Carney AL (1981) Vertebral artery surgery: historical development, basic concepts of brain hemodynamics, and clinical experience of 102 cases. In: Advances in neurology. Diagnosis and treatment of

brain ischemia, vol 30. New York, Raven Press, pp 249–282

74. Carpentier S (1961) Injury of neck as cause of vertebral artery thrombosis. J Neurosurg 18: 849–853

75. Cartlidge NEF, Whisnant JP, Elveback LR (1977) Carotid and vertebral basilar transient cerebral ischemic attacks: a community study. Rochester, Minnesota, Mayo Clin Proc 52: 117–120

76. Case MES, Archer CR, Hsieh V, Codd JE (1979) Traumatic aneurysm of vertebral artery. A case report and review of the literature. Angiology 30: 138–142

77. Castaigne P, Lhermitte F, Gautier JC, Escourolle R, Derouesne C, Der Agopian E, Popa C (1973) Arterial occlusions in the vertebro-basilar system. Brain 96: 133–154

78. Cate WR, Scott HN (1959) Cerebral ischemia of central origin: relief by subclavian vertebral artery thromboendarterectomy. Surgery 45: 19–31

79. Chiari, 1829 (1861) Cited by Chassaignac: traité clinique et pratique d'opérations chirurgicales 1: 334

80. Chiras J, Marciano S, Vega Molia J, Touboul J, Poirier B, Boris J (1985) Spontaneous dissecting aneurysm of the extracranial vertebral artery (20 cases). Neuroradiology 27: 327–333

81. Chirossel JP, Louveau A, Vasdeu A, Dreuet JG, Pasquier B, Passagia JG (1985) Les tumeurs bénignes du rachis cervical. In: Simon L, Leroux JL, Privat JM (eds), Rachis cervical et Médecine de Rééducation. Masson, Paris, pp 94–106

82. Chou SN, French LA (1965) Arteriovenous fistula of the vertebral vessels in the neck. Case reports. J Neurosurg 22: 77–80

83. Chou NS, Story JL, Seljeskog E, French LA (1967) Further experience with arteriovenous fistulas of the vertebral artery in the neck. Surgery 62: 779–788

84. Cinqualbre J, Ribiero J, Dalcher G, Mascali Y, Kieny R (1978) Fistule artério-veineuse vertébrale d'origine congénitale. A propos d'un cas. Ann Chir 32: 335–339

85. Clarisse J, Dobbelaere P, Francke JP, Julliot JP, Jomin M (1977) Superselective injection of the carotid and vertebro-basilar system using a coaxial catheter. J Neuroradiol 4: 5–11

86. Clark K, Perry MU (1956) Carotid vertebral anastomosis: an alternative technic for repair of the subclavian steal syndrome. Ann Surg 1963: 414–416

87. Comerota AJ, Cranley JJ, Katz ML (1984) Real-time B. mode carotid imaging. J Vasc Surg 1: 84–89

88. Constostavlos DL (1971) Massive subarachnoid hemorrhage due to laceration of the vertebral artery associated with fracture of the transverse process of atlas. J Forensic Sci 16: 40–56

89. Cooper DF (1980) Bone erosion of the cervical vertebrae secondary to tortuosity of the vertebral artery. J Neurosurg 53: 106–108

90. Corkill G, French BH, Michas C, Cobb CA, Mims TJ (1977) External carotid vertebral artery anastomosis for vertebro-basilar insufficiency. Surg Neurol 7: 109–115

91. Cormier JM, Laurian C (1976) Surgical management of vertebro-basilar insufficiency. J Cardiovasc Surg 11: 205–215

92. Correll JW, Stern J, Zyroff J, Wheelan M (1979) Vertebro-basilar insufficiency relieved by carotid endarteriectomy. Adv Neurosurg 2: 40–44

93. Crompton MR (1959) The visual changes in temporal (Giant cell) arteritis. Report of a case with autopsy findings. Brain 82: 377–390

94. Dandy WE (1944) Intracranial arterial aneurysm. Comstock Publishing Co., Ithaca, New York

95. Danziger J, Bloch S (1975) The widened cervical intervertebral foramen. Radiology 116: 671–674

96. Dartevelle P, Levasseur P, Rojas-Miranda A, George B, Lebrigand H, Merlier M (1984) Intérêt de la cervicotomie élargie dans les syndromes de Pancoast-Tobias. Ann Chir 38: 79–84

97. David M, Messimy R, Dilenge D, Harispe L, Metzger J (1968) Le problème des sténoses et thromboses vertébro-basilaires. A propos de 50 observations. Press Med 76: 147–150

98. Davidson KC, Welford EC, Dixon GD (1975) Traumatic vertebral artery pseudoaneurysm following chiropractic manipulation. Neuroradiology 115: 651–652

99. Deans WR, Bloch S, Leibrock I, Berman BM, Skultety PM (1982) Arteriovenous fistula in patients with neurofibromatosis. Radiology 144: 103–107

100. De Bakey ME, Simeone FA (1946) Battle injuries of the arteries in World War II. Ann Surg 123: 534–541

101. De Bakey ME, Crawford ES, Cooley DA (1965) Cerebral arterial insufficiency: one to eleven years result following arterial reconstructive operation. Ann Surg 161: 921–945

102. Debrun G, Lacour P, Caron JP, Hurth M, Comoy J, Keravel Y (1978) Detachable balloon and calibrated leak balloon techniques in the treatment of cerebral vascular lesions. J Neurosurg 49: 635–649

103. Dekleyn A, Versteegh C (1933) Über verschiedene Formen von Meniere's Syndrom. Dtsch Z Nervenheilkde 132: 157–189

104. Denny-Brown D (1960) Recurrent cerebro-vascular episodes. AMA Arch Neurol 2: 94–100

105. Deutsch HJ (1969) Aneurysm of the vertebral artery: medicine in Vietnam. Laryngoscope 79: 134–139

106. Devico DC, Farrell FW (1972) Vertebro-basilar occlusive disease in children. A recognizable entity. Arch Neurol 26: 278–281

107. Diaz FG, Ausman JI, De Los Reyes RA, Pearce J, Shroutz C, Pak H, Turcott J (1984) Surgical reconstruction of the proximal vertebral artery. J Neurosurg 61: 874–881

108. Diaz FG, Ausman JI, Shroutz, Pearce J, Tiel R (1985) Surgical reconstruction of the second portion of the vertebral artery in cerebral revascularization for stroke. Spetzler RF (ed). Thieme-Stratton, New York, pp 325–329

109. Dietrich (1831) Das Aufsuchen der Schlagadern. Neurenberg, pp 81

110. Djindjian R, Clay R, Hurth M, Vedrenne Cl (1964) Etude clinique, artériographique et anatomique d'un cas de malformation de la charnière cervico-occipitale. Press Med 72: 3013–3016

111. Djindjian R, Hurth M (1964) L'artériographie vertébrale des les malformations de la charnière cervico-occipitale. Ann Radiol 7: 887–889

112. Dodson T, Quindlen E, Crowell R, Mc Enany MT (1980) Vertebral arteriovenous fistulae following insertion of central monitoring catheters. Surgery 87: 343–346

113. Dooley JM, Smith KR (1968) Occlusion of the basilar artery in a 6-year-old boy. Neurology 18: 1034–1036

114. Dotter CT, Judkins MP (1964) Transluminal treatment of arteriosclerotic obstruction: description of a new technic and preliminary report of its applications. Circulation 30: 654–670

115. Dragon R, Saranchak H, Lakin P, Straugh G (1981) Blunt injuries to the carotid and vertebral arteries. Ann J Surg 41: 497–500

116. Duffy PE, Jacobs GB (1958) Clinical and pathological findings in vertebral artery thrombosis. Neurology 8: 862–869

117. Dumke PR, Schmidt CF (1943) Quantitative measurements of cerebral blood flow in the macaque monkey. Am J Physiol 138: 421–431

118. Early CB, Shuring AG, Hunt WB (1966) False aneurysm of the vertebral artery. A complication or radon seed implantation. Ann Surg 164: 900–904

119. Eastcott HHG, Pickering GW, Rob CG (1954) Reconstruction of internal carotid artery. Lancet 2: 994–996

120. Easton JD, Sherman DG (1977) Cervical manipulation and stroke. Stroke 8: 594–597

121. Edwards A (1969) Ehlers-Danlos syndrome with vertebral artery aneurysm. Proc R Soc Med 62: 14–16

122. Edwards WH, Mulhein JL (1984) The surgical reconstruction of the proximal subclavian and vertebral artery in vertebro-basilar arterial occlusive disease. Berguer R, Bauer R (eds). Raven Press, New York, pp 241–255

123. Elkin DC, Harris MH (1946) Arteriovenous aneurysm of the vertebral vessels. Report of ten cases. Ann Surg 124: 934–951

124. Ehrlich FE, Carey L, Kitrinos NP (1968) Congenital arteriovenous fistula between the vertebral artery and vertebral vein. Case report. J Neurosurg 29: 629–630

125. Enziger FM, Smith BH (1976) Hemangiopericytoma. An analysis of 106 cases. Hum Pathol 7: 61–82

126. Fabiani JN, Mercier JN, Ribiere N (1979) Traitement par embolisation d'une fistule artério-veineuse vertébrale congénitale. Arch Franc Pediatr 36: 34–39

127. Faeth WH, Ducker HW (1961) Arteriovenous vascular malformation of the cervical portion of the vertebral artery. A case report. Neurology 2: 492–493

128. Fairman R, Grossman R, Gonberg H (1984) A new approach to the treatment of vertebral arteriovenous fistulas. Surgery 95: 112–114

129. Faith WH, Ducker HW (1961) Arteriovenous vascular malformation of the cervical portion of the vertebral artery. Neurology (Minneap) 11: 492–493

130. Fang H (1958) A comparison of blood vessels of the brain and peripheral blood vessels. In: Wright IS, Millikan CH (eds), Cerebral vascular diseases. Grune and Stratton Inc, New York, pp 17–22

131. Feldman AJ (1984) Surgical approach to disease of the first portion of the vertebral artery. In: Vertebro-basilar arterial occlusive disease. Medical and surgical management. Raven Press, New York, pp 231–239

132. Fenger, cited by Matas

133. Fielding JW (1957) Cineroentgenography of the normal cervical spine. J Bone Joint Surg (Am) 39: 1280–1288

134. Fields WS, Zulch KJ, Maslenikou U (1972) High cervical neurinomas. Special neurologic and radiologic features. Zbl Neurochir 33: 89–100

135. Fischer C, Blanc A, Mauguière F, Courjon J (1891) Apport des potentiels évoqués auditifs précoces au diagnostic neurologique. Rev Neurol 137: 229–240

136. Fisch U (1982) Infratemporal fossa approach for glomus tumours of the temporal bone. Ann Otol Rhinol Laryngol 91: 474–479

137. Fisher CM, Karnes WE, Kubik CS (1961) Lateral medullary infarction. The pattern of vascular occlusion. J Neuropath Exp Neurol 20: 323–379

138. Fisher CM (1961) A new vascular syndrome: "The subclavian steal syndrome" N Engl J Med 265: 912–913

139. Fisher CM, Gore I, Obake N, White PD (1965) Atherosclerosis of the carotid and vertebral arteries extracranial and intracranial. J Neuropath Exp Neurol 24: 455–476

140. Fisher CM (1970) Occlusion of the vertebral arteries causing transient basilar symptoms. Arch Neurol 22: 13–19

141. Fisher CM (1975) Clinical syndrome in cerebral thrombosis, hypertensive hemorrhage and ruptured saccular aneurysm. Clin Neurosurg 22: 117–147

142. Fisher CM (1978) Ataxic hemiparesis. Arch Neurol 35: 126–128

143. Fisher CM, Ojeman RG, Roberson GH (1978) Spontaneous dissection of cervicocerebral arteries. Can J Neurol Sci 8: 9–19

144. Ford FR (1952) Syncope, vertigo, and disturbances of vision resulting from intermittent obstruction of the vertebral arteries due to a defect in the odontoid process and excessive mobility of the second cervical vertebra. Bull Hopkins Hosp 91: 168–173

145. Ford FR, Clark D (1956) Thrombosis of the basilar artery with softening in the cerebellum and brain stem due to manipulation of the neck. A report of two cases with one post-mortem examination. Reasons are given to prove that damage to the vertebral arteries is responsible. Johns Hopkins Hosp Bull 98: 37–42

146. Ford JJ, Baker WH, Ehrenhaft JL (1975) Carotid endarterectomy for non hemispheric transient ischemic attacks. Arch Surg 110: 1314–1317

147. Fowler M (1962) Two cases of basilar artery occlusion in childhood. Arch Dis Child 37: 78–82

148. Fraenckel P (1927) Gedeckte traumatische Zerreißung der gesunden Arteria basilaris. Dtsch Z Ges Gerichtl Med 10: 193–199

149. Franceschi C (1981) Explorations Doppler des voies de suppléance des artères crânio-cérébrales. J Mal Vasc 6: 89–100

150. Francke JP, Dimarino V, Pannier M, Argens on Cl, Libersa Cl (1980) Les artères vertébrales. Segments atlanto-

axoïdiens V3 et intra-crânien V4 collatérales. Anatomia Clinica 2: 229–242

151. Francke JP, Dimarino V, Pannier M, Argenson C, Libersa Cl (1981) The vertebral arteries. The V3 atlanto-axoïdal and V4 intracranial segments collaterals. Anatomia Clinica 2: 229–242

152. Frankhauser H, Kamano S, Hanmura T, Amano K, Hatnaka H (1979) Abnormal origin of the PICA. Case report. J Neurosurg 514: 569–571

153. Fraser RAR, Zimbler SM (1985) Hindbrain stroke in children caused by extracranial vertebral artery trauma. Stroke 6: 153–159

154. Fredy D, Hugonet P, Missir O, Thiebot J, Bories J (1978) Obstruction des vaisseaux cervicaux à destinée encéphalique. Problèmes hémodynamiques. Noeud de Bosniak. J Neuroradiology 5: 203–224

155. French LA, Haines GL (1950) Unilateral vertebral artery ligation: report of a case ending fatally with thrombosis of the basilar artery. J Neurosurg 7: 156–158

156. Frens DB, Petajan JH, Anderson R (1974) Fibromuscular dysplasia of the posterior cerebral artery. Stroke 5: 161–166

157. Frykolm R (1951) Lower cervical vertebral and intervertebral disc. Surgical anatomy and pathology. Acta Chir Scand 101: 345–359

158. Gabella JL, Thiebot J, Houdent G, Leonard A, Le Loet X, Deshayes P (1981) Erosion osseuse cervicale par boucle de l'artère vertébrale. Rev Rhum 48: 277–279

159. Garland D (1965) Iatrogenic vertebral arteriovenous fistula. Ann Heart J 70: 430

160. Garrido E, Garofola JH (1983) Intraluminal dilatation of the innominate artery before extracranial intracranial by-pass: case report. Neurosurgery 13: 581–583

161. Gatti JM, Juan LH, Bironne P, Glowinski J (1983) Elargissement d'un trou de conjugaison cervical par une mégadolicho artère vertébrale. Press Med 12: 2056

162. Gautier JC (1985) Vertigo in ischaemic cerebrovascular disease. In: Courbier E (ed) Basis for a classification of cerebral arterial diseases. Excerpta Medica. Current Clinical Practice. Series 22, Amsterdam, pp 111–115

163. George B, Laurian C (1979) Surgical possibilities in the third portion of the vertebral artery (above C2). VIth European Congress of Neurosurgery. Paris

164. George B, Laurian C, Derome P, Guilmet D (1979) Pontage sousclavier vertébrale en C1–C2 pour dysplasie anévrysmale. Intérêt et possibilités de l'abord chirurgical de la vertébrale en C1–C2. Neurochirurgie 25: 124–128

165. George B, Laurian C (1979) Surgical possibilities on the third portion of the vertebral artery above C2. Acta Neurochir (Wien) 28: 263–269

166. George B, Laurian C, Houdart R (1979) Lésions de l'artère vertébrale. Possibilités thérapeutiques. Indications chirurgicales Rev Neurol 135: 10–74

167. George B, Laurian C (1980) Surgical approach to the whole length of the vertebral artery with special reference to the third portion. Acta Neurochir (Wien) 51: 259–272

168. George B, Laurian C, Marshal JC (1981) Vertebro-basilar revascularization by anastomosis of subclavian or carotid artery to vertebral artery beyond C2. VIIth International Congress of Neurosurgery, Munich

169. George B, Laurian C (1981) Occlusion de l'artère vertébrale. A propos de 33 cas. Implications thérapeutiques. Neurochirurgie 273: 167–173

170. George B, Laurian C (1982) Vertebro-basilar ischemia with thrombosis of the vertebral artery. Report of 2 cases with embolism. J Neurol Neurosurg Psychiat 45: 91–93

171. George B, Laurian C (1982) Vertebro-basilar ischemia. Its relation to stenosis and occlusion of the vertebral artery. Acta Neurochir (Wien) 62: 287–295

172. George B, Laurian C, Cophignon J, Rey A (1982) Traitement des tumeurs en rapport avec l'artère vertébrale dans sa portion transversaire. Neurochirurgie 28: 173–178

173. George B (1983) Control of the vertebral artery in surgery of cervical tumours. VIIth European Neurosurgical Congress, Bruxelles

174. George B, Laurian C (1984) Chirurgie de l'artère vertébrale cervicale distale. Robert et Carrière (eds), Paris, pp 64

175. George B, Riche MC, Gaston A, Laurian C (1984) Embolisation per-opératoire des malformations artério-veineuses à partir de l'artère vertébrale. Neurochirurgie 30: 269–272

176. George B, Laurian C, Keravel Y, Cophignon J (1985) Extra-dural and hour-glass cervical neurinomas. The vertebral artery problem. Neurosurgery 16: 541–544

177. George B, Laurian C (1985) Carotid-vertebral by-pass. VIIIth International Congress of Neurological Surgery. Toronto

178. George B, Laurian C (1987) Exposure of the vertebral artery in surgical removal of cervical tumours. To be published

179. George B, Reizine D, Deffresnes D, Tran Ba Huy P (1985) Contrôle angiographique et chirurgical des pédicules nourriciers vertébraux et carotidiens des pargangliomes géants de la base du crâne et du cou. Ann Oto-Laryngol 102: 59–63

180. George B (1985) Compression extrinsèque de l'artère vertébrale. In: Simon L, Leroux JL, Privat JM (eds). Rachis cervical et Médecine de rééducation. Masson, Paris, pp 267–278

181. George B, Laurian C, Rey A, Cophignon J (1986) Indications des revascularisations de l'artère vertébrale distale. Ann Med Int 137: 108–111

182. George B (1986) Vertebral artery surgery experience. Society for Neurovascular surgery. Chicago

183. George B (1986) Revascularization of the cervical vertebral artery. In: Modern neurosurgery. Springer, Berlin Heidelberg New York Tokyo, in press

184. Geraud J, Manelfe C, Caussanel JP, Sallenave J (1973) Fistule artério-veineuse spontanée de l'artère vertébrale. Rôle éventuel de la dysplasie fibro-musculaire dans sa pathogénie. Rev Neurol 128: 206–212

185. Gerlach L (1884) Ueber die Bewegungen in den Atlasgelenken und deren Beziehungen zu der Blutströmung in den Vertebralarterien. Beitr Morphol 1: 104–117

186. Geuna E, Ogno G, Bellotti C, Formaggio G (1978) Malformations vasculaires de la vertébrale du cou. Considérations à propos d'un cas. Neuro-Chirurgie 24: 269–274

187. Giessinger JD, Gruner G, Ruge D (1972) Vertebral artery occlusion by a cervical hour-glass neurofibroma. J Neurol Neurosurg Psychiat 35: 899–902

188. Gilles FH, Bina M, Sotrel A (1979) Infantile atlanto occipital instability. The potential danger of extreme extension. Am J Dis Child 133: 30–37

189. Goldstein SJ (1982) Dissecting hematoma of the cervical vertebral artery. J Neurosurg 56: 451–454

190. Goodman SJ, Hasso A, Kirkpatrick D (1975) Treatment of vertebro-jugular fistula by balloon occlusion. J Neurosurg 43: 362–367

191. Goodman GK, Crawford KH (1983) Internuclear ophtalmoplegia following arch aortography. Neuro-radiology 25: 171–172

192. Gortvai P (1964) Insufficiency of vertebral artery treated by decompression of its cervical part. Br Med J 2: 233–234

193. Gottschau M (1885) Zwei seltene Varietäten der Stämme des Aortenbogens. Arch Anat Entwicklgesch 245–252

194. Green D, Joynt RJ (1959) Vascular accidents to the brain stem associated with neck manipulation. JAMA 170: 522–524

195. Greenberg J (1970) Spontaneous arteriovenous malformations in the cervical area. J Neurol Neurosurg Psychiat 33: 303–309

196. Grubb RL, Ratcheson RA, Raichle ME (1979) Regional cerebral blood flow and oxygen utilization in superficial temporal-middle cerebral artery anastomosis patients. J Neurosurg 50: 733–741

197. Gruntzig A, Hopff H Perkutane Rekanalisation chronischer arterieller Verschlüsse mit einem neuen Dilatationskatheter. Modifikation der Dotter Technik. Dtsch Med Wochenschr 99: 2502–2505

198. Gur D, Wolfson SK, Yonas H (1982) Progress in cerebrovascular disease: local cerebral blood flow by xenon enhanced CT 13: 750–759

199. Gustafson WA, Oldberg E (1940) Neurological significance of platybasia. Arch Neurol Psychiat 44: 1184

200. Hadley LA (1957) The covertebral articulations and cervical foramen encroachment. J Bone Joint Surg 39 A: 910–920

201. Hadley LA (1958) Tortuosity and deflection of the vertebral artery. AJR 80: 306–312

202. Hadley MN, Spetzler RF, Masferrer R, Martin MA, Carter LP (1985) Occipital artery to extradural vertebral artery bypass procedure. J Neurosurg 63: 622–625

203. Hakuba A, Komiyama M, Tsujimoto T, Soo Ahn M, Nishirmura S, Ohta T, Kitano H (1984) Transuncodiscal approach to dumb-bell tumours of the cervical spinal canal. J Neurosurg 61: 1100–1106

204. Hanus SH, Hower TD, Harter DH (1977) Vertebral artery occlusion complicating yoga exercises. Arch Neurol 34: 574–575

205. Hardin CA, Williamson WP, Streegman AT (1960) Vertebral artery insufficiency produced by cervical osteoarthritic spurs. Neurology 10: 855–858

206. Hardin CA, Poser CM (1963) Rotational obstruction of the vertebral artery due to redundancy and extralaminal cervical fascial bands. Ann Surg 158: 133–137

207. Hardin CA (1965) Vertebral artery insufficiency produced by cervical osteoarthritic spurs. Arch Surg 90: 629–633

208. Harris DJ, Fornasier VL, Livingston KE (1978) Hemangiopericytoma of the spinal canal. Report of 3 cases. J Neurosurg 49: 914–920

209. Hasegawa T, Kuboto T, Ito H, Yamamoto S (1983) Symptomatic duplication of the vertebral artery. Surg Neurol 20: 244–248

210. Hasegawa T, Ito H, Hwang WZ, Yamamoto S (1986) Single extracranial intracranial duplication of the vertebral artery. Surg Neurol 25: 369–372

211. Hasso A, Bird CR, Zinke DE, Thompson JR (1981) Fibromuscular dysplasia of the internal carotid artery: percutaneous transluminal angioplasty. AJR 136: 955–960

212. Hayes P, Gerlock AJ, Cobb CA (1980) Cervical spine trauma. A cause of vertebral artery injury. J Trauma 20: 904–905

213. Heeney DJ, Koo AH (1980) Bilateral cortical blindness associated with carotid stenosis in a patient with a persistent trigeminal artery. Case Report. J Neurosurg 52: 709–711

214. Heerschaft H, Duus P (1972) Die obstruierenden Erkrankungen der Arteria vertebralis in ihrer zervikalen Verlaufstrecke. Folia Angiologica 20: 22–32

215. Heifetz GJ (1945) Traumatic aneurysm of the first portion of the left vertebral artery. Ann Surg 122: 102–110

216. Heilbrun MP, Ratcheson RA (1972) Multiple extracranial vessel injuries following closed head and neck trauma. J Neurosurg 37: 219–223

217. Henke W (1978) Handbuch der Anatomie und Mechanik der Gelenke. Leipzig and Heidelberg 1863 (cited in White AA III, Panjabi MM Clinical biomechanics of the spine) chap. 2. JB Lippincott, Philadelphia

218. Henry AK (1966) Exposures of long bones and other surgical methode. Cited in the author's book: Extensile exposures (Wright 1927). Livingstone, Edinburgh London, pp 58–66

219. Hieshima GB, Cahan LD, Mehringer CM, Bentson JR (1975) Spontaneous arteriovenous fistulas of cerebral vessels in association with fibromuscular dysplasia. Neurosurgery 18: 454–458

220. Hill TC, Homan BL, Lovett R (1982) Initial experience with SPECT (Single photon computerized tomography) of the brain using N-isopropyl I 123 p-iodoamphetamine. Concise communication. J Nucl Med 23: 191

221. Hodes PJ, Campoy F, Riggs HE, Bly P (1953) Cerebral angiography: fundamentals in anatomy and physiology. AJR 70: 61–82

222. Hoffman HH, Kuntz A (1957) Vertebral nerves and plexus. Components, anatomical relationships and surgical complications. Arch Surg 74: 430–437

223. Holzer FJ (1955) Verschluß der Wirbelsäulenschlagader am Kopfgelenk mit nachfolgender Thrombose durch Seitwärtsdrehen des Kopfes. Eine Gefahr bei Operationen am Hals mit starker Seit-

wärtsdrehung. Dtsch Z Ges Gerichtl Med 44: 422–426

224. Hopkins LN, Budny JL (1985) A rational surgical approach to vertebro-basilar ischemia. In: Spetzler RF (ed) Cerebral revascularization for stroke. Thieme-Stratton, New York, pp 490–504

225. Houser OW, Baker HL, Sandok BA, Holley KE (1971) Cephalic arterial fibromuscular dysplasia. Radiology 101: 605–611

226. Hozawa J (1979) Peripheral vestibular disorder of cervical origin. Adv Oto-Rhino-Laryngol 25: 156–165

227. Hugenholtz H, Pokpura R, Montpetit VJA, Nelson R, Richard MT (1982) Spontaneous dissecting aneurysm of the extracranial vertebral artery. Neurosurgery 10: 96–100

228. Hugues JT (1964) Vertebral artery insufficiency in acute cervical spine trauma. Paraplegia 2: 2–14

229. Humphries AW, Beven EG, Lefevre FA, De Wolfe VS (1965) Relief of vertebrobasilar symptoms by carotid endarterectomy. Surgery 57: 48–53

230. Husni EA, Bell HS, Storer J (1966) Mechanical occlusion of the vertebral artery: a new clinical concept. JAMA 196: 475–478

231. Hutchinson EC, Yates PO (1956) The cervical portion of the vertebral artery. Brain 79: 319–331

232. Hutchinson EC, Yates PO (1957) Carotido-vertebral stenosis. Lancet I: 2, 2–8

233. Ibrahim AW, Satti MB, Ibrahim EM (1986) Extraspinal meningioma. Case report. J Neurosurg 64: 328–330

234. Imparato AM, Rites TS, Kim GE (1981) Cervical vertebral angioplasty for brain stem ischemia. Surgery 90: 892

235. Inasaki Y, Nakagawa T, Koima M (1978) Occlusion of the vertebral artery by an extradural neurinoma. Neurol Surg 6: 7, 701–705

236. Iraci G, Pardascher K, Fiore DL, Geros AM (1981) Vertebro-basilar transient ischemic attacks: an unusual clinical manifestation of a cervical aneurysmal bone cyst. Surg Neurol 16: 251–255

237. Itoh M, Shima K, Ishikawa S, Ono Y (1978) A case of cervical canal stenosis accompanied with congenital cervical fusion and extracranial occlusion of vertebral artery. A clinical and embryological study (No Shinkei Geka) Neurol Surg 6: 591–597

238. Jacob: Otoneurological examination in panic disorder and agoraphobia with panic-attacks: a pilot study. Am J Psychiatry 142: 715–720

239. Jamicson KG (1965) Vertebral arteriovenous fistula caused by angiography needle. Report of a case. J Neurosurg 23: 620–621

240. Janeway R, Toole JF, Leinbach LB, Miller HS (1966) Vertebral artery obstruction with basilar impression. An intermittent phenomenon related to head turning. Arch Neurol 15: 211–214

241. Jeanmart L, Brihaye J, Gompel C (1967) Tumeurs rares du rachis. J belge Rhum Med Phys 22: 317–332

242. Jefferson G, Bailey RA, Liverpool SK (1956) Suboccipital arterio-venous aneurysms of the vertebral artery. J Bone Joint Surg 383: 114–127

243. Jones T, Vetto R, Winterscheid L, Dillard D, Merendino A (1960) Arterial complications incident to cannulation in open-heart surgery. Ann Surg 152: 969–976

244. Jones NW, Kaufmann JCE (1976) Vertebro-basilar artery insufficiency in rheumatoïd atlanto axial subluxation. J Neurol Neurosurg Psychiat 39: 122–128

245. Juge O, Meyer JS, Sakai F (1979) Critical appraisal of cerebral blood flow measured from brain stem and cerebellar regions after 133 Xc inhalation in humans. Stroke 10: 428–437

246. Jung A, Vierling JP, Safaoui A (1964) Douze case d'arthrose cervicale inférieure. Leur traitement chirurgical par abord antérieur avec ouverture du trou transversaire et uncussectomie. Press Med 72: 3367–3372

247. Kadyi H (1886) Über die Blutgefässe des menschlichen Rückenmarkes. Anat Anz 1: 303–304

248. Kalendowsky Z, Austin J, Steele P (1975) Increased platelet aggregability in young

patients with stroke. Diagnosis and therapy. Arch Neurol 33: 13–20

249. Kamano S, Amano K, Machiyama N, Matsui T, Hatanaka H (1980) The contribution of computed tomography in the choice of anterolateral approach for treating cervical dumb-bell tumours. Neurochirurgica 23: 121–125

250. Katirji MB, Reinmuth OM, Latchaw RE (1985) Stroke due to vertebral artery injury. Arch Neurol 42: 242–248

251. Keggi KJ, Granger DP, Soutwick WO (1966) Vertebral artery insufficiency secondary to trauma and osteoarthritis of cervical spine. Yale J Biol Med 38: 471–478

252. Kempe LG (1979) Aneurysm of the V. A. In: Pia HW, Langmaid C, Zierski J (eds) Cerebral aneurysms. Advances in diagnosis and therapy. Springer, Berlin Heidelberg New York, pp 119–120

253. Kernohan JW, Sayre GP (1952) Tumors of the central nervous system. In: Atlas of tumor pathology. Sect 10, 35, and 37. Washington D.C. National Research Council. Armed Forces Institute of Pathology

254. Kernohan JW (1965) Cytology and cellular pathology of the nervous system. Penkield W (ed), New York Publ Co, pp 1013

255. Kieffer E, Rancurel G, Richard T (1984) Reconstruction of the distal cervical vertebral artery. In: Berguer R, Bauer E (eds) Vertebro-basilar arterial occlusive disease. Raven Press, New York

256. Kister SJ, Rankow RM (1966) Traumatic aneurysm of the first portion of the left vertebral artery. A case report. Plast Reconstr Surg 37: 546–549

257. Kituchi K, Kowada M (1983) New traumatic extracranial aneurysm of the V. A. Surg Neurol 19: 425–427

258. Kocher Th (1871) Ueber Verletzung und Aneurysma der Arteria vertebralis, nebst Mittheilung eines glücklich verlaufenen Falles. Arch Klin Chir (Berlin) 12: 867

259. Koga H, Austin G (1982) Regional cerebral blood flow in patients with vertebrobasilar disease. Surg Neurol 18: 466–471

260. Kojima N, Tamaki N, Fujita K, Matsumoto S (1985) Vertebral artery occlusion at the narrowed "Scalenovertebral angle". Mechanical vertebral occlusion in the distal first portion. Neurosurgery 16: 672–674

261. Kooi KA, Gilroy J (1984) Alterations of visual evoked potentials associated with vertebrobasilar occlusive disease. In: Berguer E, Bauer RB (eds) Vertebrobasilar arterial occlusive disease. Raven Press, New York, pp 95–98

262. Kormesser TW, Bergan JJ (1984) Anatomic control of vertebral arteriovenous fistula. Surgery 75: 80–86

263. Kovacs (1955) A subluxation and deformation of the cervical apophyseal joint: a contribution to the aetiology of headache. Acta Radiol 43: 1–15

264. Kowada M, Yamagushi K, Takahashi H (1972) Fenestration of the vertebral artery with review of 23 cases in Japan. Radiology 103: 343–346

265. Krayenbühl H, Yaşargil MG (1957) Die vaskulären Erkrankungen im Gebiet der Arteria vertebralis und Arteria basilaris, 38: Thieme, Stuttgart

266. Kremer M (1958) Sitting, standing and walking. Br Med J 2, part 1: 63–68, part 2: 121–126

267. Kriss FC, Schneider RC (1968) The value of vertebral angiography in the treatment of cervical neurinomas. J Neurosurg 28: 29–34

268. Krueger BR, Okazaki H (1980) Vertebrobasilar distribution. Infarction following chiropractic manipulation. Mayo Clin Proc 55: 322–332

269. Kruse F Jr (1961) Hemangiopericytoma of meninges (angioblastic meningioma of Cushing and Eisenhardt) Clinicopathologic aspects and follow-up studies in 8 cases. Neurology 11: 771–777

270. Kubik CS, Adams RD (1946) Occlusion of the basilar artery. A clinical and pathological study. Brain 69: 6–121

271. Kuhl DE, Phelps ME, Kowell AP, Metter EJ, Selin C, Winter J (1980) Effects of stroke on local cerebral metabolism and perfusion: mapping by emission computed tomography of 18 FDG and 13 NH3. Ann Neurol 8: 47–60

272. Kuhne D, Helmke K (1982) Embolization with ethibloc of vascular tumors and arterio-venous malformations in the head and neck. Neuroradiology 23: 253–258

273. Kuttner H (1917) Die Verletzungen und traumatischen Aneurysmen des Vertebralisgefäßes am Halse und ihre operative Behandlung. Beitr Klin Chir 108: 1–60

274. Labauge R, Buisson G, Boukobza M, Carrière A (1977) La dysplasie fibromusculaire des artères cervicocéphaliques. Oto Neuro Opht 49: 277–295

275. Lasjaunias P, Moret J, Theron J (1978) The so-called anterior meningeal artery of the cervical vertebral artery. Neuroradiology 17: 51–55

276. Lasjaunias P, Theron J, Moret J (1978) The occipital artery. Normal anatomy. Arteriographic aspects. Embryological significance. Neuro-Radiology 15: 31–37

277. Lasjaunias P, Braun JP, Hasso AN, Moret J, Manelfe C (1980) True and false fenestration of the vertebral artery. J Neuroradiol 7: 157–166

278. Lasjaunias P, Guilbert-Tranier F, Braun JP (1981) The pharyngo-cerebellar artery or ascending pharyngeal artery origin of the PICA. J Neuroradiol 8: 317–325

279. Lassen NA, Henriksen L, Paulson O (1981) Regional cerebral blood flow in stroke by 133 Xenon inhalation and emission tomography. Stroke 12: 284–289

280. Laurian C (1977) Traitement chirurgical des lésions athéromateuses des troncs supra-aortiques par voie extra-thoracique. Thèse de Médecine. Paris 6

281. Laurian C, George B (1979) Abord de l'artère vertébrale extracrânienne. Etude anatomique. Intérêt chirurgical. Nouv Press Med 86: 433–436

282. Laurian C, George B, Richard T, Derome P, Guilmet D (1980) Intérêt de l'abord de l'artère vertébrale dans son segment extracrânien. A propos d'un anévrysme de l'artère vertébrale en C3. J Mal Vasc 5: 149–150

283. Laurian C, George B (1982) Chirurgie de l'artère vertébrale distale. Approche par une nouvelle stratégie. Ann Chir 6: 127–135

284. Laurian C, George B, Houdart R, Cormier JM (1983) Revascularisation de l'artère vertébrale distale (3 e segment). Indication dans le traitement de l'insuffisance vertébro-basilaire. Ann Chir 375: 325–330

285. Laurian C, George B (1984) Revascularisation de l'artère vertébrale dans son 3 e segment (au dessus de C2). Ve Congrès de la Société Internationale de Chirurgie. ME de Bakey, Monte Carlo

286. Lazorthes G, Gouaze A, Santini JJ, Lazorthes Y, Laffont J (1971) Le modelage du polygone de Willis. Rôle des compressions des voies artérielles d'apport dans les mouvements de la colonne cervicale et de l'extrémité céphalique. Neurochirurgie 17: 361–378

287. Lee JF, Tindall GT, Greenfield JC, Odom GL (1965) Cerebral blood flow in the monkey. Electroencephalographic effects of temporary occlusion of the carotid and vertebral arteries at varying levels of systemic arterial pressure. J Neurosurg 719–726

288. Lenzi GL, Frackowiak RS, Jones T (1982) Cerebral oxygen metabolism and blood flow in human cerebral infarction. J Cereb Blood Flow Metab 2: 321–335

289. Lester J (1966) Arteriovenous fistula after percutaneous vertebral angiography. Acta Radiol 5: 337–340

290. Lie TA (1972) Congenital malformations of the carotid and vertebral arterial systems including persistent anastomosis. In: Vinken PJ, Bruyn GW (eds) Handbook of clinical neurology, vol 12. Elsevier, New York, pp 289–339

291. Liéou YC (1928) Syndrome sympathique cervical postérieur et arthrite chronique de la colonne vertébrale cervicale (Etude clinique et radiologique). Thèse Med Strasbourg

292. Linde LM, Fonkolsrud EW, Wilson GH, Batzdorf G (1970) Traumatic vertebral arterio-venous fistula in a child. JAMA 213: 1465–1468

293. Love JG, Dodge HWJr (1952) Dumb-bell (hour-glass) neurofibroma affecting the spinal cord. Surg Gynecol Obstet 94: 161–172

294. Lyness SS, Simeone (1978) Vascular complications of upper cervical spine injuries. Orthop Clin N Amer 9: 1029–1038

295. Lynn GE, Gilroy J (1984) Auditory evoked potentials in vertebro-basilar arterial occlusive disease. In: Berguer R, Bauer RB (eds) Vertebrobasilar arterial occlusive disease. Raven Press, New York, pp 85–94

296. Macke A, Macke-Ribert C (1978) L'artère carotide interne. Etude anatomique et microradiographique. Exploration endoluminale. Thèse Med, Lille, pp 76

297. Maisonneuve, Favrot (1852) Journal des connaissances médico-chirurgicales. 2 s, vol 11, pp 181

298. Makins GH (1919) On gunshot injuries to the blood vessels. William and Co, New York, p 7

299. Malik GK, Chhabra DK (1982) Internal carotid and vertebral artery occlusion in pediatric stroke. Indian Pediatr 19: 99–100

300. Mant AK (1972) Traumatic subarachnoid haemorrhage following blows to the neck. J Forensic Sci Soc 12: 567–572

301. Mapstone T, Spetzler RF (1956) Vertebrobasilar insufficiency secondary to vertebral artery occlusion from a fibrous band. J Neurosurg 4: 581–583

302. Margolis MT, Newton TH (1972) Borderlands of the normal and abnormal PICA. Acta Radiol (Diagn) 13: 163–176

303. Margolis MT, Newton TH (1974) The PICA. In: Newton TH, Potts DG (eds) Radiology of the skull and brain, Vol 2, Book 2. CV Mosby, St Louis, pp 1710–1774

304. Marks RL, Freed MM (1973) Non penetrating injuries of the neck and cerebrovascular accident. Arch Neurol 28: 412–414

305. Maroun FB, Mangau MA, Cornel G, Jacob JC (1983) Balloon occlusion of traumatic arteriovenous fistula. Surg Neurol 19: 122–125

306. Marshall J (1964) The natural history of transient ischemic cerebro-vascular attacks. QJ Med 33: 309–324

307. Martin MJ, Whisnant JP, Sayre (1960) Occlusive vascular disease in the extracranial cerebral circulation. Arch Neurol 3: 530–538

308. Mas JL, Goeau C, Bousser MG, Chiras J, Verret JM, Touboul PJ (1985) Spontaneous dissecting aneurysms of the internal carotid and vertebral arteries. Two case reports. Stroke 16: 125–129

309. Matas R (1888) Traumatic aneurysm of the left brachial artery. Incision and partial excision of the sac with recovery. Med News 53: 462–466

310. Matas R (1893) Traumatisms and traumatic aneurysms of the vertebral artery, and their surgical treatment with report of a cured case. Ann Surg 18: 477–516

311. Mathey J, Cormier JM (1957) Fistule artério-veineuse congénitale du segment cervical des vaisseaux vertébraux. Ann Chir 22: 307–314

312. Mathias K, Staiger J, Thron A, Spillner F, Heiss HW, Konrad-Graf S (1980) Perkutane Katheteragioplastik der Arteria subclavia. Dtsch Med Wochenschr 105: 16–18

313. Matsunaga T, Sano M, Yamamoto K, Kubo T (1979) Vestibular neuronal function during ischemia, response of vestibular neurons to vertebral and carotid occlusion in rabbits. Adv Otorhinolaryngol 25: 184–191

314. Mc Lean JM, Wright RM, Henderson JP, Lister JR (1985) Vertebral artery rupture associated with closed head injury. J Neurosurg 62: 135–138

315. Meier DE, Brink BE, Fry WJ (1981) Vertebral artery trauma. Acute recognition and treatment. Arch Surg 116: 236–239

316. Merland JJ, Riche MC, George B, Laurian C, Picard L (1979) Current trends in the combined radiological and surgical management of vascular malformations, tumors, dysplasias involving the vertebral artery. J Neuro-Radiology 6: 269–286

317. Mettinger KL, Ericson K (1982) Fibromuscular dysplasia and the brain. Observations on angiographic, clinical and genetic characteristics. Stroke 13: 46–52

318. Mettinger KL (1982) Fibromuscular dysplasia and the brain. Current concept of the disease. Stroke 13: 53–58

319. Meyer JS, Sheeha S, Bauer RB (1960) An arteriographic study of cerebro-vascular disease in man. 1. Stenosis and occlusion of the vertebral basilar arterial system. Arch Neurol 2: 27–45

320. Meyer WW (1964) Über die rhythmische Lokalisation der atherosklerotischen Herde im cervicalen Abschnitt der Vertebralarterie. Beitr Path Anat 24: 130–136

321. Meyer JS, Yoshida K, Sakamoto K (1967) Autonomic control of cerebral blood flow measured by electromagnetic flowmeters. Neurology 17: 638–648

322. Meyer JS, Nakajima S, Okabe T (1982) Redistribution of cerebral blood flow following STA-MCA by-pass in patients with hemispheric ischemia. Stroke 13: 774–784

323. Miller RG, Burton R (1974) Stroke following chiropractic manipulation of the spine. JAMA 229: 189–190

324. Miller RE, Hieshma GB, Giannotta SL, Grinnell US, Mehringer CM, Kerin DS (1984) Acute traumatic vertebral arteriovenous fistula: balloon occlusion with the use of a controlateral approach. Neurosurgery 14: 225–229

325. Millikan CH, Siekert RG (1955) Studies in cerebrovascular disease. 1: The syndrome of intermittent insufficiency of the basilar arterial system. Proc Mayo Clin 30: 61–68

326. Mills CM, Brant-Zawadski M, Crooks LE, Kaufman L (1983) Nuclear magnetic resonance: principles of blood flow imaging. AJNR 4: 1161–1166

327. Mitchell GAG (1956) Cardiovascular innervation. Livingstone, London, pp 146–172

328. Mitchell OC, Netsky MC (1962) Anatomic and angiographic study of the vertebral basilar arterial system in the dog. Am J Anat 110: 187–198

329. Mitchell JRA, Schwarz CJ (1965) Arterial disease. Blackwell, Oxford

330. Mizukami M, Tomita T, Mine T, Mihara H (1972) By-pass anomaly of the vertebral artery associated with cerebral aneurysm and arteriovenous malformation. J Neurosurg 37: 204–209

331. Moniz E (1927) L'encéphalographie artérielle, son importance dans la localisation des tumeurs cérébrales. Rev Neurol 2: 72–81

332. Moore RS, Russell WF, Parent AD, Parker JL, Smith RR (1982) Percutaneous transluminal angioplasty in subclavian steal syndrome: recurrent stenosis and retreatment in two patients. Neurosurgery 11: 512–517

333. Morelli RJ (1967) An angiographic complication of vertebral arteriovenous fistula. J Neurol Neurosurg Psychiat 30: 264–266

334. Moret J, Lasjaunias P, Doyon P (1979) Occipital approach for treatment of arteriovenous malformation of the vertebral artery by balloon occlusion. Neuroradiology 17: 269–273

335. Mortarjemme A, Keiffer JW, Zuska AJ (1981) Percutaneous transluminal angioplasty of the vertebral arteries. Radiology 139: 715–717

336. Mortarjemme A, Keiffer JW, Zuska AJ (1982) Percutaneous translumina angioplasty of the brachiocephalic arteries. AJR 138: 457–462

337. Moscow NP, Newton TH (1975) Angiographic features of hypervascular neurinomas of the head and neck. Neuroradiology 114: 635–640

338. Murray DS (1957) Post-traumatic thrombosis of the internal carotid and vertebral arteries after non penetrating injuries of the neck. Br J Surg 44: 556–561

339. Nagashima C (1970) Surgical treatment of vertebral artery insufficiency caused by cervical spondylosis. J Neurosurg 32: 512–521

340. Nagashima C, Iwama K, Sakata E, Miki Y (1970) Effects of temporary occlusion of a vertebral artery on the human vestibular system. J Neurosurg 33: 388–394

341. Nagashima C, Iwana K (1972) Electrical stimulation of the steallate ganglion and the vertebral nerve. J Neurosurg 36: 756–762

342. Nagashima C, Iwasaki T, Kawanuma S, Sakaguchi A, Kamisasa A, Suzuki K (1977) Traumatic arteriovenous fistula of the vertebral artery with spinal cord symptoms. Case report. J Neurosurg 46: 681–687

343. Nagashima C (1985) Vertebral artery insufficiency and cervical spondylosis. In: Fein JM, Flamm ES (eds) Cerebrovascular surgery, vol 2, Chap 12. Springer, New York, pp 529–555

344. Nagawara J, Usami S, Takeda T (1982) Cerebral blood flow measurement in carotid and vertebrobasilar artery territory by direct injection of 133 Xe. 25th Japanese

Symposium for cerebral blood flow and metabolism, Tokyo

345. Nagler W (1973) Vertebral artery obstruction by hyperextension of the neck. Report of three cases. Arch Phys Med Rehabil 54: 237–240

346. Naritomi H, Sakai F, Meyer JS (1979) Pathogenesis of transient ischemic attacks within the vertebrobasilar arterial system. Arch Neurol 36: 121–128

347. Nay HE, Nahser HC, Mehdron JM, Gerhard H, Scharafinski W, Jorg J, Engel W (1985) Value of multimodality evoked potentials in patients with cerebral ischemia. In: Spetzler RF, Carter LP, Selman WR, Martin NA (eds) Cerebral revascularization for stroke. 6. Thieme Stratton, New York, pp 29–36

348. Noel P, Desment JE (1975) Somatosensory cerebral evoked potentials after vascular lesions of the brain stem and diencephalon. Brain 98: 113–128

349. Norman JA, Schmidt KW, Grow JB (1950) Congenital arteriovenous fistula of the cervical vertebral vessels with heart failure in an infant. J Pediat 36: 598–604

350. Nubourgh Y, Noterman J, Baleriaux-Waha D, Ebinger G, Flament-Durand J (1979) Osteochondrome vertébral solitaire avec syndrome de compression medullaire. Neurochirurgie 25: 134–137

351. Nurick S (1963) Vertebral artery compression due to recurrent subluxation or cervical vertebra. Guy's Hosp Rep 112: 152–158

352. O'Brien P, Brasfield RD (1965) Hemangiopericytoma. Cancer 18: 249–252

353. Oertel O (1922) Über die Persistenz embryonaler Vernichtungen zwischen der A. Carotis interna und der A. vertebralis cerebralis. Dtsch Med Wochenschr 48: 1264

354. Ogilvic W (1940) Extracranial aneurysm of the vertebral artery. Guy's Hosp Rep 90: 178–179

355. Ojeman RG, Fischer CM, Rich JC (1972) Spontaneous dissecting aneurysms of the internal carotid artery. Stroke 3: 434–440

356. Okawara S, Nibbelinik D (1974) Vertebral artery occlusion following hyperextension and rotation of the head. Stroke 5: 640–643

357. Oljenick I (1917) Über die Unterbindung der Arteria vertebralis. Zbl Chir 44: 1067–1069

358. Olson RW, Baker HL, Svien HJ (1963) Arteriovenous fistula: a complication of vertebral angiography. Report of a case. J Neurosurg 20: 73–75

359. Osborn AG, Anderson RE (1977) Angiographic spectrum of cervical and intracranial fibromuscular dysplasia. Stroke 8: 617–626

360. Outchi H, Ohara I (1973) Extracranial abnormalities of the vertebral artery detected by selective arteriography. J Cardiovasc Surg 18: 250–261

361. Ouvrier RA, Hopkins IJ (1970) Occlusive disease of the vertebro-basilar arterial system in childhood. Develop Med Child Neurol 12: 186–192

362. Padget DH (1948) The development of cranial arteries in the human embryo. Contrib Embryol 32: 205–262

363. Padget DH (1954) Designation of the embryonic intersegmental arteries in the reference to the vertebral artery and subclavian stem. Anat Rec 119: 349–356

364. Paillas JE, Serratrice C, Legre J (1963) Les tumeurs primitives du rachis. Masson, Paris, pp 70–72

365. Pamela F, Beaugerie L, Couturier M, Duval G, Gaudy JH (1983) Syndrome de déafférentation motrice par thrombose du tronc basilaire après manipulation vertébrale. Press Med 12: 1548

366. Parkinson D, Reddy V, Ross RT (1979) Congenital anastomosis between the vertebral artery and internal carotid artery in the neck. Case report. J Neurosurg 51: 697–699

367. Pascual-Castroviego I, Pascual-Pascual JI, Mulas F, Roche C, Tendero A (1977) Bilateral obstruction of the vertebral arteries in a three year old child. Develop Med Child Neurol 19: 232–238

368. Paul GA, Shaw CA, Wray LM (1980) True traumatic aneurysm of the vertebral artery. Case report. J Neurosurg 53: 101–105

369. Pentecost M, Stanley P, Takahashi M, Isaacs H (1981) Aneurysms of the aorta and subclavian and vertebral arteries in neurofibromatosis. Am J Dis Child 135: 475–477

370. Perrig H (1931) Zur Anatomie, Klinik und Therapie der Verletzungen und Aneurysmen der Arteria vertebralis. Bruns Beitr Klin Chir 154: 272–307

371. Philippe N, Floret D, Rosenberg D, Monnet P (1974) Obstruction des deux carotides internes et de la vertébrale gauche chez un nourrisson de 17 mois. Ann Pediat 21: 251–256

372. Philipson J (1956) Arteriovenöse Fistel nach Punktion der Arteria vertebralis für cerebrale Angiographie. Opusc Med (Stock) 1: 49

373. Picard L, Marshal JC, George B, Laurian C, Muller G, Roland J, Gengler L, Lepoire J (1981) Traitement radical d'une fistule vertébrale multi-pédiculaire par abord combiné séquentiel endo et exovasculaire. Rev Oto Neuro Ophtalmo 53: 167–176

374. Pilz P (1982) Idiopathische Medianekrose intrakranieller und zervikaler Arterien. Wien Klin Wochenschr 94: 455–458

375. Pitlyk PJ, Dockery MB, Miller RH (1965) Hemangiopericytoma of the spinal cord. Report of three cases. Neurology 15: 649–653

376. Powers SR, Drislane TM, Nevins S (1961) Intermittent vertebral artery compression: a new syndrome. Surgery 49: 257–264

377. Pratt-Thomas HR, Berger KE (1947) Cerebellar and spinal injuries after chiropractic manipulation. JAMA 133: 600–603

378. Putney FJ, Moran JJ, Thomas GK (1964) Neurogenic tumors of the head and neck. Laryngoscope 74: 1037–1059

379. Quatromoni JC, Hohnson JM, Wood MD (1979) Vertebral arteriovenous fistulas. Am J Surg 138: 907–911

380. Radojevic S, Negovanovic B (1963) La gouttière et les anneaux osseux de l'artère vertébrale de l'atlas. Acta Anat 55: 186–194

381. Rainer WG, Quianzon EP, Liggett MS, Newby JP, Bloomquist CD (1970) Surgical considerations in the treatment of vertebrobasilar arterial insufficiency. Am J Surg 120: 594–597

382. Rao TS, Sethi PK (1975) Persistent proatlantal artery with carotid vertebral anastomosis. Case report. J Neurosurg 43: 499–501

383. Rappaport I, Rappaport J (1977) Congenital arteriovenous fistula of the maxillo-facial region. Am J Surg 134: 39–46

384. Recordier AN (1966) Agenesis of one vertebral artery with malformation of cervical occipital joint. Rheumatology 18: 353–355

385. Reddy SVR, Karnes WE, Earnest IV F, Sundt TM (1981) Spontaneous extracranial vertebral arteriovenous fistula with fibromuscular dysplasia. J Neurosurg 54: 399–402

386. Reivich M, Holling HE, Roberts B, Toole JF (1961) Reversal of blood flow through the vertebral artery and its effect on cerebral circulation. N Engl J Med 265: 878–885

387. Reizine D, Laouti M, Guimaraens L, Riche MC, Merland JJ (1985) Vertebral arteriovenous fistulas. Clinical presentation. Angiographical appearance and endovascular treatment. A review of twenty five cases. Ann Radiol 28: 425–438

388. Rinaldi I (1972) The value of pre-operative angiography in the surgical management of cervical hour-glass neurofibroma. J Neurosurg 36: 97–101

389. Ringel SP, Harrison SH, Norenberg MD, Austin JH (1977) Fibromuscular dysplasia: multiple "spontaneous" dissecting aneurysms of the major cervical arteries. Ann Neurol 1: 301–304

390. Ritter VH, Grossman K, Basche S, Heerklotz I, Schiffmann R, Schumann E (1982) Die perkutane transluminale Angioplastik (PTA) von Aortenbogenasten. Fortschr Rontgenstr 136: 365–370

391. Robb-Smith AHT, Penny Backer J (1952) In: British encyclopedia of medical practice—2nd edition, vol 10. Butterworth, London, pp 549

392. Robinson HS (1966) Rheumatoid arthritis: atlanto-axial subluxation. Can Med Ass J 94: 470–477

393. Robles J (1968) Congenital arteriovenous malformation of the vertebral vessels in the neck. Case report. J Neurosurg 29: 206–208

394. Rogers L, Weeney PH (1979) Stroke: a neurologic complication of Wrestling. A case of brain stem stroke in a 17-year-old athlete. Ann J Sports Med 7: 352–354

395. Rogers LA (1983) Acute subdural hematoma and death following lateral cervical

spinal puncture. Case report. J Neurosurg 58: 284–286

396. Roon AJ, Ehrenfeld WK, Cocke PD (1979) Vertebral artery reconstruction. Am J Surg 138: 29–34

397. Roper PR, Guinto FC, Wolma FJ (1984) Post-traumatic vertebral artery aneurysm and arteriovenous fistula. A case report. Surgery 96: 556–559

398. Roski RA, Spetzler RF, Hopkins LN (1982) Occipital artery to posterior inferior cerebellar artery by-pass for vertebro-basilar ischemia. Neurosurgery 10: 44–49

399. Rossi P, Passariello R, Simonetti G (1978) Control of a traumatic vertebral arteriovenous fistula by a modified. Gianturco coil embolus system. AJR 131: 331–333

400. Rothman SL, Pratt AG, Kier EL, Allen WE (1974) Traumatic vertebral carotid jugular arterio-venous aneurysm. Case report. J Neurosurg 41: 92–96

401. Rougerie J (1973) Les compressions médullaires non traumatique de l'enfant. Masson, Paris, pp 218

402. Roualdes G, Lartigue C, Boudigue MD, Van der Marcq P, Drouineau J, Desplat A, Bataille B (1985) Dissection de l'artère vertébrale dans sa portion extra-crânienne après un match de tennis. Masson, Paris, pp 14, 860

403. Roy Camille R, Thibierge M, Metzger J (1982) Exploration d'une lacune de l'axis chez une patiente cervicalgique. Nouv Press Med 11: 453–454

404. Rubinstein LJ (1972) Tumors of the central nervous system. Atlas of tumor pathology: second series, fascicle, section 6. Armed Forces Institute of Pathology, Wahington, D.C., pp 186–190 (400 p)

405. Ryan GMS, Cope S (1955) Cervical vertigo. Lancet 2: 1355–1358

406. Samson Y, Baron JC, Bousser MG (1985) Regional hemodynamic and metabolic consequences of temporosylvian anastomosis: study of 15 patients by position emission tomography. Neurochirurgie 31: 31–36

407. Samsom LJ (1836) Des hémorragies traumatiques. J Baillière, Paris, pp 352

408. Sarter K, Freckmann N, Boker DK (1980) Related anomalies of origin of left vertebral artery and left thyroïd arteries. Report of 3 cases. Neurorad 19: 27–30

409. Schellhas KP, Latchaw RE, Wendling LR, Gold LHA (1980) Vertebral injuries following cervical manipulation. JAMA 244: 1450–1453

410. Schmidt CF, Pierson JC (1934) The intrinsic regulation of the blood vessels of the medulla oblongata. Am J Physiol 108: 241–263

411. Schmitt HP (1976) Rupturen und Thrombosen der Arteria vertebralis nach gedeckten mechanischen Insulten. Schweiz Arch Neurol Neurochir Psychiatr 119: 363–379

412. Schneider RC, Crosby EC (1959) Vascular insufficiency of brain stem and spinal cord in spinal trauma. Neurology (Minneap) 9: 643–656

413. Schneider RC, Schemm GW (1961) Vertebral artery insufficiency in acute and chronic spinal trauma. J Neurosurg 18: 348–360

414. Schneider RC, Gosch HH, Taren JA (1972) Blood vessel trauma following head and neck injuries. Chir Neurosurg 19: 312–354

415. Schott B, Bouillat G, Tommasi M, Goutelle A (1965) Pathologie artérielle du système vertébro-basilaire. Rapport du Congrès de Psychiatrie et de Neurologie de Langue Française. Masson, Paris, 216 p

416. Schubiger O, Yaşargil MG (1978) Extracranial vertebral aneurysm with neurofibromatosis. Neuroradiology 15: 171–173

417. Schwartz CJ, Mitchell JR (1961) Atheroma of the carotid and vertebral artery systems. Br Med J 2: 1057–1063

418. Selecki BR (1969) The effects of rotation of the atlas on the axis: experimental work. Med J Anst 1: 1012–1015

419. Senter HJ, Long ET (1983) Subclavian to distal vertebral artery by-pass. Case report. J Neurosurg 58: 607–610

420. Senter HJ, Bittar SM, Long ET (1985) Revascularization of the extracranial vertebral artery at any level without cross-clamping. J Neurosurg 62: 334–339

421. Sheehan S, Bauer RB, Meyer JS (1960) Vertebral artery compression in cervical spondylosis. Arteriographic demonstra-

tion during life of vertebral artery insufficiency due to rotation and extension of the neck. Neurology 10: 968–986

422. Sher MH, Meyer MI, Leuhardt HF et al (1966) Arteriovenous fistula involving the vertebral artery, report of three cases. Ann Surg 408–413

423. Sherman DG, Hart RG, Easton JD (1981) Abrupt change in head position and cerebral infarction. Stroke 12: 2–6

424. Shintani A, Zervas NT (1972) Consequence of ligation of the veretebral artery. J Neurosurg 36: 447–450

425. Shumacker HB (1946) Arteriovenous fistulas of the cervical portion of the vertebral vessels. Surg Gynecol Obstet 83: 625

426. Shumacker HB, Carter KL (1946) Arteriovenous fistulas and arterial aneurysms in Military Personnel. Surgery 20: 9–25

427. Shumacker HB, Campbell RL, Heimburger RF (1966) Operative treatment of vertebral arteriovenous fistulas. J Trauma 6: 3–19

428. Sigel B, Coelho JCU, Flanigan DP (1982) Detection of vascular defects during operation by imaging ultrasound. Ann Surg 196: 473–481

429. Simeone FA, Goldberg HI (1968) Thrombosis of vertebral artery from hyperextension injury to neck. J Neurosurg 29: 540–544

430. Singer WD, Haller JS, Wolpert SM (1975) Occlusive vertebro-basilar artery disease associated with cervical spine anomaly. Am J Child 129: 492–495

431. Six EG, Stringer WL, Cowley AR (1981) Post-traumatic bilateral vertebral artery occlusion. Case report. J Neurosurg 54: 814–817

432. Skinhoj E, Lassen NA, Hoedt-Rasmussen K (1964) Cerebellar blood flow in man. Arch Neurol 10: 464–467

433. Skopakoff C (1964) Über die Variabilität der Abzweigung der Arteria subclavia und ihrer Hauptäste. Anat Anz 115: 393–402

434. Smith RA, Estridge MN (1962) Neurologic complications of head and neck manipulations. JAMA 182: 528–531

435. Smith RS, Moore TS, Russell WF (1983) Transluminal angioplasty of the cerebral circulation. Clin Neurosurg 3110: 117–134

436. Smyth AW (1869) A case of successful ligature of the innominate artery. New Orleans. J Med 22: 464–469

437. So EL, Took JF, Dalal P, Moody DM (1981) Cephalic fibromuscular dysplasia in 32 patients. Arch Neurol 38: 619–622

438. Spetzler RF, Modic M, Bonstelle C (1980) Spontaneous opening of large occipital vertebral artery anastomosis during embolization. Case report. J Neurosurg 53: 849–850

439. Spetzler RF, Zabramski JM, Kaufman B, Yeung MN (1983) Acute NMR changes during middle cerebral artery occlusion: a preliminary study in primates. Stroke 14: 185–191

440. Stanley JC, Fry WJ, Seeger JF, Hoffman GL, Gabrielson TO (1974) Extracranial internal carotid and vertebral artery fibrodysplasia. Arch Surg 109: 215–222

441. Starr A, Hamilton AE (1976) Correlation between confirmed sites of neurological lesions and abnormalities of far-field auditory brain stem responses. Electroencephalogr Clin Neurophysiol 41: 595–608

442. Stecken J, Jan M, Lapierre F, M Bouyou D (1983) Fistule artério-veineuse vertébrale post-artériographique. Neurochirurgie 29: 161–165

443. Steimle R, Bonneville JF, Aboulrazzak A, Akkari MEl (1978) Quadriplègie traumatique et thrombose vertébrale. Neurochirurgie 24: 275–278

444. Stein BM, Mc Cormick WF, Rodriguez JN, Taveras JM (1962) Post-mortem angiography of cerebral vascular system. Arch Neurol 7: 545–558

445. Stringer WL, Kelly DL Jr (1980) Traumatic dissection of the extracraniàl internal carotid artery. Neurosurgery 6: 123–130

446. Suen JY, Boellner SW, Araos CA, Boop WC (1972) Congenital arteriovenous fistula of the vertebral artery and internal jugular vein. J Pediat 80: 837–838

447. Suetching RL, French LA (1955) Posterior inferior cerebellar artery syndrome following a fracture of the cervical vertebra. J Neurosurg 12: 187–189

448. Sugar O, Holden LB, Powell CB (1949) Vertebral angiography. AJR 61: 166–182

449. Sullivan HG, Harbison JW, Vines FS, Becker D (1975) Embolic posterior cerebral artery occlusion secondary to spondylitic vertebral artery compression. J Neurosurg 43: 818–822

450. Sundt T, Whisnant J, Piepgras D, Campbell J, Homan C (1978) Intracranial by-pass grafts for vertebral basilar ischemia. Mayo Clin Proc 53: 12–18

451. Sundt TM Jr, Smith HC, Campbell JK, Vliestra RE, Cucchiara RF, Stanson AW (1980) Transluminal angioplasty for basilar artery stenosis. Mayo Clin Proc 55: 673–680

452. Sutton D (1950) Anomalous carotid-basilar anastomosis. Br J Radiol 23: 617–619

453. Suzuki S (1979) Angiographic aspects of anomalies of vertebral artery. Clin Radiol 24: 3–14

454. Symonds CP (1927) Cervical rib. Thrombosis of subclavian artery. Contralateral hemiplegia of sudden onset, probably embolic. Proc R Soc Med 20 (part 3): 1244–1245

455. Takahashi M, Kananami H, Watanabe N (1970) Fenestration of the extracranial vertebral artery. Radiology 96: 359–360

456. Tanaka Y, Hara H, Mamose G, Kobayaschi S, Kobayaschi S, Sugiat K (1983) Proatlantal intersegmental artery and trigeminal artery associated with an aneurysm. J Neurosurg 59: 520–523

457. Tatlow WF, Tissington J, Bammer HG (1957) Syndrome of vertebral artery compression. Neurology 7: 331–341

458. Taylor AR, Chakravorty BC (1964) Clinical syndromes associated with basilar impression. Arch Neurol 10: 475

459. Theron J, Courtheoux P, Henriet JP, Pelouze G, Derlon JM, Maiza D (1984) Angioplasty of supra-aortic arteries. Neuroradiology 11: 181–200

460. Thevenet A, Ruotolo C (1984) Surgical repair of vertebral artery stenoses. J Cardiovasc Surg 25: 101–110

461. Thomas GK, Anderson KN, Hain RD, Merendino KA (1959) The significance of anomalous vertebral basilar artery communications in operation on the heart and great vessels. Surgery 46: 747–752

462. Thompson JE, Eilber F, Baker JD (1979) Vertebral artery aneurysm. Case report and review of literature. Surgery 85: 583–585

463. Toole JF, Tucker SH (1960) Influence of head position upon cerebral circulation. Arch Neurol 2: 616–620

464. Tasi FY, Mahon J, Woodruff JV, Roach JP (1975) Congenital absence of bilateral vertebral arteries with occipital basilar anastomosis. Am J Roentgenol Rad Ther Nucl Med 124: 281–286

465. Tsukamoto S, Hori Y, Ursumi S, Tanigake T, Horrike N, Otani R (1981) Proatlantal intersegmental artery with absence of bilateral vertebral arteries. Case report. J Neurosurg 54: 122–125

466. Tsuji HK, Redington JV, Kay JH (1968) Vertebral arteriovenous fistula. J Thor Cardiovasc Surg 55: 746–753

467. Uziel A, Benezech J (1978) Auditory brainstem responses in comatose patients: relationship with brain stem reflexes and level of coma. Electroencephalogr Clin Neurophysiol 45: 515–524

468. Vasin NI, Loshakov VA, Kornienki VN (1977) Clinical picture of cranio-cerebral trauma combined with trauma to the cervical region of the spine. Zh Vopr Neurokhir 1: 14–18

469. Velpeau A (1839) Nouveaux éléments du médecine opératoire, Tome 2, pp 221

470. Vencken LM (1970) Les fistules artério-veineuses par ponction directe. Neurochir 16: 539–542

471. Verbiest H (1968) Intracranial and cervical arterio-venous aneurysms of the carotid and vertebral arteries. Report of a series of 12 personal cases. Johns Hopkins Med 122: 350–357

472. Verbiest H (1968) A lateral approach to the cervical spine: technique and indications. J Neurosurg 28: 191–203

473. Verbiest H (1970) La chirurgie antérieure et latérale du rachis cervical. Neurochirurgie 16 [Suppl] n° 2: 212 p

474. Verbiest H (1973) Anterolateral operations for fracture or dislocations of the cervical spine due to injuries or previous surgical interventions. Clin Neurosurg 20, chap 27: 334–366

475. Viteck JJ, Morwetz RB (1982) Percuta-
     neous transluminal angioplasty of the
     external carotid artery: preliminary report.
     AJNR 3: 541–546

476. Vlajic I, Distelmaier P (1978) Traumen der
     Halswirbelsäule und Kompression der
     Vertebralarterien. Neurochirurgia 21:
     122–127

477. Voordecker G, Chanoine F, Flament-
     Durand J (1972) Arterite giganto-
     cellulaire atteignant les artères vertébrales.
     Acta Neurol Belg 72: 385–394

478. Vorstrup S, Hesmmingen R, Henriksen L,
     Lindewald H, Engell HL, Lassen NA
     (1983) Regional cerebral blood flow in
     patient with transient ischemic attacks
     studied by Xenon 133 inhalation and emis-
     sion tomography. Stroke 14: 903–910

479. Wackenheim A, Babin E (1969) Extra-
     transversal course of the vertebral artery; a
     little known anomaly capable of interfering
     with various tests of cervical compression.
     Press Med 77: 1213–1214

480. Waga S, Handa J, Terauta T, Honda H
     (1974) Traumatic vertebral arteriovenous
     fistula. Surg Neurol 2: 279–282

481. Wagner M (1963) Vertebral artery insuf-
     ficiency. Arch Surg 87: 885–886

482. Walsh JW, Stevens DB, Young AB (1983)
     Traumatic paraplegia in children without
     contiguous spinal fracture or dislocation.
     Neurosurgery 124: 439–444

483. Walt AJ (1984) The story of vertebrobas-
     ilar surgery. In: Berguer R, Bauer RB
     (eds) Vertebro-basilar arterial occlusive
     disease. Raven Press, New York, pp 225–
     230

484. Watanabe M, Irino T, Taneda M (1981)
     Measurements of cerebral blood flow in
     vertebrobasilar artery territory deter-
     mined by direct injection of 133 Xe. Clin-
     ical application for posterior fossa stroke.
     Jpn J Stroke 3: 268–274

485. Webb WR, Burford TH (1952) Gangrene
     of arm following use of the subclavian
     artery in pulmosystemic (Blalock) anas-
     tomosis. J Thorac Surg 23: 199–207

486. Webb FWS, Hickman JA, Brew StJ (1968)
     Death from vertebral artery thrombosis in
     rheumatoid arthritis. Br Med J 2: 537–538

487. Weinberg PE, Flom RA (1973) Traumatic
     vertebral arteriovenous fistula. Surg
     Neurol 1: 162–167

488. Weinstein PR, Brant-Zawadski M, Mills C
     (1985) Nuclear magnetic resonance imag-
     ing in cerebral ischemia. Basic principles
     and early experience. In: Spetzler RF,
     Carter LP, Selman WR, Martin NA (eds)
     Cerebral revascularization for stroke, vol
     19. Thieme Stratton, New York, pp 106–
     112

489. Welch DM, Coleman RE, Hardin WB,
     Siegel BA (1975) Brain scanning in
     cerebral vascular disease: a reappraisal.
     Stroke 6: 136–141

490. Wellinger Cl (1975) Le chordome
     rachidien. Revue de la Littérature depuis
     1960. Rev Rhum 42: 109–116, 145, 204,
     287–295

491. Wells RP, Smith RR (1982) Fibromuscular
     dysplasia of the internal carotid artery. A
     long term follow-up. Neurosurgery 10: 39–
     43

492. Wilckbom GI, Williamson MR (1980)
     Anomalous foramen transversarium of C 2
     simulating erosion of bone. Neurorad 19:
     43–46

493. Wilkinson IMS (1972) The vertebral
     artery. Extracranial and intracranial
     structure. Arch Neurol 27: 392–396

494. Wilkinson IMS, Russel RWR (1972)
     Arteries of the head and neck in giant cell
     arteritis. A pathological study to show the
     pattern of arterial involvement. Arch
     Neurol 27: 378–391

495. Williams D, Wilson TG (1962) Diagnosis
     of major and minor syndromes of basilar
     insufficiency. Brain 85: 741–774

496. Willie EJ, Ehrenfeld WK (1970) Surgical
     techniques in extracranial occlusive
     cerebro-vascular disease. Diagnosis and
     management. Saunders Company, Lon-
     don, pp 184–213

497. Wolff K (1928) Traumatische Zerreißung
     der gesunden Arteria vertebralis an der
     Hirnbasis. Dtsch Z Ges Gerichtl Med 22:
     464–467

498. Wollschlaeger G, Wollschlaeger PB (1974)
     The circle of Willis. In: Newton TH, Potts
     DG (eds) Radiology of the skull and brain:
     angiography vol 2, Book 2, Chap 58. CV
     Mosby Co, St Louis, pp 1171–1201

499. Wu KK, Hoak JC (1975) Increased platelet aggregates in patients with transient ischemic attacks. Stroke 60: 521–524

500. Yagamata S, Terauta T, Yumitori K, Nakamura K (1985) Percutaneous transluminal angioplasty for cerebral ischemic diseases. In: Spetzler RF, Carter LP, Selman WR, Martin NA (eds) Cerebral revascularization for stroke, vol 98. Thieme Stratton, New York, pp 598–602

501. Yates PO (1959) Birth trauma to the vertebral arteries. Arch Dis Child 34: 436–441

502. Zimmerman AW, Kumar AJ, Gadoth N, Hodges FJ (1978) Traumatic vertebrobasilar occlusion disease in childhood. Neurology 28: 185–188

SUBJECT INDEX

Druck: A. Holzhausens Nfg., Universitätsbuchdrucker

JIRO SUZUKI

TREATMENT OF CEREBRAL INFARCTION

EXPERIMENTAL AND CLINICAL STUDY

1987. 240 partly colored figures. XIV, 380 pages.
Cloth DM 165,–, öS 1160,– ISBN 3-211-81933-9

CONTENTS: Introduction. – Experimental Study: Experimental Models – Histological Study – Cerebral Blood Flow – Ischemic Brain Edema – Cerebral Metabolism and Free Radical Pathology – The Development of New Brain Protective Agents. – Clinical Study: Epidemiology and Symptomatology – Diagnostic Techniques – Medical and Surgical Treatments of Cerebral Infarction. Revascularization in the Acute Stage. – Appendixes: Temporary Occlusion of Trunk Arteries of the Brain During Surgery – The Pathology of Cerebral Vasospasms and Its Treatment – Surgical Therapy for Moyamoya Disease. – References. – Subject Index.

Among the developed nations, Cerebrovascular Disease (CVD) ranks among the top three causes of death and must therefore be regarded as a major health hazard. Although a gradual decrease in the incidence of hemorrhagic CVD has been observed, the number of ischemic CVDs still increases steadily, partly due to higher longevity. Therefore the development of techniques for the prevention and treatment of ischemic diseases of the brain is of utmost importance.

The causes of ischemic CVD are well known, but there remain considerable uncertainties concerning the nature of the gradual intracerebral changes which occur after the ischemic attack. The volume introduces the most recent developments concerning cerebral infarction, reviewing the present state-of-knowledge and the author's own extensive research which resulted in a significant advance in the treatment of the acute stage cerebral infarct, the "Sendai Cocktail", a combination of Mannitol, Vitamin E, Steroids and Phenytoin.

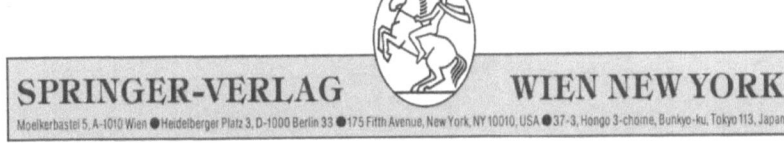

SPRINGER-VERLAG **WIEN NEW YORK**

Moelkerbastei 5, A-1010 Wien ● Heidelberger Platz 3, D-1000 Berlin 33 ● 175 Fifth Avenue, New York, NY 10010, USA ● 37-3, Hongo 3-chome, Bunkyo-ku, Tokyo 113, Japan